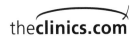

PEDIATRIC CLINICS
OF NORTH AMERICA

Pediatric Hematology

GUEST EDITORS
Max J. Coppes, MD, PhD, MBA
Russell E. Ware, MD, PhD

April 2008 • Volume 55 • Number 2

SAUNDERS

An Imprint of Elsevier, Inc.
PHILADELPHIA   LONDON   TORONTO   MONTREAL   SYDNEY   TOKYO

W.B. SAUNDERS COMPANY
A Division of Elsevier Inc.

1600 John F. Kennedy Boulevard • Suite 1800 • Philadelphia, Pennsylvania 19103

http://www.theclinics.com

THE PEDIATRIC CLINICS OF NORTH AMERICA
April 2008
Editor: Carla Holloway

Volume 55, Number 2
ISSN 0031-3955
ISBN-13: 978-1-4160-5791-8
ISBN-10: 1-4160-5791-9

The ideas and opinions expressed in *The Pediatric Clinics of North America* do not necessarily reflect those of the Publisher. The Publisher does not assume any responsibility for any injury and/or damage to persons or property arising out of or related to any use of the material contained in this periodical. The reader is advised to check the appropriate medical literature and the product information currently provided by the manufacturer of each drug to be administered to verify the dosage, the method and duration of administration, or contraindications. It is the responsibility of the treating physician or other health care professional, relying on independent experience and knowledge of the patient, to determine drug dosages and the best treatment for the patient. Mention of any product in this issue should not be construed as endorsement by the contributors, editors, or the Publisher of the product or manufacturers' claims.

The Pediatric Clinics of North America (ISSN 0031-3955) is published bi-monthly by Elsevier Inc. 360 Park Avenue South, New York, NY 10010-1710. Months of publication are February, April, June, August, October, and December. Business and Editorial Offices: 1600 John F. Kennedy Blvd., Suite 1800, Philadelphia, PA 19103-2899. Customer Service Office: 6277 Sea Harbor Drive, Orlando, FL 32887-4800. Periodicals postage paid at New York, NY and additional mailing offices. Subscription prices are $149.00 per year (US individuals), $315.00 per year (US institutions), $202.00 per year (Canadian individuals), $411.00 per year (Canadian institutions), $226.00 per year (international individuals), $411.00 per year (international institutions), $72.00 per year (US students), $119.00 per year (Canadian students), and $119.00 per year (foreign students). To receive students/resident rare, orders must be accompanied by name of affiliated institution, date of term, and the signature of program/residency coordinator on institution letterhead. Orders will be billed at individual rate until proof of status is received. Foreign air speed delivery is included in all Clinics subscription prices. All prices are subject to change without notice. POSTMASTER: Send address changes to *The Pediatric Clinics of North America*, Elsevier Journals Customer Service, 6277 Sea Harbor Drive, Orlando, FL 32887-4800. **Customer Service: 1-800-654-2452 (US). From outside of the United States, call 1-407-563-6020. Fax: 1-407-363-9661. E-mail: JournalsCustomerService-usa@elsevier.com.**

The Pediatric Clinics of North America is also published in Spanish by McGraw-Hill Inter-americana Editores S.A., Mexico City, Mexico; in Portuguese by Riechmann and Affonso Editores, Rua Comandante Coelho 1085, CEP 21250, Rio de Janeiro, Brazil; and in Greek by Althayia SA, Athens, Greece.

The Pediatric Clinics of North America is covered in *Index Medicus*, *Excerpta Medica*, *Current Contents*, *Current Contents/Clinical Medicine*, *Science Citation Index*, *ASCA*, *ISI/BIOMED*, and *BIOSIS*.

Printed in the United States of America.

GOAL STATEMENT

The goal of the *Pediatric Clinics of North America* is to keep practicing physicians and residents up to date with current clinical practice in pediatrics by providing timely articles reviewing the state-of-the-art in patient care.

ACCREDITATION

The *Pediatric Clinics of North America* is planned and implemented in accordance with the Essential Areas and Policies of the Accreditation Council for Continuing Medical Education (ACCME) through the joint sponsorship of the University of Virginia School of Medicine and Elsevier. The University of Virginia School of Medicine is accredited by the ACCME to provide continuing medical education for physicians.

The University of Virginia School of Medicine designates this educational activity for a maximum of 15 *AMA PRA Category 1 Credits*™. Physicians should only claim credit commensurate with the extent of their participation in the activity.

The American Medical Association has determined that physicians not licensed in the US who participate in this CME activity are eligible for 15 *AMA PRA Category 1 Credits*™.

Credit can be earned by reading the text material, taking the CME examination online at http://www.theclinics.com/home/cme, and completing the evaluation. After taking the test, you will be required to review any and all incorrect answers. Following completion of the test and evaluation, your credit will be awarded and you may print your certificate.

FACULTY DISCLOSURE/CONFLICT OF INTEREST

The University of Virginia School of Medicine, as an ACCME accredited provider, endorses and strives to comply with the Accreditation Council for Continuing Medical Education (ACCME) Standards of Commercial Support, Commonwealth of Virginia statutes, University of Virginia policies and procedures, and associated federal and private regulations and guidelines on the need for disclosure and monitoring of proprietary and financial interests that may affect the scientific integrity and balance of content delivered in continuing medical education activities under our auspices.

The University of Virginia School of Medicine requires that all CME activities accredited through this institution be developed independently and be scientifically rigorous, balanced and objective in the presentation/discussion of its content, theories and practices.

All authors/editors participating in an accredited CME activity are expected to disclose to the readers relevant financial relationships with commercial entities occurring within the past 12 months (such as grants or research support, employee, consultant, stock holder, member of speakers bureau, etc.). The University of Virginia School of Medicine will employ appropriate mechanisms to resolve potential conflicts of interest to maintain the standards of fair and balanced education to the reader. Questions about specific strategies can be directed to the Office of Continuing Medical Education, University of Virginia School of Medicine, Charlottesville, Virginia.

The authors/editors listed below have identified no financial or professional relationships for themselves or their spouse/partner:
Denise M. Adams, MD; Timothy J. Bernard, MD; Melody J. Cunningham, MD; Ross Fasano, MD, PhD; Neil A. Goldenberg, MD; Matthew M. Heeney, MD; Carla Holloway (Acquisitions Editor); Paula D. James, MD; David Lillicrap, MD; Henry E. Rice, MD; Jeremy Robertson, MD; Nidra I. Rodriguez, MD; Elizabeth T. Tracy, MD; Russell E. Ware, MD, PhD (Guest Editor); and Mary Sue Wentzel, RN.

The authors/editors listed below identified the following professional or financial affiliations for themselves or their spouse/partner:
Victor Blanchette, FRCP serves on the Bayer Corporation International Haemophilia Advisory Board and the Amgen AMG 531 Advisory Board. He is also on the Baxter BioScience Corporation Global Steering Committee for the Protein-Free Recombination Factor VIII (rAHF PFM).
Paula Bolton-Maggs, DM, FRCP serves on the Advisory Committee for Glaxo Smith Kline.
Max J. Coppes, MD, PhD, MBA (Guest Editor) is a consultant for Eisai.
W. Keith Hoots, MD is an independent contractor for Grifols, Wyeth, Boxter, Bayer, ZLB Behring, and NovoNordisk, and serves on the Speaker's Bureau for Baxter and NovoNordisk.
Janet L. Kwiatkowski, MD, MSCE has served as a site PI co co-investigator for Novartis.
Naomi L.C. Luban, MD is a consultant for Westat.
Sarah H. O'Brien, MD, MSc spouse is on the Speaker's bureau for CORIA.

Disclosure of Discussion of Non-FDA Approved Uses for Pharmaceutical and/or Medical Devices:
The University of Virginia School of Medicine, as an ACCME provider, requires that all authors identify and disclose any "off label" uses for pharmaceutical and medical device products. The University of Virginia School of Medicine recommends that each physician fully review all the available data on new products or procedures prior to clinical use.

TO ENROLL

To enroll in the *Pediatric Clinics of North America* Continuing Medical Education program, call customer service at 1-800-654-2452 or visit us online at www.theclinics.com/home/cme. The CME program is available to subscribers for an additional fee of $195.00.

GUEST EDITORS

MAX J. COPPES, MD, PhD, MBA, Executive Director, Center for Cancer and Blood Disorders, Children's National Medical Center; and Professor of Oncology, Medicine, and Pediatrics, Georgetown University, Washington, DC

RUSSELL E. WARE, MD, PhD, Lemuel W. Diggs Chair in Hematology, Member, and Chair, Department of Hematology, St. Jude's Children Research Hospital; and Professor of Pediatrics, University of Tennessee Health Sciences Center, Memphis, Tennessee

CONTRIBUTORS

DENISE M. ADAMS, MD, Associate Professor, Division of Hematology/Oncology, Cincinnati Children's Hospital Medical Center, University of Cincinnati; and Medical Director, Hemangioma and Vascular Malformation Center, Cincinnati Children's Hospital Medical Center, Cincinnati, Ohio

TIMOTHY J. BERNARD, MD, Assistant Professor of Pediatrics, Department of Child Neurology; Co-Director, Pediatric Stroke Program, University of Colorado and The Children's Hospital; and Mountain States Regional Hemophilia and Thrombosis Center, Aurora, Colorado

VICTOR BLANCHETTE, FRCP, Chief, Division of Hematology/Oncology, The Hospital for Sick Children; and Department of Pediatrics, University of Toronto, Toronto, Ontario, Canada

PAULA BOLTON-MAGGS, DM, FRCP, University Department of Hematology, Manchester Royal Infirmary, Manchester, United Kingdom

MELODY J. CUNNINGHAM, MD, Assistant Professor, Harvard Medical School; and Director, Thalassemia Research Program, Division of Hematology/Oncology, Children's Hospital Boston, Boston, Massachusetts

ROSS FASANO, MD, Department of Hematology/Oncology, Children's National Medical Center; and Department of Pediatrics, The George Washington University Medical Center, Washington, DC

NEIL A. GOLDENBERG, MD, Assistant Professor of Pediatrics and Medicine; Co-Director, Pediatric Stroke Program, University of Colorado and The Children's Hospital; and Associate Director, Mountain States Regional Hemophilia and Thrombosis Center, Aurora, Colorado

MATTHEW M. HEENEY, MD, Instructor of Pediatrics, Harvard Medical School; and Division of Hematology/Oncology, Children's Hospital Boston, Boston, Massachusetts

W. KEITH HOOTS, MD, Professor, Division of Pediatrics, Hematology Section, The University of Texas Health Sciences Center; and Medical Director, Gulf States Hemophilia and Thrombophilia Center, Houston, Texas

PAULA D. JAMES, MD, Assistant Professor, Department of Medicine, Queen's University, Kingston, Ontario, Canada

JANET L. KWIATKOWSKI, MD, MSCE, Assistant Professor of Pediatrics, University of Pennsylvania School of Medicine; and Attending Hematologist, The Children's Hospital of Philadelphia, Division of Hematology, Philadelphia, Pennsylvania

DAVID LILLICRAP, MD, Professor, Department of Pathology and Molecular Medicine, Queen's University, Kingston, Ontario, Canada

NAOMI L.C. LUBAN, MD, Chief, Laboratory Medicine and Pathology; Director, Transfusion Medicine/The Edward J. Miller Donor Center; Senior Attending, Department of Hematology/Oncology; Associate Program Director, Pediatric Clinical Research Center; and Vice Chair of Academic Affairs, Department of Pediatrics, Children's National Medical Center; Professor, Pediatrics and Pathology, The George Washington University Medical Center, Washington, DC

SARAH H. O'BRIEN, MD, MSc, Assistant Professor, Hematology/Oncology, Nationwide Children's Hospital/The Ohio State University; and Center for Innovation in Pediatric Practice, The Research Institute at Nationwide Children's Hospital, Columbus, Ohio

HENRY E. RICE, MD, Associate Professor and Chief, Division of Pediatric Surgery, Department of Surgery, Duke University Medical Center, Durham, North Carolina

JEREMY ROBERTSON, MD, Clinical Fellow, Division of Hematology/Oncology, Hospital for Sick Children, Toronto, Ontario, Canada

NIDRA I. RODRIGUEZ, MD, Assistant Professor, Division of Pediatrics, Hematology Section, The University of Texas Health Sciences Center; and Assistant Professor, Gulf States Hemophilia and Thrombophilia Center, Houston, Texas

ELISABETH T. TRACY, MD, Division of General Surgery, Department of Surgery, Duke University Medical Center, Durham, North Carolina

RUSSELL E. WARE, MD, PhD, Lemuel W. Diggs Chair in Hematology, Member, and Chair, Department of Hematology, St. Jude's Children Research Hospital; and Professor of Pediatrics, University of Tennessee Health Sciences Center, Memphis, Tennessee

MARY SUE WENTZEL, RN, Research Nurse, Hemangioma and Vascular Malformation Center, Division of Hematology/Oncology, Cincinnati Children's Hospital Medical Center, Cincinnati, Ohio

CONTENTS

important that the condition be recognized and diagnosed. This article reviews the pathophysiology of the condition, the current classification scheme, and the available treatments, highlighting issues specific to the pediatric population.

Childhood Immune Thrombocytopenic Purpura: Diagnosis and Management
Victor Blanchette and Paula Bolton-Maggs

Immune thrombocytopenic purpura (ITP) is an autoimmune disorder characterized by a low circulating platelet count caused by destruction of antibody-sensitized platelets in the reticuloendothelial system. ITP can be classified as childhood versus adult, acute versus chronic, and primary versus secondary. Persistence of thrombocytopenia defines the chronic form of the disorder. Secondary causes of ITP include collagen vascular disorders, immune deficiencies, and some chronic infections. This review focuses on the diagnosis and management of children who have acute and chronic ITP. Emphasis is placed on areas of controversy and new therapies.

Blood Component Therapy
Ross Fasano and Naomi L.C. Luban

Blood component transfusion is integral in the treatment of infants and children by pediatricians, surgeons, intensivists, and hematologists/oncologists. Technologic advances in blood collection, separation, anticoagulation, and preservation have resulted in component preparation of red blood cells, platelets, white blood cells, and plasma, which are superior to whole blood used in the past. Advances in donor selection, infectious disease testing, leukoreduction filters, and gamma irradiation have made products safer. Physicians prescribing blood components should have a basic understanding of indications (and contraindications) and be cognizant of methods of preparation, proper storage conditions, and requirements for modification of blood products to prevent potential adverse effects.

Update on Thalassemia: Clinical Care and Complications
Melody J. Cunningham

β-Thalassemia, originally named Cooley anemia, is an inherited blood disease. Various types of thalassemia are inherited anemias caused by mutations at the globin gene loci on chromosomes 16 and 11, affecting the production of α- or β-globin protein, respectively. The combination of early diagnosis, improvements in monitoring for organ complications, and advances in supportive care have enabled many patients who have severe thalassemia syndromes to live productive, active lives well into adulthood.

FORTHCOMING ISSUES

June 2008

Pediatric Critical Care
James P. Orlowski, MD, FAAP, FCCP, FCCM,
Guest Editor

August 2008

Pediatric Resuscitation
Steve Schexnayder, MD,
and Arno Zaritsky, MD, *Guest Editors*

October 2008

Developmental Disabilities: Part I
Donald E. Greydanus, MD, FAAP, FSAM,
Dilip R. Patel, MD, FAACPDM, FAAP, FSAM, FACSM,
and Helen D. Pratt, PhD, *Guest Editors*

RECENT ISSUES

February 2008

Pediatric Oncology
Max J. Coppes, MD, PhD, MBA,
and Jeffrey S. Dome, MD, *Guest Editors*

December 2007

Complementary and Alternative Medicine
Lawrence D. Rosen, MD, FAAP,
and David S. Riley, MD, *Guest Editors*

October 2007

Pediatric Palliative Care
Tammy I. Kang, MD, David Munson, MD,
and Jeffrey C. Klick, MD, *Guest Editors*

THE CLINICS ARE NOW AVAILABLE ONLINE!

Access your subscription at
www.theclinics.com

Preface

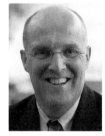 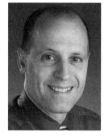

Max J. Coppes, MD, PhD, MBA   Russell E. Ware, MD, PhD
Guest Editors

For many decades, the subspecialties of pediatric hematology and pediatric oncology have been practiced by the same individuals. Today in many institutions this still occurs, either because the size of the institution does not allow the recruitment of sufficient pediatric hematologists and oncologists to allow for separate services, or because the practitioners themselves, trained in a combined hematology/oncology program, are disinclined to give up part of what they trained to do. Other institutions with sufficient interest and resources, including ours, have come to the realization that the knowledge base and experience to function optimally as a pediatric hematologist or oncologist mandate a separation in the same manner as the care for children requiring stem cell transplantation is now relegated primarily to pediatric bone marrow transplantation physicians. The formal separation of pediatric hematology and oncology allows specialists to focus on specific hematologic disorders such as sickle cell disease, transfusion medicine, or clotting disorders, to study their pathophysiology in detail, to establish collaborative research studies to optimize treatment, and to develop novel therapeutic approaches. We believe that a focused approach is required to further develop this exciting field of medicine. This issue of *Pediatric Clinics of North America* affirms the fact that pediatric hematology has evolved in a multifaceted and often complex specialty on its own. For example, managing patients with hemophilia who have inhibitors is not always easy, whereas optimally treating the increased number of young patients who develop a venous thromboembolism requires specialized expertise and experience, and really requires the involvement of a knowledgeable specialist.

doi:10.1016/j.pcl.2008.02.004   *pediatric.theclinics.com*

Unlike pediatric oncology, where most treatments are directed or have been established by prospective randomized clinical trials, the management of many primary hematologic conditions in children lacks such guidance. For some conditions, most notably sickle cell disease and, more recently, disorders of hemostasis, the lack of insight gained through prospective clinical trials is currently being addressed, but for other hematologic conditions, some of which are very rare, pediatric hematologists need to determine management based on a review of the literature and experience. Assessing the value of publications is not always a trivial matter and we have therefore included an article that specifically deals with making management decisions when so-called "solid" information is unavailable.

The articles selected for this issue of *Pediatric Clinics of North America* cover aspects that most pediatricians deal with on a regular basis (eg, immune thrombocytopenic purpura [ITP], vascular malformations, and transfusions), but which continue to pose challenges with regard to optimal management. Other articles deal with hematologic disorders in children who most often are managed by pediatric hematologists for their hematological condition (eg, stroke, thalassemia, hereditary spherocytosis, and sickle cell disease), but are also followed by pediatricians or general practitioners for overall health care management. In either case, the authors contributing to this issue have done an excellent job in providing a relevant update on hematologic disorders that affect many children worldwide.

As some authors indicate, we anticipate that the future of pediatric hematology will include a better understanding of the biology that leads to hematologic diseases as well as interdisciplinary multi-institutional (and, on occasion, international) trials to further improve life expectancy and/or quality of life of children affected by these hematologic disorders.

Max J. Coppes, MD, PhD, MBA
Center for Cancer and Blood Disorders
Children's National Medical Center
Washington, DC, USA

Georgetown University
Washington, DC, USA

E-mail address: MCoppes@cnmc.org

Russell E. Ware, MD, PhD
Department of Hematology
St. Jude Children's Research Hospital
Memphis, TN, USA

University of Tennessee Health Science Center
Memphis, TN, USA

E-mail address: russell.ware@stjude.org

ELSEVIER
SAUNDERS

PEDIATRIC CLINICS
OF NORTH AMERICA

Pediatr Clin N Am 55 (2008) 287–304

Decision Analysis in Pediatric Hematology

Sarah H. O'Brien, MD, MSc[a,b,*]

[a]Center for Innovation in Pediatric Practice, The Research Institute at Nationwide
Children's Hospital, 700 Children's Drive, Columbus, OH 43205, USA
[b]Division of Pediatric Hematology/Oncology, Nationwide Children's Hospital/The
Ohio State University, 700 Children's Drive, Columbus, OH 43205, USA

Every day, physicians must make decisions regarding which medical interventions benefit their patients most. For example, a 5-year-old healthy girl presents to an emergency department with a 1-day history of bruising and petechiae. History, physical examination, and initial laboratory studies all are consistent with a diagnosis of immune thrombocytopenic purpura (ITP). The hematologist on call has several decisions to make. Should the child be admitted to the hospital or discharged home? Should the child receive therapy or simply be observed? If the child receives therapy, should it be immune globulin, anti-D, or steroids? There are no results of large clinical trials available to guide or provide definitive answers to any one of these questions. Instead, the hematologist must weigh the risks and benefits of each potential management strategy and choose a course of action that he or she believes is "the right thing to do."

Performing large randomized controlled trials to answer every clinical question in medicine is not feasible, particularly in pediatric hematology, a field of many rare diseases. Rather, hematologists need to be able to evaluate and synthesize the literature that is available—observational cohort studies, administrative or claims data, or small clinical trials—regarding a particular clinical dilemma. Several formal methods have been developed to evaluate and combine data from diverse sources addressing clinical questions that have not or cannot be answered by traditional clinical trials. Systematic reviews, such as the Cochrane reviews, use a well-defined and uniform approach to identify all relevant studies addressing a particular

* Center for Innovation in Pediatric Practice, The Research Institute at Nationwide Children's Hospital, 700 Children's Drive, Columbus, OH 43205.
   E-mail address: sarah.obrien@nationwidechildrens.org

0031-3955/08/$ - see front matter © 2008 Elsevier Inc. All rights reserved.
doi:10.1016/j.pcl.2008.01.004
pediatric.theclinics.com

research question. The results of eligible studies are displayed and, when appropriate, summary estimates of the overall results are calculated [1]. Meta-analysis, which can be performed only if the results of studies are similar enough, refers to the statistical aspects of a systematic review, in which summary effect estimates and variance from several similar studies, statistical tests of heterogeneity, and estimates of publication bias are calculated. Formal methods of grading clinical recommendations often are used in clinical practice guidelines, taking into account the risk-benefit ratio of the treatment under consideration and the methodologic quality of the underlying evidence [2]. Decision analysis is another method of combining data from multiple sources.

For many physicians, the phrase, "decision analysis," may refer to an esoteric research technique involving complicated mathematics and perhaps some smoke and mirrors. In reality, clinicians use the techniques of decision analysis in almost every patient encounter. Clinical decision analysis is the application of explicit, quantitative methods to analyze decision making under conditions of uncertainty [3]. The technique originally was developed in the 1940s and used initially in financial and government sectors [4]. In decision analysis, an investigator structures a clinical problem into a decision tree representing the temporal sequence of possible clinical events. Next, data are collected to estimate the probability of each event and the expected risks and benefits of each strategy. The decision tree then is analyzed to identify which strategy has the highest expected value and, therefore, the preferred course of action. Decision analysis can be used to analyze many different types of decisions in medicine, such as determining whether or not to screen for a disease, choosing a testing strategy, or selecting an intervention. Models also can be built from many different perspectives, from individual patients or families to third-party payers to society as a whole.

The possibilities for using decision analysis to address clinical dilemmas in pediatric hematology are nearly endless. Which of the following is the preferred strategy: Chronic transfusions versus hydroxyurea for prevention of stroke in sickle cell disease? Partial versus complete splenectomy in patients who have hereditary spherocytosis? Six weeks or 3 months of anticoagulation for a central line–related deep venous thrombosis (DVT)? This review first outlines the basic steps of decision analysis: choosing a research question, building a decision tree, filling the tree with probabilities and outcome measures, and analyzing and interpreting the results. This outline is followed by a discussion of how quality of life is measured in decision analysis and the challenges of obtaining these measurements in the pediatric population. Several decision analyses published in the field of pediatric hematology and recommendations on evaluating and judging the decision analysis literature are described. Finally, the limitations of decision analysis are discussed and readers are directed to additional resources on learning about and performing decision analysis.

The basic steps of decision analysis

The decision analysis approach entails four basic steps, as described by Weinstein and Fineberg [3] in their seminal textbook, *Clinical Decision Analysis*. These steps are (1) identifying and defining the scope of a problem and population of interest; (2) structuring a problem over time in the form of a decision tree; (3) characterizing the information (probabilities, costs, and utilities) needed to fill in the decision tree; and (4) choosing the preferred course of action.

Identify and define the scope of a problem and population of interest

Decision analysis is appropriate for a given research question if two conditions are met: (1) there is uncertainty about the appropriate clinical strategy for a given health state and (2) there is a meaningful tradeoff in the problem [5]. For example, performing a decision analysis of chronic transfusion versus observation in sickle cell patients who have abnormal transcranial Doppler velocities is not appropriate, as the multicenter Stroke Prevention Trial in Sickle Cell Anemia (STOP) clearly demonstrated that children randomized to receive chronic transfusions had significantly fewer primary strokes [6]. Likewise, a decision analysis comparing ultrasonography to venography for the diagnosis of DVT in the central upper venous system is not meaningful if the only variable of interest is the number of DVTs detected, for venography is already known to be the more sensitive test [7]. If the additional costs of venography and the invasiveness of the procedure are factored into the analysis, however, the tradeoff of risks and benefits becomes meaningful.

Once a research question is chosen, it is critical to define precisely the patient population of interest, the clinical strategies being compared, and the primary and secondary outcomes of interest, just as would be expected in the design of a prospective randomized, clinical trial. These determinations guide an investigator's choice of model design. For example, when comparing prophylaxis strategies for the management of severe hemophilia, an investigator could choose a decision analysis model with the incidence of hemorrhagic events as the primary outcome of interest. Alternatively, an investigator could choose a cost-effectiveness model with the cost per hemorrhagic event avoided as the primary outcome. Depending on the type of model chosen, the analysis and subsequent preferred course of action are quite different.

Structure a problem over time in the form of a decision tree

Once a study population and research question are defined, the problem is structured in the form of a decision tree. A variety of commercial software packages are available to assist with tree construction and data analysis [8]. The decision tree is constructed as a series of nodes connected by branches, with a horizontal orientation and flowing from left to right (Fig. 1). The tree always begins with a square decision node, which in this example represents

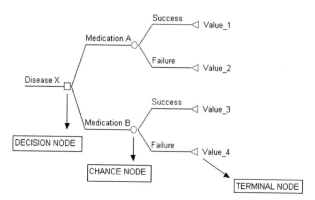

Fig. 1. Basic structure and components of a decision analysis tree.

the decision to prescribe Medication A or Medication B for a patient who has Disease X. The circular nodes are chance nodes and represent events beyond the control of the clinician, in this case the probability of treating Disease X successfully with Medication A or B. In reality, each strategy often is associated with multiple chance nodes. These chance nodes must represent all possible clinical events of interest, such as treatment success or failure, side effects, complications, and mortality. Finally, the triangular nodes are terminal (or outcome) nodes and represent the health outcomes and costs associated with the full sequence of events in that particular pathway.

A simple tree model is useful for research questions involving short periods of time, such as a comparison of treatment strategies for the initial presentation of ITP or a comparison of DVT prophylaxis strategies after a pelvic fracture. A Markov model, alternatively, is a useful tool for depicting a clinical problem involving risks that are ongoing or changing over time [9]. Markov models assume that patients always are in one of a finite number of mutually exclusive health states, referred to as Markov states (Fig. 2). During each time cycle of the model (a week, month, year, and so forth), patients remain in their original health state or transition to a different state, depending on the probability of those events. In Fig. 2, two anticoagulation strategies are compared for a patient who has DVT. In this clinical scenario, four possible health states are described. The patient can be anticoagulated and well, can experience a major bleed as a side effect of anticoagulation, can experience a recurrent DVT as a failure of anticoagulation, or can die from a thrombotic event, bleed, or other cause. The Markov model continues to cycle until stopping criteria are met—the death of all patients or the passage of a given amount of time.

Characterize probabilities, costs, and utilities of the decision tree

Model estimation involves assigning probability estimates to each chance node in the decision tree and cost and utility estimates to each pathway.

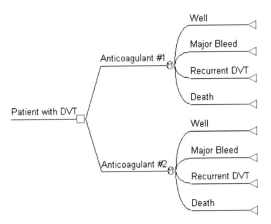

Fig. 2. Basic structure and components of a Markov model, using the example of a patient who has DVT who can be treated with anticoagulant #1 or #2. Four possible Markov, or health, states are included.

Usually, the exact probabilities cannot be estimated with certainty. Therefore, the values that estimate the probabilities best are used in the original, or base-case, analysis. In sensitivity analysis (discussed later), each probability is varied over an estimated range. A rigorous literature search is performed using a hierarchy of sources (case series → large cohort studies → prospective randomized trials → systematic reviews), and the quality and applicability of each source should be determined [10]. Probabilities must be assigned to each branch emanating from a chance node, and for each chance node, the sum of the probabilities must be equal to 1. In some cases there may be insufficient data in the medical literature to inform every chance node in a decision analysis model. Investigators then may turn to expert or personal opinion to generate a probability estimate. Although these estimates certainly can be rigorously tested later in sensitivity analysis, the need to use them does decrease the validity of the technique.

Once the optimal strategy is identified in a decision analysis study, costs can be added to the model to understand the cost-effectiveness or cost-utility of that strategy compared with others. When performing a cost-effectiveness analysis, an investigator should capture all health care use costs and the productivity loss of patients' caregivers [11]. It also is important to differentiate cost data from charge data. Actual cost data always are preferred in decision analysis models, as charge data can be arbitrary and often depend highly on a third-party payer or treatment setting. A popular source for medication costs is the *Drug Topics Red Book*, an annual reference reporting the average wholesale price of prescription and over-the-counter medications [12]. In the United States, Medicare and Medicaid reimbursement data often are considered the best estimate of health care costs. Average hospitalization costs can be derived from Medicare and Medicaid diagnosis-related groups, laboratory costs can be obtained from the Clinical Diagnostic Laboratory Fee Schedule, and the costs of physician visits, tests, and procedures can be estimated using Healthcare Common Procedure Coding System codes. More information about these data sources and the Physician Fee Schedule Search can be found at the Centers for Medicare and Medicaid Services Web site [13]. In 1996, the Panel on Cost-Effectiveness in Health and Medicine published consensus-based recommendations for the conduct of cost-effectiveness analyses [14]. This document is an excellent resource that addresses the proper methodology for measuring costs and health consequences, incorporating time preferences and discounting, and handling uncertainty in cost-effectiveness analyses.

Economic evaluations that take a societal point of view, as recommended by the Panel on Cost-Effectiveness in Health and Medicine, must include the indirect costs of health care. These costs include patient transportation expenses for office and laboratory visits and costs for patient time. Productivity losses, or costs for time, are yet to be well described for children and adolescents. A common technique for estimating the costs of adult patient and parent time is to base these costs on the average hourly wage of a United States non–farm production worker, published annually by the United States Department of Labor, Bureau of Labor Statistics [15].

Although usually considered under the umbrella term of "cost-effectiveness analyses," it is important to distinguish cost-effectiveness from cost-utility analyses. Both studies measure costs in the same manner; it is the benefits that are measured in different metrics [16]. In a cost-effectiveness analysis, costs all are related to a single, common effect. For example, an investigator could compare ultrasonography to venography in terms of number of upper extremity DVTs detected or primary versus secondary hemophilia prophylaxis in terms of number of joint bleeds. In a cost-utility analysis, outcomes are measured in terms of the value placed on the outcome rather than the outcome itself, which usually is expressed as quality-adjusted life-years (QALYs). Total QALYs are calculated for each strategy by multiplying the time spent in a state of health by the utility value of that particular health state. Utilities represent a patient's preference for a particular health state and can range from 0 (death) to 1 (perfect health). There are two main advantages to the use of QALYs as an outcome measure: (1) the measure combines length of life and quality of life into a single outcome and (2) the measure allows direct comparison of health benefits across different diseases, patient populations, and studies [17].

Utilities can be measured in several different ways. An investigator can measure utilities directly for the decision analysis model by performing a choice-based valuation technique, such as the standard gamble or time trade-off method, in a representative sample of the general population. In the standard gamble, the respondent is asked to consider one health state with a certain outcome and one that involves a gamble between two additional health states. The probability of the gamble is varied until the respondent has no preference for either alternative. For example, a respondent could be asked, "If you had to live with blindness for the rest of your life, would you undergo an eye surgery with a 5% chance of immediate death but a 95% chance of restoring perfect vision?" The respondent may choose the surgery, live with the blindness, or state that it is too hard to make a decision at those particular probabilities.

In time trade-off, the respondent is given a choice between two health states and asked to decide how many years of life he would be willing to give up to achieve the healthier state. For example, a respondent could be asked, "In exchange for 10 years of poor health with sickle cell disease, would you accept 9 years of perfect health with new drug therapy X?" The respondent can choose to accept or not accept that amount of time. Detailed descriptions and simulated interviews using each of these techniques can be found in *Methods for the Economic Evaluation of Health Care Programs* [18]. On-line demonstrations are also available [19]. Standard gamble and time trade-off exercises, however, are time consuming and complex tasks. They are challenging to use particularly in pediatric research because they require a lengthy attention span and a minimum sixth-grade reading skills level.

An alternative method of measuring utilities directly is to use a pre-scored multiattribute health status classification system, such as the Health Utilities Index or the EuroQol-5D [18,19]. Formulas have been developed to calculate utilities using patient responses to these generic quality-of-life instruments. These instruments are easier and faster to administer and require less advanced reading levels. The EuroQol-5D consists of five questions regarding a patient's mobility, self-care, usual activities, pain/discomfort, and anxiety/depression. In the mobility question, for example, a patient may choose between the following options: (1) I have no problems in walking about; (2) I have some problems in walking about; and (3) I am confined to bed.

Options also exist for cost-effectiveness analysts unable to collect primary utility data. In an effort to increase consistency in cost-utility analyses, Gold and colleagues [20] have developed an "off-the-shelf" source of utility values for hundreds of health states. These investigators derived and conducted preliminary validation on a set of utilities for chronic conditions using nationally representative data from the National Health Interview Survey and the Healthy People 2000 years of healthy life measure. The list often is referred to as the Health and Activities Limitation Index. In another step toward the goal of developing a national repository of utility weights, Tengs and Wallace [21] gathered 1000 health-related quality-of-life estimates from publicly available source documents in a comprehensive review.

Choose the preferred course of action (model analysis)

In a base-case analysis, an investigator uses the "best estimate" for each probability, cost, and utility variable in the model. This analysis, therefore, contains the values an analyst believes are closest to the actual state of affairs. Analyzing a decision tree involves comparing the overall benefits expected from choosing each strategy, defined as the expected utility [22]. For example, in Fig. 1, assume that Medication A has an 80% chance of success and, therefore, a 20% chance of failure. If the medication succeeds, the patient has perfect health or a utility of 1. If the medication fails, the patient remains ill and has a utility of 0.7. The expected utility for this chance node is the sum of the product of each of the probabilities multiplied by its utility, or $(0.8 \times 1) + (0.2 \times 0.7) = 0.94$. This process is repeated for every chance node, moving from right to left. The process is called folding back or rolling back and typically performed using decision analysis software. The expected utility can be measured using any scale an analyst chooses: number of blood transfusions, gain in life expectancy, or quality of life (utilities), as chosen in this example. Details on the rolling back process can be found in several reviews [10,23,24].

The end result of rolling back is that each clinical strategy in the model is assigned a final value. In a decision analysis for which morbidity or mortality is the primary outcome measure, the strategy with the lowest value is the preferred option. If QALYs are the primary outcome measure, the strategy with the highest value is preferred. In a cost-effectiveness analysis (the most common type of decision analysis), the software program presents each clinical strategy in ascending order by total cost and compares the strategies using an incremental cost-effectiveness ratio. This ratio is defined as the extra cost of a strategy divided by its extra clinical benefit as compared with the next least expensive strategy. Any strategy that costs more but is less effective than an alternative strategy is considered dominated and removed from further consideration. Although there is no absolute threshold for cost-effectiveness, incremental cost-effectiveness ratios of less than $50,000 to $100,000 per healthy life year (QALY) gained typically are considered cost effective [25]. These proposed ratios, more than 20 years old, however, have not been adjusted for inflation and have not been considered independently for the pediatric population [26].

In most decision analysis studies, there is some uncertainty about the inputs used in model construction. Sensitivity analysis, always performed after the base-case analysis, is an important tool for handling the uncertainty inherent in any decision analysis model and evaluates the effect of alternative assumptions on the final result. In this process, the probabilities, costs, and utilities of a model can be changed systematically, and the results of the analysis are recalculated multiple times. For example, in Fig. 1, the probability of treatment success with Medication A can be changed from 80% to 50%, 90%, or any other number chosen by the analyst. If changing a variable over a reasonable range of values changes the preferred strategy, the model is considered sensitive to that variable. Typically, a model is sensitive to variation of some parameters and insensitive to variation of others. A model that is insensitive to variation of most parameters is a robust model.

The simplest method of assessing the uncertainty of a decision analysis is a one-way sensitivity analysis, in which each model input is varied one at a time. An investigator typically uses ranges suggested by the published literature or adds and subtracts 50% to 100% from the base-case estimates. For example, in a cost-utility analysis of therapies for ITP, the 2005 wholesale price of anti-D immune globulin for a 20-kg child ($81) was used in the base-case analysis [27]. This value was varied, however, from $40 to $120 during sensitivity analysis. The investigators found that even if the price of anti-D could be reduced by 50%, prednisone is still the more cost-effective strategy. The results of one-way sensitivity analysis often are displayed in the form of a tornado diagram. In the hypothetical example of a tornado diagram (illustrated in Fig. 3), one-way sensitivity analysis reveals that the model is sensitive to variations in the utility of the painful health state and the cost of medication, less so to the utility of wellness, and quite insensitive to variation in the probability of hospitalization.

Although beyond the scope of this introductory review, probabilistic sensitivity analysis, which allows for the simultaneous variation of multiple parameters, is becoming a standard part of decision analyses [28]. Briefly, each probability, cost, and utility value is assigned a range of possible values over a specified distribution. All parameters then are varied simultaneously through random draws from each distribution, incremental cost-effectiveness ratios are calculated, and the process is repeated thousands of times. These results can be expressed in several different formats and allow for conclusions, such as, "Medication X is the most cost-effective strategy in 95% of simulations." Analysts can use sensitivity analyses to calculate cost-effectiveness thresholds, or frontiers. These exercises allow for conclusions,

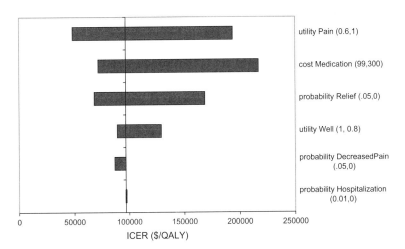

Fig. 3. The results of a one-way sensitivity analysis displayed in a tornado figure. Numbers in parentheses indicate the range of each one-way sensitivity analysis. ICER, incremental cost-effectiveness ratio, expressed as cost per additional QALY.

such as, "Observation for ITP patients is the most cost-effective strategy, unless the incidence of intracranial hemorrhage is greater than 5%."

Published examples of decision analyses in pediatric hematology

Over the past decade, several decision analyses have been performed that address clinical dilemmas in pediatric hematology. A comprehensive list is in Table 1, but three examples warrant further discussion.

Management options for inhibitors in hemophilia include eradicating the inhibitor via immune tolerance induction or treating bleeding episodes with large quantities of hemostatic agents. In a study by Colowick and colleagues [29], the investigators constructed a decision analysis model to compare the expected clinical outcomes and costs over a lifetime for a typical 5 year old who has severe factor VIII deficiency and high inhibitor levels. Only the costs of factor concentrates were considered rather than the full complement of direct and indirect health care costs, as recommended by the Panel on Cost-Effectiveness. The investigators stated, however, that they considered only factor costs because many studies have demonstrated that factor concentrates account for 80% to 90% of total costs in managing patients who have hemophilia in inpatient and outpatient settings. Because the timeline of interest is a lifetime, the investigators appropriately used a Markov model. The patient could experience one of seven possible health states: three short-term (acute bleed) states, three chronic joint disease states, and death. In this model, the immune tolerance strategy was cost saving and clinically superior, costing $1.7 million less and providing 4.6 additional life-years for each patient. Because decision analysis has the advantage of being able to consider any timeframe, this study was able to show that an intervention that is extremely expensive upfront actually is cost saving when considered over a child's lifetime.

To date, no clinical trial has examined whether or not patients who have sickle cell disease and a high risk for stroke would have better outcomes with a chronic transfusion program or bone marrow transplantation (BMT). In a study by Nietert and coworkers [30], decision analysis was used to compare the number of QALYs experienced by patients who had abnormal cerebral flow velocities treated with periodic blood transfusions (PBT) or BMT. One weakness of this study is that although QALYs were the major outcome of interest, utility estimates were based solely on the opinion of two of the investigators because of the absence of direct reports of quality of life from sickle cell patients. Although the investigators noted that their estimates were within the ranges of the Health and Activities Limitation Index measurements for other chronic diseases, this study would have been strengthened by obtaining some utility measurements from patients who had sickle cell anemia and their families. In a recent study of therapy preferences and decision making among the parents of children who had severe sickle cell anemia, PBT and BMT were viewed as similarly efficacious treatments, but BMT was viewed as a more dangerous treatment [31]. Because a lifetime timeframe was considered, a Markov model was constructed. Patients managed with BMT could expect 16 QALYs as compared with 15.7 QALYs for patients receiving PBT; however, the variation around these estimates was large. Patients compliant with PBT therapy and iron chelation could expect the best outcomes (19.2 QALYs). Based on their results, the authors recommended that abnormal cerebral blood flow velocity alone should not be considered an indication for BMT in sickle cell disease. This study would have been strengthened by including costs in the model, especially as the difference in QALYs was small between the clinical strategies.

The need to perform a bone marrow aspiration (BMA) before using steroids for the treatment of ITP remains controversial because of the concern that a diagnosis of leukemia could be missed. Unlike the prior two examples, which compared treatment strategies, a study by Klaassen and colleagues [32] evaluated three possible screening strategies using a simple decision tree. The population of interest was children ages 6 months to 18 years presenting with acute-onset petechiae and bruising, idiopathic thrombocytopenia, and no peripheral blasts. The three strategies were (1) initial BMA in all patients, (2) initial BMA only in patients at high risk (thrombocytopenia combined with anemia or leukopenia), and (3) empiric steroid therapy for all patients who did not have initial BMA. Costs were not considered in this model, and the primary outcome was total QALYs. Utilities for the various health states were determined by interviews with 10 health care providers and included time trade-off tasks, a rating scale task, and the Health Utilities Index. Model results indicated excellent and similar life expectancies with all three strategies, with total QALYs ranging from only 69.64 to 69.65. Even if initial BMA was performed only in high-risk patients, the analysis demonstrated that only seven missed cases of leukemia would occur in a population of 100,000 children presenting with thrombocytopenia. The investigators concluded that if the history, physical examination, and peripheral blood smear are determined by a pediatric hematologist to be consistent with ITP, an initial BMA is not compulsory before starting steroids. This study is an example of how decision analysis models never can match the complexity of "real-life" medicine. Although the model included the most significant complication of a missed diagnosis of leukemia, the altered chance of survival for patients, it cannot account for the more intangible complications, such as emotional stress for patients and families, decreased trust in the patient-doctor relationship, and possible legal implications of a missed diagnosis.

The Centre for Reviews and Dissemination at The University of York maintains a publicly available, free-of-charge database of economic evaluations [33]. This is an excellent resource to use when searching for

Table 1
Examples of recently published studies using decision analysis to address conditions of uncertainty in pediatric hematology

Author	Decision	Strategies compared	Primary outcomes	Results and conclusions
Allen et al [39]	Treatment of zidovudine-related anemia in HIV-infected children	(1) Recombinant human erythropoietin (r-HuEPO) (2) Monthly transfusions	Costs over 1 year	r-HuEPO costs $1373 per transfusion episode averted.
Colowick et al [29]	Management of high-titer inhibitors in a 5-year-old child who has severe factor VIII deficiency	(1) Immune tolerance induction (2) Treat bleeding with large quantities of factor	Total lifetime costs and lifetime expectancy	Immune tolerance led to increased life expectancy (4.6 years per patient) and decreased costs ($1.7 million per patient).
Killie et al [40]	Screening strategies for neonatal alloimmune thrombocytopenia	(1) Screening pregnant women (2) No screening	QALYs and costs	In 100,000 women, screening and subsequent treatment led to 220 extra QALYs and decreased costs by 1.7 million euros.
Klaassen et al [32]	Initial management of child over 6 months old who has idiopathic thrombocytopenia and no blasts on peripheral smear	(1) BMA in all patients (2) BMA in high-risk patients (3) No BMA	QALYs	BMA did not significantly change overall QALYs (<4-day difference between strategies) and should not be mandatory in every ITP patient before starting steroids.
Mazumdar et al [41]	Stroke prevention in sickle cell anemia using transcranial Doppler and chronic transfusion	Six strategies differing by frequency of Doppler screening and duration of chronic transfusions	Number of ischemic strokes prevented	Optimal strategy was annual screening from 2–10 years, with monthly transfusions in high-risk children until 18 years.

Study	Clinical question	Strategies	Outcome measure	Results
Nietert et al [30]	Treatment of sickle cell patients who have increased cerebral blood velocity	(1) BMT (2) PBT	QALYs	Neither BMT (16 QALYs) nor PBT (15.7) can be considered "best treatment." Abnormal cerebral blood flow velocity should not be the only criterion for BMT.
O'Brien et al [27]	Treatment of acute ITP	(1) Intravenous immunoglobulin (IVIG) (2) Anti-D (3) Methylprednisolone (4) Prednisone	Cost per day of severe thrombocytopenia avoided	Predisone and anti-D are the most cost-effective strategies. Compared to prednisone, anti-D costs $7600/day of severe thrombocytopenia avoided.
Panepinto et al [42]	Neonatal screening for sickle cell disease	(1) No screening (2) Targeted screening of African Americans (3) Universal screening	Cost per additional year of life saved	Targeted screening of African Americans, compared with no screening, costs only $6700 per year of life saved.
Thung and Grobman [43]	Antepartum treatment of neonatal alloimmune thrombocytopenia	(1) IVIG and corticosteroids as indicated by fetal blood sampling (2) Empiric IVIG	Marginal cost per QALY gained	Empiric IVIG has a favorable cost-effectiveness ratio of $32,700 per QALY gained.

cost-effectiveness and cost-utility analyses. The database describes each study and appraises study quality, strengths, and weaknesses.

Evaluating the decision analysis literature

The number of published decision analysis articles has increased steadily over the past 2 decades. Also, the demand for economic evaluations in health care has increased the use of modeling tools to assess the cost-effectiveness of new drug therapies and treatment strategies [11]. Therefore, it is important for all physicians to be able to analyze the results of these studies critically. An excellent guide to interpreting a clinical decision analysis has been published by Richardson and Detsky, as part of the *Users' Guides to the Medical Literature* series in the *Journal of the American Medical Association* [22,34]. This section briefly summarizes those recommendations.

First, readers must be able to assess the validity of a decision analysis model. The structure of any decision tree should mirror as closely as possible a real-life clinical dilemma. All available and important clinical strategies should be considered, and the strategies need to have competing benefits and risks in order for the dilemma to be meaningful and worth studying. Just as with a systematic review, the investigators of a clinical decision analysis should describe how they searched and reviewed the literature to estimate probabilities, and this methodology should be explicit and reproducible. Analysts should describe how they judged the quality of the available data and if and how any data were transformed. For example, 5-year DVT recurrence rates may have been adjusted to fit a model with a 2-year timeline. Investigators also should report the source of cost and utility estimates. The most credible utility ratings come from the following sources: (1) direct measurements from a large group of patients who had the disease in question or the general public or (2) published studies of quality-of-life ratings from patients who had the disease in question. Finally, readers always should assess how the investigators determined the impact of uncertainty in the model. All probability, cost, and utility estimates should be tested in at least a one-way sensitivity analysis, and readers should take note of which variables, if any, altered the optimal strategy. The more robust the model, the more confident readers can be that a recommended strategy is in fact the optimal choice.

In the second part of the series, Richardson and Detsky [22] describe how to interpret the results and generalizability of a clinical decision analysis. In a decision analysis, any one clinical strategy can be chosen as a preferred strategy or there may be a toss-up between two or more strategies. Readers must decide if the difference between strategies is important clinically. Previous studies have suggested that a gain in life expectancy or QALYs of 2 or more months can be considered significant [35,36]. Another rule of thumb in decision analysis, as discussed previously, is that an intervention costing less than $50,000 to $100,000 per QALY gained typically is considered cost effective. Finally, readers need to ensure that their patients are similar to the hypothetical patients in the decision analysis model or at least the populations included in the sensitivity analysis and must consider whether or not the patient utility values used in a model are similar to the health preferences and values held by their own patient populations.

Readers of a decision analysis study need to be aware of the limitations inherent in this type of research [37]. The complexity of any disease process in real life is higher than can be expressed in a decision analysis model. More complex and sophisticated models are being developed, but the more complex the model, the more data are required. The lack of data for clinical probabilities, long-term effects, and patient utilities is a major limitation to model building, particularly in pediatrics. Finally, most models are built from only one perspective, for example, a patient, third-party payer, or heath policy maker. Finding the "true" optimal clinical strategy often may require taking all of these perspectives under consideration.

Summary

Decision analysis is the application of explicit, quantitative methods to analyze decisions under conditions of uncertainty [34]. This method is a valuable tool for addressing clinical dilemmas in pediatric hematology for which traditional clinical studies may be impractical or even impossible. Decision analysis also can help inform the design of future clinical research by identifying key probability values in the sensitivity analysis that affect model results strongly. Models that are extremely sensitive to patient utility values emphasize the need for increased quality-of-life research in a particular disease state. As with any research method, there are strengths and weaknesses associated with decision analysis. The more accurate and unbiased the estimates of probabilities and outcomes that go into the model, the stronger the desired results. With the current emphasis on costs in the health care system, pediatric hematologists need to be aware of the methodology of economic evaluations, such as cost-effectiveness and cost-utility analyses, and be able to interpret the results of these studies.

Several excellent review articles and textbooks have been published on the topic of decision analysis [5,9,10,14,18,22–24,34]. Many universities offer introductory courses in cost-effectiveness and decision analysis through their master's degree programs in public health, health administration, or clinical research. The Society for Medical Decision Making and the International Society for Pharmacoeconomics and Outcomes Research offer introductory short courses coinciding with their annual meetings. Recognizing that many beginning decision analysis investigators may not have a mentor at their own institution, the Society for Medical Decision Making has started a year-long mentorship program for junior investigators. This program starts with a one-on-one meeting with a senior investigator during the annual meeting. Finally, decision analysis software companies may offer introductory courses for new users. Tree Age Software offers a 1-day training course several times a year focused on new investigators in the health care field [38]. All these resources provide excellent opportunities for interested readers to learn more about decision analysis and receive introductory training in this increasingly important research technique.

Glossary of terms

Base-case Analysis: a model analysis that uses the best estimate for each variable in the model, uses the estimates that the investigator believes are closest to the actual state of affairs

Clinical Practice Guidelines: a group process used to generate clinical recommendations; techniques include informal peer committees, nominal group techniques, the Delphi method, and expert or nonexpert consensus conferences

Cost-effectiveness Analysis: costs are related to a single, common effect that may differ in magnitude between the clinical strategies being compared (i.e. cost per DVT averted, cost per life saved)

Cost-utility Analysis: allows for quality of life adjustments to the clinical outcomes, strategies are compared using the outcome of quality-adjusted life-year (QALY)

Decision Analysis: the application of explicit, quantitative methods to analyze decision making under conditions of uncertainty

Folding or Rolling Back: the process of analyzing a decision tree, comparing the overall benefits expected from choosing each strategy

Markov Model: a type of decision analysis ideal for modeling clinical problems with ongoing risks, the patient transitions between a finite number of health states referred to as Markov states

Meta-analysis: the statistical aspects of a systematic review, includes calculating summary effect estimates and variance, statistical tests of heterogeneity and statistical estimates of publication bias

Quality-Adjusted Life-Year (QALY): the number of years spent in a particular health state multiplied by the utility of that health state

Robust model: a decision analysis model that is insensitive to variation of most parameters during the sensitivity analysis

Sensitivity Analysis: the process of repeatedly folding back a decision tree using different values for probability, cost, and utility variables. In one-way sensitivity analysis, each model input is varied one at a time. Probabilistic sensitivity analysis allows for simultaneous variation of multiple parameters.

Systematic Reviews: a well-defined and uniform approach to identifying all relevant studies addressing the same research question, displaying the results of eligible studies, and if appropriate, calculating summary estimates

Utility: a person's preference for a particular health state ranging from 0 (death) to 1 (perfect health); measured using a quality of life instrument, direct ratings, or choice-based valuation technique (standard gamble, time trade-off)

Acknowledgments

Special thanks to Dr. Kelly Kelleher for his thoughtful review of this article and to Ms. Christine Riley for her administrative support.

References

[1] Hulley SB. Research using existing data: secondary data analysis, ancillary studies, and systematic reviews. In: Hulley SB, Cummings SR, Browner WS, editors. Designing clinical research. 2nd edition. Philadelphia: Lippincott Williams & Wilkins; 2001. p. 195–212.

[2] Cook DJ, Greengold NL, Ellrodt AG, et al. The relation between systematic reviews and practice guidelines. Ann Intern Med 1997;127:210–6.

[3] Weinstein MC, Fineberg HV. Clinical decision analysis. Philadelphia: W.B. Saunders; 1980.

[4] Albert DA. Decision theory in medicine: a review and critique. Milbank Mem Fund Q Health Soc 1978;56:362–401.

[5] Detsky AS, Naglie G, Krahn MD, et al. Primer on medical decision analysis: part 1–getting started. Med Decis Making 1997;17:123–5.

[6] Adams RJ, McKie VC, Hsu L, et al. Prevention of a first stroke by transfusions in children with sickle cell anemia and abnormal results on transcranial Doppler ultrasonography. N Engl J Med 1998;339:5–11.

[7] Male C, Chait P, Ginsberg JS, et al. Comparison of venography and ultrasound for the diagnosis of asymptomatic deep vein thrombosis in the upper body in children: results of the PARKAA study. Prophylactic antithrombin replacement in kids with all treated with asparaginase. Thromb Haemost 2002;87:593–8.

[8] Maxwell D. Improving hard decisions: biennial survey of decision analysis software offers side-by-side comparison of critical O.R. tools. OR/MS Today, 2006;33(6).

[9] Sonnenberg FA, Beck JR. Markov models in medical decision making: a practical guide. Med Decis Making 1993;13:322–38.

[10] Burd RS, Sonnenberg FA. Decision analysis: a basic overview for the pediatric surgeon. Semin Pediatr Surg 2002;11:46–54.

[11] Bohn RL, Colowick AB, Avorn J. Probabilities, costs, and outcomes: methodological issues in modelling haemophilia treatment. Haemophilia 1999;5:374–7.

[12] Drug topics red book. Montvale (NY): Medical Economics; 2006.

[13] US Department of Health and Human Services. Centers for Medicare and Medicaid services. Available at: http://www.cms.hhs.gov. Accessed February 14, 2008.

[14] Weinstein MC, Siegel JE, Gold MR, et al. Recommendations of the panel on cost-effectiveness in health and medicine. JAMA 1996;276:1253–8.

[15] US Department of Labor. Bureau of Labor Statistics data. Available at: http://www.bls.gov/data/home.htm. Accessed February 14, 2008.

[16] Drummond M. Basic types of economic evaluation. In: Drummond MF, Obrien B, Stoddard GL, et al, editors. Methods for the economic evaluation of health care programmes. 2nd edition. Oxford (UK): Oxford University Press; 1997. p. 6–26.

[17] Griebsch I, Coast J, Brown J. Quality-adjusted life-years lack quality in pediatric care: a critical review of published cost-utility studies in child health. Pediatrics 2005;115:e600–14.

[18] Drummond MF, O'Brien B, Stoddart GL, et al. Methods for the economic evaluation of health care programmes. 2nd edition. Oxford (England); New York: Oxford University Press; 1997.

[19] Health Decision Strategies, LLC. Decision tools, questionnaires, and surveys. Available at: http://www.healthstrategy.com/objectiv.htm. Accessed February 15, 2008.

[20] Gold MR, Franks P, McCoy KI, et al. Toward consistency in cost-utility analyses: using national measures to create condition-specific values. Med Care 1998;36:778–92.

[21] Tengs TO, Wallace A. One thousand health-related quality-of-life estimates. Med Care 2000;38:583–637.

[22] Richardson WS, Detsky AS. Users' guides to the medical literature. VII. How to use a clinical decision analysis. B. What are the results and will they help me in caring for my patients? Evidence based medicine working group. JAMA 1995;273:1610–3.

[23] Weinstein MC, Fineberg HV. Clinical decision analysis. Philadelphia: W.B. Saunders; 1980.

[24] Elkin EB, Vickers AJ, Kattan MW. Primer: using decision analysis to improve clinical decision making in urology. Nat Clin Pract Urol 2006;3:439–48.

[25] Hirth RA, Chernew ME, Miller E, et al. Willingness to pay for a quality-adjusted life year: in search of a standard. Med Decis Making 2000;20:332–42.

[26] Ubel PA, Hirth RA, Chernew ME, et al. What is the price of life and why doesn't it increase at the rate of inflation? Arch Intern Med 2003;163:1637–41.

[27] O'Brien SH, Ritchey AK, Smith KJ. A cost-utility analysis of treatment for acute childhood idiopathic thrombocytopenic purpura (ITP). Pediatr Blood Cancer 2007;48:173–80.

[28] Briggs AH, Goeree R, Blackhouse G, et al. Probabilistic analysis of cost-effectiveness models: choosing between treatment strategies for gastroesophageal reflux disease. Med Decis Making 2002;22:290–308.

[29] Colowick AB, Bohn RL, Avorn J, et al. Immune tolerance induction in hemophilia patients with inhibitors: costly can be cheaper. Blood 2000;96:1698–702.

[30] Nietert PJ, Abboud MR, Silverstein MD, et al. Bone marrow transplantation versus periodic prophylactic blood transfusion in sickle cell patients at high risk of ischemic stroke: a decision analysis. Blood 2000;95:3057–64.

[31] Hankins J, Hinds P, Day S, et al. Therapy preference and decision-making among patients with severe sickle cell anemia and their families. Pediatr Blood Cancer 2007;48:705–10.

[32] Klaassen RJ, Doyle JJ, Krahn MD, et al. Initial bone marrow aspiration in childhood idiopathic thrombocytopenia: decision analysis. J Pediatr Hematol Oncol 2001;23:511–8.

[33] Centre for Review and Dissemination. National Health Service economic evaluation database. Available at: http://www.york.ac.uk/ubst/crd/crddatabases.htm. Accessed February 15, 2008.

[34] Richardson WS, Detsky AS. Users' guides to the medical literature. VII. How to use a clinical decision analysis. A. Are the results of the study valid? Evidence-based medicine working group. JAMA 1995;273:1292–5.

[35] Naimark D, Naglie G, Detsky AS. The meaning of life expectancy: what is a clinically significant gain? J Gen Intern Med 1994;9:702–7.

[36] Tsevat J, Weinstein MC, Williams LW, et al. Expected gains in life expectancy from various coronary heart disease risk factor modifications. Circulation 1991;83:1194–201.

[37] Goel V. Decision analysis: applications and limitations. The health services research group. CMAJ 1992;147:413–7.

[38] TreeAge Software, Inc. TreeAge software training. Available at: http://server.treeage.com/treeagepro/training/index.asp. Accessed February 17, 2008.

[39] Allen UD, Kirby MA, Goeree R. Cost-effectiveness of recombinant human erythropoietin versus transfusions in the treatment of zidovudine-related anemia in HIV-infected children. Pediatr AIDS HIV Infect 1997;8:4–11.

[40] Killie MK, Kjeldsen-Kragh J, Husebekk A, et al. Cost-effectiveness of antenatal screening for neonatal alloimmune thrombocytopenia. BJOG 2007;114:588–95.

[41] Mazumdar M, Heeney MM, Sox CM, et al. Preventing stroke among children with sickle cell anemia: an analysis of strategies that involve transcranial Doppler testing and chronic transfusion. Pediatrics 2007;120:e1107–16.

[42] Panepinto JA, Magid D, Rewers MJ, et al. Universal versus targeted screening of infants for sickle cell disease: a cost-effectiveness analysis. J Pediatr 2000;136:201–8.

[43] Thung SF, Grobman WA. The cost effectiveness of empiric intravenous immunoglobulin for the antepartum treatment of fetal and neonatal alloimmune thrombocytopenia. Am J Obstet Gynecol 2005;193:1094–9.

ELSEVIER
SAUNDERS

PEDIATRIC CLINICS
OF NORTH AMERICA

Pediatr Clin N Am 55 (2008) 305–322

Venous Thromboembolism in Children

Neil A. Goldenberg, MD[a,b,*],
Timothy J. Bernard, MD[a,b,c]

[a]*Mountain States Regional Hemophilia and Thrombosis Center, P.O. Box 6507,*
Mail-Stop F-416, Aurora, CO 80045-0507, USA
[b]*Pediatric Stroke Program, University of Colorado and The Children's Hospital,*
13123 East 16th Avenue, Aurora, CO 80045, USA
[c]*Department of Child Neurology, University of Colorado and The Children's Hospital,*
13123 East 16th Avenue, Aurora, CO 80045, USA

With improved pediatric survival from serious underlying illnesses, greater use of invasive vascular procedures and devices, and a growing (albeit still suboptimal) awareness that vascular events do occur among the young, venous thromboembolism (VTE) increasingly is recognized as a critical pediatric concern. The focus of this review is on providing background on etiology and epidemiology in this disorder, followed by an in-depth discussion of approaches to the clinical characterization, diagnostic evaluation, and management of pediatric VTE. Prognostic indicators and long-term outcomes are considered, with emphasis placed on available evidence underlying present knowledge and key questions for further investigation.

Characterization

VTE is classified clinically by various relevant descriptors, including first episode versus recurrent, symptomatic versus asymptomatic, acute versus chronic (a distinction that can be difficult at times), veno-occlusive versus nonocclusive, and idiopathic versus risk associated. This last category includes clinical prothrombotic risk factors (eg, exogenous estrogen administration, indwelling central venous catheter, and reduced mobility) and blood-based thrombophilic conditions (eg, transient or persistent

---

* Corresponding author. Mountain States Regional Hemophilia and Thrombosis Center, P.O. Box 6507, Mail-Stop F-416, Aurora, CO 80045-0507.
E-mail address: neil.goldenberg@uchsc.edu (N.A. Goldenberg).

0031-3955/08/$ - see front matter © 2008 Elsevier Inc. All rights reserved.
doi:10.1016/j.pcl.2008.01.003   *pediatric.theclinics.com*

antiphospholipid antibodies [APAs], acquired or congenital anticoagulant deficiencies, and factor V Leiden or prothrombin G20210A mutations); the latter are discussed in greater detail later. Because of the frequency of indwelling central venous catheters as a major clinical risk factor for VTE in children, VTE also may be classified as catheter-related thromboembolism (CRT) versus non-CRT. VTEs also are distinguished anatomically by vascular type (ie, venous versus arterial); vascular distribution (eg, distal lower extremity versus proximal lower extremity versus central or superficial versus deep vasculature); and organ system affected, if applicable (eg, cerebral sinovenous thrombosis [CSVT] or pulmonary embolism). The use of systematic nomenclature and precise descriptors for VTE assists in optimizing clinical care and in evaluating clinical research evidence in the field.

Epidemiology

Several years ago, registry data revealed an estimated cumulative incidence of 0.07 per 10,000 (5.3 per 10,000 hospitalizations) for extremity deep venous thrombosis (DVT) or pulmonary embolism (PE) among non-neonatal Canadian children [1] and an incidence rate of 0.14 per 10,000 Dutch children per year for VTE in general [2]. More recently, an evaluation of the National Hospital Discharge Survey and census data for VTE in the United States disclosed an overall incidence rate of 0.49 per 10,000 per year [3].

Epidemiologic data have revealed that the age distribution of the incidence rate for VTE in children is bimodal, with peak rates in the neonatal period and adolescence. The Dutch registry, for example, indicated a VTE incidence rate of 14.5 per 10,000 per year in the neonatal period, approximately 100 times greater than the overall rate in childhood [2], whereas the VTE-specific incidence rate in the United States among adolescents 15 to 17 years of age was determined as 1.1 per 10,000 per year, a rate nearly threefold that observed overall in children [3].

Etiology

The pathogenesis of VTE readily can be appreciated by considering the Virchow triad, consisting of venous stasis, endothelial damage, and the hypercoagulable state. In children, greater than 90% of VTEs are risk associated [2,4,5] (compared with approximately 60% in adults), with risk factors often disclosed from more than one component of this triad. Specific examples of VTE risk factors in children are shown in Fig. 1. One of the most common clinical prothrombotic risk factors in childhood is an indwelling central venous catheter. More than 50% of cases of DVT in children and more than 80% of cases in newborns occur in association with central venous catheters [1,6]. The presence of an indwelling central venous

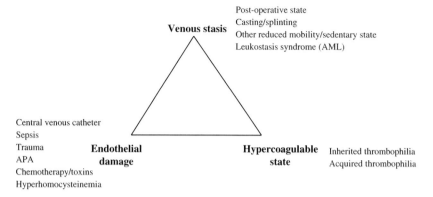

Fig. 1. Clinical prothrombotic risk factors: the Virchow triad applied to VTE in children.

catheter, underlying malignancy or disorder for which bone marrow transplantation was undertaken, and congenital cardiac disease and its corrective surgery all were highly prevalent in the Canadian pediatric thrombosis registry [4], whereas underlying infectious illness and the presence of an indwelling central venous cathether were identified as pervasive clinical risk factors in a recent cohort study analysis from the United States [5]. It is likely that differences in the composition of referral populations contribute strongly to differences in the composition of VTE etiologies across major pediatric thrombosis centers.

With regard to the third component of the Virchow triad, the hypercoagulable state, blood-based risk factors for VTE in children include inherited and acquired thrombophilic conditions and markers of coagulation activation (discussed later). Potent thrombophilic conditions (eg, APAs) in children frequently are acquired and, more rarely, may be congenital (eg, severe anticoagulant deficiencies). By contrast, mild congenital thrombophilia traits (eg, the factor V Leiden and prothrombin G20210A mutations) are common in white populations, with prevalences of approximately 5% and 2%, respectively. Thrombophilia potentially can be caused by any alteration in the hemostatic balance that increases thrombin production, enhances platelet activation or aggregation, mediates endothelial activation or damage, or inhibits fibrinolysis. Common examples of acquired thrombophilia in children include increased factor VIII activity with significant infection and inflammatory states, anticoagulant deficiencies resulting from consumption in bacterial sepsis and disseminated intravascular coagulation (DIC) or production of inhibitory antibodies in acute viral infection, and parainfectious development of APAs. To provide an appreciation of the magnitude of VTE risk increase associated with several congenital or genetically influenced thrombophilia traits, population-based VTE risk estimates derived from the adult literature are shown in Table 1. As seen in Table 1, the addition of standard-dose estrogen oral contraceptive pill to an

Table 1
Venous thromboembolism risk estimates for selected thrombophilia traits and conditions

Trait/condition	Venous thromboembolism risk estimate (× baseline)
Hyperhomocysteinemia	2.5
Prothrombin 20,210 mutation, heterozygous	3
Oral contraceptive pill (tandard dose estrogen)	4
Factor V Leiden mutation, heterozygous	2–7
OCP + factor V Leiden mutation, heterozygous	35
Factor V Leiden mutation, homozygous	80

underlying heterozygous factor V Leiden (in large part by virtue of a "double-hit" to the protein C pathway) substantially increases the risk for VTE from a baseline risk of 15 per 10,000 women in the United States, ages 15 to 17, per year [3] to a risk of more than 500 per 10,000 (or 5%) per year.

Clinical presentation

The degree of clinical suspicion for acute VTE in children should be influenced principally by (1) clinical prothrombotic risk factors and family history of early VTE or other vascular disease elicited on thorough interview; (2) known thrombophilia traits and risk factors; and (3) clinical signs and symptoms. The signs and symptoms of VTE depend on anatomic location and organ system affected and are influenced by characteristics of veno-occlusiveness and chronicity. The classic manifestation of acute extremity DVT is painful unilateral limb swelling. The lack of other physical examination findings (eg, Homans' sign or presence of a palpable cord in the popliteal fossa) should not reduce the clinical index of suspicion of DVT. In upper extremity DVT with extension into, and occlusion of, the superior vena cava (SVC), signs and symptoms may include swelling of neck and face, bilateral periorbital edema, and headache. PE classically is manifest by sudden-onset, unexplained shortness of breath with pleuritic chest pain. When PE is proximal or extensive bilaterally in the distal pulmonary arterial tree, hypoxemia often is demonstrated. Associated right heart failure may manifest with hepatomegaly or peripheral edema. Proximal PE and especially saddle embolus can present with cyanosis or sudden collapse. In many cases, however, PE may be asymptomatic or produce only subtle symptoms in children [7–10], especially when involving limited segmental branches of the pulmonary arteries. In one retrospective series, only 50% of affected children had clinical symptoms attributable to PE [8]. Acute CSVT may present with unusually severe and persistent headache, blurred vision, neurologic signs (eg, cranial nerve palsy and papilledema), or seizures. The classic findings in renal vein thrombosis (RVT) are hematuria and thrombocytopenia, sometimes associated with uremia (especially when bilateral). Presenting signs include oliguria (especially when bilateral) and, in the neonatal period (the time at which RVT is most common during childhood), a flank mass that often is palpable on examination. RVT in older children often is associated with nephrotic syndrome (a risk factor for VTE in general) and, hence, may present with associated stigmata of peripheral and periorbital edema when diagnosed at presentation of nephrosis [11]. Thrombocytopenia may be a presenting manifestation not only of RVT but also of an intracardiac (eg, right atrial) thrombus, especially as in cases of CRT associated with sepsis and DIC. Portal vein thrombosis characteristically presents with splenomegaly and is associated with thrombocytopenia and, often, anemia; gastrointestinal bleeding at presentation typically signals the presence of gastroesophageal varices as a result of portal hypertension. Internal jugular vein thrombosis may manifest with neck pain or swelling and, in the Lemierre syndrome, also is associated classically with fever, trismus, and a palpable mass in the lateral triangle of the neck. Isolated intracardiac thrombosis in association with cardiac surgery or central venous catheter placement most often is asymptomatic.

Chronic VTE may be diagnosed incidentally without signs or symptoms (as sometimes occurs for CSVT during unrelated brain imaging) or, alternatively, may present with signs and symptoms of chronic venous obstruction or post-thrombotic syndrome (PTS) secondary to central venous or extremity thrombosis, including limb pain and edema, dilated superficial collateral veins, venous stasis dermatitis, or frank ulceration of the skin.

Diagnostic evaluation

Radiologic imaging

Historically, venography has been the gold standard for diagnosis of venous thrombosis but limited by its invasiveness. In recent years, this modality has experienced a diminishing role with the development of effective noninvasive or minimally invasive radiologic imaging techniques. Radiologic imaging is used not only to confirm the clinical diagnosis of VTE but also to define the extent and occlusiveness of thrombosis. For suspected DVT of the distal or proximal lower extremity, compression ultrasonography with Doppler imaging typically is used for objective confirmation. When the thrombus may affect or extend into deep pelvic or abdominal veins, CT or MRI often is required. In suspected DVT of the upper extremity, compression ultrasound with Doppler effectively evaluates the limb, but other modalities (eg, echocardiography, CT, and MRI) are needed to disclose involvement of more central vasculature (eg, right atrial thrombosis and SVC thrombosis). In the case of asymptomatic nonocclusive extremity DVT, conventional venography may be used as an alternative to CT or MRI. To establish a diagnosis of DVT of the jugular venous system (such as in suspected cases of the Lemierre syndrome) [12], compression ultrasound with Doppler imaging typically is used.

PE in children commonly is disclosed by spiral CT or, alternatively, ventilation-perfusion scan, the latter generally is suboptimal in cases wherein other lung pathology exists and at centers wherein availability of (and expertise with) this modality is limited. CSVT typically is diagnosed by standard CT or CT venography or, alternatively, MRI or MR venography. The diagnosis of RVT most often is made clinically in neonates and supported by Doppler ultrasound findings of intrarenal vascular resistive indices; however, in some cases a discrete thrombus may be suggested by Doppler ultrasound (especially when extending into the inferior vena cava [IVC]) or disclosed further via MR venography. When RVT occurs in older children, Doppler ultrasound or CT often is diagnostic. Similarly, portal vein thrombosis typically is visualized by Doppler ultrasound or CT.

When new-onset venous thrombosis is evaluated in patients in areas of anatomic abnormality of the venous system (eg, extensive collateral venous circulation due to a prior VTE episode, May-Thurner anomaly, or atretic IVC with azygous continuation), more sensitive methods, such as CT venography or magnetic resonance (MR) venography, often are required to delineate the vascular anatomy adequately and the presence, extent, and occlusiveness of thrombosis. In some cases, conventional venography may be required.

MR venography is more expensive than CT venography, typically requires sedation in children less than 8 years of age or those who are developmentally delayed or very anxious, and its feasibility during acute VTE evaluation may be limited by availability of MR-trained technologists. MR venography offers a significant advantage over CT venography, however, in that it provides diagnostic sensitivity at least as great as CT venography, without engendering the significant radiation exposure of the latter modality.

Laboratory evaluation

Diagnostic laboratory evaluation for pediatric acute VTE includes a complete blood count, comprehensive thrombophilia evaluation (discussed previously), and beta-hCG testing in postmenarchal women. Additional laboratory studies may be warranted depending on associated medical conditions and VTE involvement of specific organ systems. Table 2 summarizes a panel of thrombophilia traits and markers identified as risk factors for VTE in pediatric studies and recommended by the Scientific and Standardization Committee Subcommitee on Perinatal and Pediatric Haemostasis of the International Society on Thrombosis and Haemostasis for the diagnostic laboratory evaluation of acute VTE in children [13]. The panel is comprised of testing for states of anticoagulant (eg, protein C, protein S, and antithrombin) deficiency and procoagulant (eg, factor VIII) excess, mediators of hypercoagulablity or endothelial damage (eg, APAs, lipoprotein(a), and homocysteine), and markers of coagulation activation (eg, D-dimer).

Treatment

A summary of conventional antithrombotic agents and corresponding target anticoagulant levels, based on recent pediatric recommendations

Table 2
Thrombophilic conditions and markers tested during comprehensive diagnostic laboratory evaluation of acute venous thromboembolism in children

Condition/marker	Testing methods
Genetic	
Factor V Leiden polymorphism	PCR
Prothrombin G20210A polymorphism	PCR
Elevated plasma lipoprotein(a) concentration[a]	ELISA
Acquired or genetic	
Antithrombin deficiency	Chromogenic (functional) assay
Protein C deficiency	Chromogenic (functional) assay
Protein S deficiency	ELISA for free (ie, functionally active) protein S antigen
Elevated plasma factor VIII activity[b]	One-stage clotting assay (aPTT-based)
Hyperhomocysteinemia	Mass spectroscopy
APAs	ELISA for anticardiolipin and anti-β2-glycoprotein I IgG and IgM; clotting assay (dilute Russell viper venom time or aPTT-based phospholipid neutralization method) for LA
DIC	Includes platelet count, fibrinogen by clotting method (Clauss), and D-dimer by semiquantitative or quantitative immunoassay (eg, latex agglutination)
Activated protein C resistance	Clotting assay (aPTT based)

[a] Although desginated here as genetic, lipoprotein(a) also may be elevated as part of the acute phase response.

[b] Noted as worthy of consideration in original International Society on Thrombosis and Haemostasis recommendations [13]; this since has been shown a prognostic marker in pediatric thrombosis [6]. Additional testing involving the fibrinolytic system and systemic inflammatory response also is noted as worthy of consideration.

[14], is provided in Table 3 for initial (ie, acute phase) and extended (ie, subacute phase) treatment. Conventional anticoagulants attenuate hypercoagulability, decreasing the risk for thrombus progression and embolism, and rely on intrinsic fibrinolytic mechanisms to dissolve the thrombus over time. The conventional anticoagulants used most commonly in children include heparins and warfarin. Heparins, including unfractionated heparin (UFH) and low molecular weight heparin (LMWH), enhance the activity of antithrombin, an intrinsic anticoagulant protein that serves as a key inhibitor of thrombin. Warfarin acts through antagonism of vitamin K, thereby interfering with γ-carboxylation of the vitamin K–dependent procoagulant factors II, VII, IX, and X and intrinsic anticoagulant proteins C and S.

Initial anticoagulant therapy (ie, acute phase) for VTE in children uses UFH or LMWH. LMWH increasingly is used as a first-line agent for initial anticoagulant therapy in children given the relative ease of subcutaneous over intravenous administration, the decreased need for blood monitoring

Table 3
Recommended intensities and durations of conventional antithrombotic therapies in children, by etiology and treatment agent

Episode	Agents and target anticoagulant activities		Duration of therapy, by etiology
	Initial treatment	Extended treatment	
First	UFH 0.3–0.7 anti-Xa U/mL	Warfarin INR 2.0–3.0	Resolved risk factor: 3–6 months
	LMWH 0.5–1.0 anti-Xa U/mL	LMWH 0.5–1.0 anti-Xa U/mL	No known clinical risk factor: 6–12 months
			Chronic clinical risk factor: 12 months
			Potent congenital thrombophilia: indefinite
Recurrent	UFH 0.3–0.7 anti-Xa U/mL	Warfarin INR 2.0–3.0	Resolved risk factor: 6–12 months
	LMWH 0.5–1.0 anti-Xa U/mL	LMWH 0.5–1.0 anti-Xa U/mL	No known clinical risk factor: 12 months
			Chronic clinical risk factor: indefinite
			Potent congenital thrombophilia: indefinite

of anticoagulant efficacy, and a decreased risk for the development of heparin-induced thrombocytopenia (HIT). UFH (which has a shorter half-life than LMWH) typically is preferred in circumstances of heightened bleeding risk or labile acute clinical status, given the rapid extinction of anticoagulant effect after cessation of the drug. In addition, UFH often is used for acute VTE therapy in the setting of significant impairment or lability in renal function because of the relatively greater renal elimination of LMWH. Common initial maintenance dosing for UFH in non-neonatal children begins with an intravenous loading dose (50 to 75 U/kg) followed by a continuous intravenous infusion (15 to 25 U/kg per hour). In full-term neonates, a maintenance dose (up to 50 U/kg per hour) may be required, especially if the clinical condition is complicated by antithrombin consumption. The starting dose for the LMWH enoxaparin in non-neonatal children commonly ranges between 1.0 and 1.25 mg/kg subcutaneously on an every-12-hour schedule; no bolus dose is given. In full-term neonates, a higher dose of enoxaparin (1.5 mg/kg) typically is necessary [15]. Some recent research has investigated whether once-daily enoxaparin dosing may be suitable for acute VTE therapy in children. For the LMWH dalteparin, initial maintenance dosing of 100–150 antifactor Xa (anti-Xa) U/kg seems appropriate based on available pediatric data [16]; however, further studies are warranted (with more robust representation of all age groups within the pediatric age range) to determine the optimal intensity and frequency of dosing of dalteparin. Heparin therapy, UFH or LMWH, is monitored most accurately by anti-Xa activity. Anti-Xa level is obtained 6 to 8 hours after initiation of UFH infusion and 4 hours after one of the first few doses of LMWH. Clinical laboratories must be made aware of the type of heparin administered so that the appropriate assay standard (eg, UFH or enoxaparin) is used. For UFH, the therapeutic range is 0.3 to 0.7 anti-Xa activity U/mL, whereas for LMWH the therapeutic range is 0.5 to 1.0 U/mL. When the anti-Xa assay is not available, the activated partial thromboplastin time (aPTT) may be used (with a goal aPTT of 60–85 seconds or approximately 1.5–2 times the upper limit of age-appropriate normal values); however, this approach is suboptimal especially in the pediatric age group, in which transient APAs are common and may alter the clotting endpoint. One study of pediatric heparin monitoring demonstrated inaccuracy of aPTT approximately 30% of the time [17]. When dosed by weight in childhood, LMWH does not require frequent monitoring, but anti-Xa activity should be evaluated with changes in renal function. In addition, in cases of acute VTE in which acquired antithrombin deficiency is related to consumption in acute infection or inflammation, anti-Xa activity may rise as antithrombin levels normalize with resolution of the acute illness; in this circumstance, follow-up evaluation of anti-Xa activity is warranted in the subacute period.

The recommended duration of heparinization of 5 to 10 days during the initial therapy for acute VTE has been extrapolated from adult data [18]. UFH treatment rarely is maintained beyond the acute period, given the risk for osteoporosis with extended administration [14] and the inconvenience of continuous intravenous administration. Although adult data suggest efficacy of subcutaneous administration of UFH for acute VTE [19], this has been evaluated only for the acute therapy period before extended therapy with warfarin, and the appropriateness of such an approach in children is not established.

Extended anticoagulant therapy (ie, subacute phase) for VTE in children may use LMWH or warfarin. For warfarin anticoagulation, warfarin may be started during the acute phase; however, because severe congenital deficiencies involving the protein C pathway can present as VTE in early childhood and are associated with warfarin skin necrosis, warfarinization ideally should be initiated only after therapeutic anticoagulation is achieved with a heparin agent. Warfarin is available in tablet form in a variety of doses (eg, 5 mg, 2 mg, or 1 mg) and as an oral liquid formulation at many pediatric tertiary care hospitals. Commonly, the starting dose for warfarin in children is 0.1 mg/kg orally once daily. Warfarin is monitored by international normalized ratio (INR), derived from the measured prothrombin time. The therapeutic INR range for warfarin anticoagulation in VTE is 2.0 to 3.0. Recent adult data do not agree with the historical evidence for maintaining a higher INR (2.5–3.5) in the presence of an APA; however, pediatric data are lacking with regard to optimal dose intensity and duration in children who have APA syndrome. The INR typically is checked after the first 5 days of initiation of (or dosing change in) warfarin therapy and weekly thereafter until stable; gradually, less frequent monitoring often is feasible, with continued stability. The INR also should be evaluated at the time of any bleeding manifestations or increased bruising. Warfarin must be discontinued at least 5 days before invasive procedures, with an INR obtained preprocedurally. Often, an anticoagulant transition (bridge) to LMWH can be performed. The development of pediatric anticoagulation monitoring and transition algorithms can assist in optimizing patient care.

Pediatric recommendations for the duration of antithrombotic therapy in acute VTE [14] largely are derived from evidence in adult trials. For first-episode VTE in children in the absence of potent chronic thrombophilia (eg, APA syndrome, homozygous anticoagulant deficiency, and homozygous factor V Leiden or prothrombin G20210A), the recommended duration of anticoagulant therapy is 3 to 6 months in the presence of an underlying reversible risk factor (eg, postoperative VTE), 6 to 12 months when idiopathic, and 12 months to lifelong when a chronic risk factor persists (eg, systemic lupus erythematosus [SLE]). Recurrent VTE is treated for 6 to 12 months in the presence of an underlying reversible risk factor, 12 months to lifelong when idiopathic, and lifelong when a chronic risk factor persists. In the setting of APA syndrome or potent congenital thrombophilia, the treatment duration for first-episode VTE often is indefinite. Some evidence suggests that children who have SLE and persistence of the lupus anticoagulant (LA) have a 16- to 25-fold greater risk for VTEs than children who have SLE and no LA [20]. In children who have primary (ie, idiopathic) or secondary (ie, associated with SLE or other underlying chronic inflammatory condition) APA syndrome, however, it is possible that the autoimmune disease will become quiescent in later years, such that the benefit of continued therapeutic anticoagulation as secondary VTE prophylaxis may be re-evaluated. Some experts recommend consideration of low-dose anticoagulation as secondary VTE prophylaxis after a conventional 3- to 6-month course of therapeutic anticoagulation for VTE in children who have SLE and who have APA syndrome [21]. Such low-dose anticoagulation might, for example, consist of enoxaparin 1.0–1.5 mg/kg subcutaneously once daily, enoxaparin 0.5 mg/kg subcutaneously twice daily, or daily warfarin with a goal INR of approximately 1.5. Further study to optimize the intensity and duration of therapy or secondary prophylaxis for VTE in children who have APA syndrome urgently is needed, however, especially given the recent evidence in adult VTE that secondary prophylaxis with low-dose warfarin not only may offer little risk reduction beyond no anticoagulation but also is associated with bleeding complications despite a reduced warfarin dose [22,23].

Thrombolytic approaches are gaining increasing attention and use during acute VTE therapy in children, particularly in patients who have hemodynamically significant PE or extensive limb-threatening VTE. Unlike conventional anticoagulants, which attenuate hypercoagulability, thrombolytics promote fibrinolysis directly. Tissue-type plasminogen activator is an intrinsic activator of the fibrinolytic system and is administered as a recombinant agent by various routes (eg, systemic bolus, systemic short-duration infusion, systemic low-dose continuous infusion, or local catheter-directed infusion with or without interventional mechanical thrombectomy/thrombolysis). A recent cohort study analysis of children who had acute lower extremity DVT and who had an a priori high risk for poor post-thrombotic outcomes by virtue of completely veno-occlusive thrombus and plasma FVIII activity greater than 150 U/dL or D-dimer concentration greater than 500 ng/mL revealed that a thrombolysis regimen followed by standard anticoagulation may reduce the risk for PTS substantially compared with standard anticoagulation alone [24]. Further investigation in clinical trials is necessary to confirm these findings.

Other antithrombotic agents include factor Xa inhibitors and direct thrombin inhibitors. Factor Xa inhibitors, including fondaparinux, inhibit the activation of factor X, thereby inhibiting thrombin indirectly. Direct thrombin inhibitors, by contrast, inhibit thrombin directly via its active site or by binding to its target on fibrin and include such drugs as hirudin, recombinant hirudins (eg, lepirudin), and argatroban, all of which are administered intravenously. Intravenous direct thrombin inhibitors are indicated for the treatment of HIT, in particular HIT with associated acute thrombosis, and are used in patients who have a history of HIT. The aforementioned factor Xa inhibitors and direct thrombin inhibitors routinely are monitored by aPTT, with the therapeutic goal ranging from a 1.5- to 3.0-fold aPTT prolongation. A variety of factor Xa inhibitors and oral direct thrombin inhibitors are undergoing preclinical development or evaluation in adult clinical trials.

Other products may have antithrombotic roles in selected circumstances but await demonstration of efficacy in clinical trials. For example, plasma replacement with protein C concentrate is a useful adjunctive therapy to conventional anticoagulant for VTE or purpura fulminans because of microvascular thrombosis in severe congenital protein C deficiency [25–28] and may play a beneficial role in the treatment of purpura fulminans resulting from microvascular thrombosis in children who have sepsis, in particular meningococcemia [29–31]. In addition, case series suggest a role for antithrombin replacement in prevention of VTE in children and young adults who have congenital severe antihrombin deficiency [32] for the prevention of L-asparaginase–associated VTE in pediatric acute lymphoblastic leukemia [33,34] and as combination therapy with defibrotide in the prevention and treatment of hepatic sinusoidal obstruction syndrome (formerly termed veno-occlusive disease) in children undergoing hematopoietic stem cell transplantation [35]. The potential benefit for VTE risk reduction using a regimen of antithrombin replacement combined with daily prophylactic LMWH during induction and consolidation phases of therapy in acute lymphoblastic leukemia also is suggested by a historically controlled cohort study of the BFM 2000 protocol experience in Europe [36]. As discussed previously, antithrombin replacement also may be worthy of consideration in patients who have acute VTE and are undergoing heparinization in whom significant antithrombin deficiency prevents the achievement of therapeutic anti-Xa levels (ie, heparin "resistance"). This may be the case in nephrotic syndrome–associated VTE. Additionally, neonates who have clinical conditions complicated by antithrombin consumption in particular are predisposed to such heparin "resistance" because of a physiologic relative deficiency of this key intrinsic thrombin inhibitor.

The use of vena caval filters should be considered in children of appropriate size in whom recurrent VTE (especially PE) occurs on therapeutic anticoagulation in the presence of a persistent prothrombotic risk factor. In addition, temporary vena caval filters may be considered during times of especially heightened risk for PE. With regard to long-standing vena caval filters, although a case series has suggested that these devices are effective when used with concomitant therapeutic anticoagluation for primary and secondary prevention of PE in teens [37], the impact of such nonretrievable devices on the vena cava of developing children is not well studied, and experience with surgical removal of permanent vena caval filters is limited. Consequently, the use of nonretrievable vena caval filters in pediatrics should be undertaken with great caution.

Outcomes

Complications of VTEs can occur acutely and over the long term. Short-term adverse outcomes include major hemorrhagic complications of antithrombotic interventions and of the thrombotic event itself (eg, post-thrombotic hemorrhage in the brain, testis, or adrenal gland); early recurrent VTE (including DVT and PE); SVC syndrome in DVT of the upper venous system; acute renal insufficiency in RVT; catheter-related sepsis, PE, and catheter malfunction (sometimes necessitating surgical replacement) in CRT; severe acute venous insufficiency leading to venous infarction with limb gangrene in rare cases of occlusive DVT involving the extremities; and death from hemodynamic instability in extensive intracardiac thrombosis or proximal PE. Given the long-term risks for recurrence, disease sequelae, and functional impairment, however, VTE arguably is best considered a chronic disorder in children. Long-term adverse outcomes in pediatric VTE recently have been reviewed [38] and include recurrent VTE; chronic hypertension and renal insufficiency in RVT; variceal hemorrhage in portal vein thrombosis; chronic SVC syndrome in CRT involving SVC occlusion; loss of availability for venous access in recurrent or extensive CRT of the upper venous system; and development of the PTS, a condition of chronic venous insufficiency after DVT. The manifestations of PTS may include edema, visibly dilated superficial collateral veins (Fig. 2A), venous stasis dermatitis (see Fig. 2B), and (in the most severe cases) venous stasis ulcers.

Registry [1,4,39] and cohort study [5] data in pediatric VTE of all types indicate that children seem to have a lower risk for recurrent thromboembolism than adults (cumulative incidences at 1 to 2 years of 6% to 11% versus

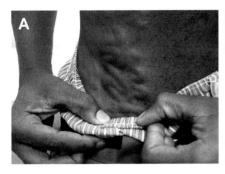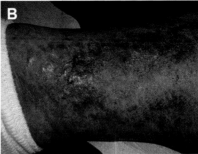

Fig. 2. PTS: dilated collateral superficial venous circulation and venous stasis dermatitis. (*A*) Dilated collaterals in a 14-year-old boy who had ileofemoral to IVC DVT. (*B*) Stasis dermatitis in a 13-year-old boy who had iliofemoral to IVC DVT.

12% to 22%, respectively) [40,41]. The risk for PTS in children who have DVT of the limbs, however, seems at least as great as that in adults (cumulative incidences at 1 to 2 years of 33% to 70% [2,5] versus 29%, respectively [41]). In addition, a German cohort study of children who had spontaneous VTE (ie, VTE in the absence of identified clinical risk factors), the cumulative incidence of recurrent VTE at a median follow-up time of 7 years was 21% [42], suggesting that, in this subgroup of pediatric VTE, the risk for recurrent events is long-lived. Although VTE-specific mortality in children is low, ranging from 0% to 2% [43,44], considerably higher all-cause mortality reflects the severity of underlying conditions (eg, sepsis, cancer, and congenital cardiac disease) in pediatric VTE. Neonate-specific outcomes data in pediatric non-RVT VTE reflect an all-cause mortality of 12% to 18% [6,45,46], including one series of premature infants who had CRT treated with enoxaparin [46]. With regard to major bleeding complications occurring during the anticoagulation period, frequencies in children range from 0% to 9% [5,43] in recent studies.

As indicated previously, outcomes of VTE in children may differ among specific anatomic sites. In a Canadian study of CRT in children from 1990 to 1996 [47], VTE-specific mortality was 4% among all children and 20% among those children in whom CRT was complicated by PE. No major bleeding episodes were observed. At a median follow-up of 2 years, the cumulative incidence of symptomatic recurrent VTE was 6.5%, and PTS developed in 9% of children. In other series of RVT [48–52] (primarily among neonates), VTE-related death has been uncommon, and the cumulative incidence of recurrent VTE ranged from 0% to 4%. The cumulative incidence of chronic hypertension in RVT in these studies was reported at 22% to 33%. For CSVT, the pediatric literature reflects a VTE-specific mortality ranging from 4% to 20%, with a cumulative incidence of recurrent VTE of 8% for neonatal CSVT cases and 17% for CSVT occurring in older children [53–56]. Long-term neurologic sequelae were noted in 17% to 26% of neonatal CSVT cases and the cumulative incidence of such sequelae in child-hood (ie, non-neonatal) CSVT ranged widely between 8% and 47%. In the aforementioned pediatric series of RVT and CSVT, the proportion of chil-dren who received anticoagulation and the duration of the anticoagulation course varied considerably across studies. With regard to portal vein throm-bosis, few pediatric series reporting outcomes have been published; however, it seems that the risk for developing recurrent gastrovariceal bleeding in this population is substantial, occurring in many cases even after surgical inter-ventions have been undertaken to reduce portal hypertension [57]. For PE in childhood, long-term outcomes, such as chronic pulmonary hypertension and pulmonary function, have yet to be established.

An additional VTE outcome of interest is residual thrombus burden. To date, data (principally in adults) suggest that the persistence of thrombosis after a therapeutic course of anticoagulation of appropriate duration does not increase the risk for recurrent VTE, including PE, appreciably. Some ev-idence [58] indicates, however, that persistent thrombosis is associated with the development of venous valvular insufficiency, an important risk factor for (albeit an imperfect correlate of) [59] the development of PTS. The prev-alence of residual thrombosis despite adequate anticolagulation in neonatal VTE has ranged from 12% in a small series of premature newborns who had CRT [46] to 62% in full-term neonatal VTE survivors [4]. Among primarily older children, the prevalence of persistent thrombosis has ranged broadly from 37% to 68% in the few longitudinal studies that have used systematic radiologic evaluation of thrombus evolution [5,16].

The ability to predict clinically relevant long-term outcomes of VTE at di-agnosis and during the acute and subacute phases of treatment is essential to establishing a future risk-stratified approach to antithrombotic management in children. Early work defined strong associations of homozygous anticoag-ulant deficiencies and APA syndrome with recurrent VTE. Over the past sev-eral years, the presence of multiple thromophilia traits has been identified as prognostic for recurrent VTE [42], and the radiologic finding of complete veno-occlusion at diagnosis of DVT is associated with an increased risk for persistent thrombosis [60] (which, in turn, is associated with the development of venous valvular insufficiency [58], as discussed previously). Most recently, plasma FVIII activity greater than 150 U/dL and D-dimer concentration greater than 500 ng/mL at the time of diagnosis of VTE in children and after 3 to 6 months of standard anticoagulation are shown to predict a composite adverse thrombotic outcome, characterized by persistent thrombosis, recur-rent VTE, or the development of PTS [5], adding to evidence for the prognostic usefulness of these markers in adult VTE [61–63].

Future directions

VTE has emerged in recent years as a critical pediatric concern with acute and chronic sequelae. Important and highly clinically relevant questions on its etiology, pathogenesis, and natural history remain to be addressed via collaborative cohort studies. For example, what are the mechanisms by which distinct APA mediate the prothrombotic state and, in turn, confer distinct risks for relevant outcomes of thrombus progression, recurrence, and embolism? Do criteria for APA syndrome established in adults—and the implications for indefinite anticoagulation—readily apply to children? Pediatric recommendations for antithrombotic management in acute VTE in general are derived largely from evidence from adult trials. The ability to predict clinically relevant long-term outcomes of pediatric VTE at diagnosis and during the acute and subacute phases of treatment, however, is essential to establishing a risk-stratified approach to antithrombotic management specific to children. Key evidence in this area is beginning to emerge. Using such evidence, multicenter randomized controlled trials are proposed (or already are underway) to evaluate the duration of standard anticoagulant therapy for first-episode VTE in children who do not have an increased a priori risk for recurrent VTE and PTS and to investigate thrombolytic therapeutic approaches in children who have acute DVT of the proximal lower extremities and who are at high risk for adverse outcomes. Finally, increased regulatory emphasis for devoted pediatric study of agents newly approved in adult populations promises to add diversity to the available antithrombotic strategies for pediatric VTE in the future. New agents will be important particularly in rare but life-threatening circumstances, such as catastrophic APA syndrome and HIT, for which alternative approaches to conventional anticoagulants are needed.

References

[1] Andrew M, David M, Adams M, et al. Venous thromboembolic complications (VTE) in children: first analyses of the Canadian Registry of VTE. Blood 1994;83:1251–7.

[2] van Ommen CH, Heijboer H, Buller HR, et al. Venous thromboembolism in childhood: a prospective two-year registry in the Netherlands. J Pediatr 2001;139:676–81.

[3] Stein PD, Kayali R, Olson RE, et al. Incidence of venous thromboembolism in infants and children: data from the National Hospital Discharge Survey. J Pediatr 2004;145:563–5.

[4] Monagle P, Adams M, Mahoney M, et al. Outcome of pediatric thromboembolic disease: a report from the Canadian Childhood Thrombophilia Registry. Pediatr Res 2000;47: 763–6.

[5] Goldenberg NA, Knapp-Clevenger R, Manco-Johnson MJ, et al. Elevated plasma factor VIII and D-dimer levels as predictors of poor outcomes of thrombosis in children. N Engl J Med 2004;351:1081–8.

[6] Schmidt B, Andrew M. Neonatal thrombosis: report of a prospective Canadian and international registry. Pediatrics 1995;96:939–43.

[7] David M, Andrew M. Venous thromboembolic complications in children. J Pediatr 1993; 123:337–46.

[8] Buck JR, Connor RH, Cook WW, et al. Pulmonary embolism in children. J Pediatr Surg 1981;16:385–91.

[9] Van Ommen CH, Peters M. Acute pulmonary embolism in childhood. Thromb Res 2006; 118(1):13–25.

[10] Hoyer PF, Gonda S, Barthels M, et al. Thromboembolic complications in children with nephritic syndrome. Risk and incidence. Acta Paediatr Scand 1986;75:804–10.

[11] Lewy PR, Jao W. Nephrotic syndrome in association with renal vein thrombosis in infancy. J Pediatr 1974;85:359–65.

[12] Goldenberg NA, Knapp-Clevenger R, Hays T, et al. Lemierre's and Lemierre's-like syndromes in children: survival and thromboembolic outcomes. Pediatrics 2005;116:e543–8.

[13] Manco-Johnson MJ, Grabowski EF, Hellgreen M, et al. Laboratory testing for thrombophilia in pediatric patients. On behalf of the Subcommittee for Perinatal and Pediatric Thrombosis of the Scientific and Standardization Committee of the International Society on Threombosis and Haemostasis (ISTH). Thromb Haemost 2002;88:155–6.

[14] Monagle P, Chan A, Massicotte P, et al. Antithrombotic therapy in children: the Seventh ACCP Conference on Antithrombotic and Thrombotic Therapy. Chest 2004;126(Suppl 3): 645S–87S.

[15] Manco-Johnson M. How I treat venous thrombosis in children. Blood 2006;107:21–9.

[16] Nohe N, Flemmer A, Rumler R, et al. The low molecular weight heparin dalteparin for prophylaxis and therapy of thrombosis in childhood: a report on 48 cases. Eur J Pediatr 1999; 158:S134–9.

[17] Andrew M, Marzinotto V, Massicotte P, et al. Heparin therapy in pediatric patients: a prospective cohort study. Pediatr Res 1994;35:78–83.

[18] Hull RD, Raskob GE, Rosenbloom D, et al. Heparin for 5 days as compared with 10 days in the initial treatment of proximal venous thrombosis. N Engl J Med 1990;322:1260–4.

[19] Kearon C, Ginsberg JS, Julina JA, et al. Comparison of fixed-dose weight-adjusted unfractionated heparin and low-molecular-weight heparin for acute treatment of venous thromboembolism. JAMA 2006;296:935–42.

[20] Berube C, Mitchell L, Silverman E, et al. The relationship of antiphospholipid antibodies to thromboembolic events in pediatric patients with systemic lupus erythematosus: a cross-sectional study. Pediatr Res 1998;44:351–6.

[21] Monagle P, Andrew M. Acquired disorders of hemostasis. In: Nathan DG, Stuart H, Orkin A, editors. Nathan and Oski's hematology of infancy and childhood. 6th edition. Philadelpia: Saunders; 2003.

[22] Kearon C, Ginsberg JS, Kovacs MJ, et al. Comparison of low-intensity warfarin therapy with conventional-intensity warfarin therapy for long-term prevention of recurrent venous thromboembolism. N Engl J Med 2003;349:631–9.

[23] Kovacs MJ. Long-term low-dose warfarin use is effective in the prevention of recurrent venous thromboembolism: no. J Thromb Haemost 2004;2:1041–3.

[24] Goldenberg NA, Knapp-Clevenger R, Durham JD, et al. A thrombolytic regimen for high-risk deep venous thrombosis may substantially reduce the risk of post-thrombotic syndrome in children. Blood 2007;110:45–53.

[25] Vukovich T, Auberger K, Weil J, et al. Replacement therapy for a homozygous protein C deficiency state using a concentrate of human protein C and S. Br J Haematol 1988;70:435–40.

[26] Dreyfus M, Masterson M, David M, et al. Replacement therapy with a monoclonal antibody purified protein C concentrate in newborns with severe congenital protein C deficiency. Semin Thromb Hemost 1995;21:371–81.

[27] Dreyfus M, Magny JF, Bridey F, et al. Treatment of homozygous protein C deficiency and neonatal purpura fulminans with a purified protein C concentrate. N Engl J Med 1991;325: 1565–8.

[28] Muller FM, Ehrenthal W, Hafner G, et al. Purpura fulminans in severe congenital protein C deficiency: monitoring of treatment with protein C concentrate. Eur J Pediatr 1996;155:20–5.

[29] de Kleijn ED, de Groot R, Hack CE, et al. Activation of protein C following infusion of protein C concentrate in children with severe meningococcal sepsis and purpura fulminans: a randomized, double-blinded, placebo-controlled, dose-finding study. Crit Care Med 2003;31:1839–47.

[30] Ettingshausen CE, Veldmann A, Beeg T, et al. Replacement therapy with protein C concentrate in infants and adolescents with meningococcal sepsis and purpura fulminans. Semin Thromb Hemost 1999;25:537–41.

[31] Rivard GE, David M, Farrell C, et al. Treatment of purpura fulminans in meningococcemia with protein C concentrate. J Pediatr 1995;126(4):646–52.

[32] Konkle BA, Bauer KA, Weinstein R, et al. Use of recombinant human antithrombin in patients with congenital antithrombin deficiency undergoing surgical procedures. Transfusion 2003;43:390–4.

[33] Zaunschirm A, Muntean W. Correction of hemostatic imbalances induced by L-asparaginase therapy in children with acute lymphoblastic leukemia. Pediatr Hematol Oncol 1986; 3:19–25.

[34] Mitchell L, Andrew M, Hanna K, et al. Trend to efficacy and safety using antithrombin concentrate in prevention of thrombosis in children receiving L-asparaginase for acute lymphoblastic leukemia. Results of the PARKAA study. Thromb Haemost 2003;90: 235–44.

[35] Haussmann U, Fischer J, Eber S, et al. Hepatic veno-occlusive disease in pediatric stem cell transplantation: impact of pre-emptive antithrombin III replacement and combin antithrombin III/defibrotide therapy. Haematologica 2006;91:795–800.

[36] Meister B, Kropshofer G, Klein-Franke A, et al. Comparison of low-molecular-weight heparin and antithrombin versus antithrombin alone for the prevention of thrombosis in children with acute lymphoblastic leukemia. Pediatr Blood Cancer 2008;50(2):298–303.

[37] Cahn MD, Rohrer MJ, Martella MB, et al. Long-term follow-up of Greenfield inferior vena cava filter placement in children. J Vasc Surg 2001;34:820–5.

[38] Goldenberg NA. Long-term outcomes of venous thrombosis in children. Curr Opin Hematol 2005;12:370–6.

[39] van Ommen CH, Heijboer H, van den Dool EJ, et al. Pediatric venous thromboembolic disease in one single center: congenital prothrombotic disorders and the clinical outcome. J Thromb Haemost 2003;1:2516–22.

[40] Bick RL. Prothrombin G20210A mutation, antithombin, heparin cofactor II, protein C, and protein S defects. Hematol Oncol Clin North Am 2003;17:9–36.

[41] Prandoni P, Lensing AW, Cogo A, et al. The long-term clinical course of acute deep venous thrombosis. Ann Intern Med 1996;125:1–7.

[42] Nowak-Göttl U, Junker R, Kruez W, et al. Risk of recurrent venous thrombosis in children with combined prothrombotic risk factors. Blood 2001;97:858–62.

[43] Massicotte P, Julian JA, Gent M, et al. An open label randomized controlled trial of low molecular weight heparin compared to heparin and Coumadin for the treatment of venous thromboembolic events in children: the REVIVE trial. Thromb Res 2003;109: 85–92.

[44] Oren H, Devecioglu O, Ertem M, et al. Analysis of pediatric thrombotic patients in Turkey. Pediatr Hematol Oncol 2004;21:573–83.

[45] Nowak-Göttl U, Von Kries R, Gobel U. Neonatal symptomatic thromboembolism in Germany: two year survey. Arch Dis Child Fetal Neonatal Ed 1997;76:F163–7.

[46] Michaels LA, Gurian M, Hagyi T, et al. Low molecular weight heparin in the treatment of venous and arterial thromboses in the premature infant. Pediatrics 2004;114:703–7.

[47] Massicotte MP, Dix D, Monagle P, et al. Central venous catheter related thrombosis in children: analysis of the Canadian Registry of Venous Thromboembolic Complications. J Pediatr 1998;133:770–6.

[48] Mocan H, Beattie TJ, Murphy AV, et al. Renal venous thrombosis in infancy: long-term follow-up. Pediatr Nephrol 1991;5:45–9.

[49] Nuss R, Hays T, Manco-Johnson M. Efficacy and safety of heparin anticoagulation for neonatal renal vein thrombosis. Am J Pediatr Hematol Oncol 1994;16:127–31.

[50] Keidan I, Lotan D, Gazit G, et al. Early neonatal renal venous thrombosis: long-term outcome. Acta Paediatr 1994;83:1225–7.

[51] Kuhle S, Massicotte P, Chan A, et al. A case series of 72 neonates with renal vein thrombosis: data from the 1-800-NO-CLOTS Registry. Thromb Haemost 2004;92:929–33.

[52] Kosch A, Kuwertz-Broking E, Heller C, et al. Renal venous thrombosis in neonates: pro-thrombotic risk factors and long-term follow-up. Blood 2004;104:1356–60.

[53] deVeber G, Andrew M, Adams C, et al. Cerebral sinovenous thrombosis in children. N Engl J Med 2001;345:417–23.

[54] deVeber GA, MacGregor D, Curtis R, et al. Neurologic outcome in survivors of childhood arterial ischemic stroke and sinovenous thrombosis. J Child Neurol 2000;15:316–24.

[55] Kenet G, Waldman D, Lubetsky A, et al. Paediatric cerebral sinus vein thrombosis. Thromb Haemost 2004;92:713–8.

[56] De Schryver EL, Blom I, Braun KP, et al. Long-term prognosis of cerebral venous sinus thrombosis in childhood. Dev Med Child Neurol 2004;46:514–9.

[57] Gurakan F, Eren M, Kocak N, et al. Extrahepatic portal vein thrombosis in children: etiology and long-term follow-up. J Clin Gastroenterol 2004;38:368–72.

[58] Meissner MH, Manzo RA, Bergelin RO, et al. Deep venous insufficiency: the relationship between lysis and subsequent reflux. J Vasc Surg 1993;18:596–605.

[59] Kahn SR, Dsmarais S, Ducruet T, et al. Comparison of the Villalta and Ginsberg clinical scales to diagnose the post-thrombotic syndrome: correlation with patient-reported disease burden and venous valvular reflux. J Thromb Haemost 2006;4:907–8.

[60] Revel-Vilk S, Sharathkumar A, Massicotte P, et al. Natural history of arterial and venous thrombosis in children treated with low molecular weight heparin: a longitudinal study by ultrasound. J Thromb Haemost 2004;2:42–6.

[61] Kyrle PA, Minar E, Hirschl M, et al. High plasma levels of factor VIII and the risk of recurrent venous thromboembolism. N Engl J Med 2000;343:457–62.

[62] Palareti G, Legnani C, Cosmi B, et al. Risk of venous thromboembolism recurrence: high negative predictive value of D-dimer performed after oral anticoagulation is stopped. Thromb Haemost 2002;87:7–12.

[63] Eichinger S, Minar E, Bialonczyk C, et al. D-dimer levels and risk of recurrent venous thromboembolism. JAMA 2003;290:1071–4.

ELSEVIER
SAUNDERS

PEDIATRIC CLINICS
OF NORTH AMERICA

Pediatr Clin N Am 55 (2008) 323–338

Pediatric Arterial Ischemic Stroke

Timothy J. Bernard, MD[a,b,c,*],
Neil A. Goldenberg, MD[a,b]

[a]*Mountain States Regional Hemophilia and Thrombosis Center, P.O. Box 6507, Mail-Stop F-416, Aurora, CO 80045-0507, USA*
[b]*Pediatric Stroke Program, University of Colorado and The Children's Hospital, 13123 East 16th Avenue, Aurora, CO 80045, USA*
[c]*Department of Child Neurology, University of Colorado and The Children's Hospital, 13123 East 16th Avenue, Aurora, CO 80045-0507, USA*

Arterial ischemic stroke (AIS) is a rare, but increasingly recognized, disorder in children. Research in this area suggests that risk factors, outcomes, and even presentation are different from those of adult stroke. In particular, prothrombotic abnormalities and large vessel arteriopathies that are nonatherosclerotic seem to play a large role in the pathogenesis of childhood AIS. The purpose of this review is first to examine the epidemiology and etiologies of neonatal and childhood AIS and then provide a detailed discussion of approaches to the clinical characterization, diagnostic evaluation, and management of this disorder in pediatric patients. Long-term outcomes of recurrent AIS and neuromotor, speech, cognitive, and behavioral deficits are considered. Emphasis is on available evidence underlying current knowledge and key questions for further investigation.

Characterization

AIS is characterized by a clinical presentation consistent with stroke combined with radiographic evidence of ischemia or infarction in a known arterial distribution. Unless otherwise specified, throughout this article the term, "stroke," is used synonymously with AIS. AIS in pediatrics is divided into two main categories: neonatal AIS and childhood (non-neonatal) AIS. Neonatal AIS is defined as any ischemic stroke occurring within the first 28 days of life and is subdivided further into prenatal, perinatal, and

* Corresponding author. Department of Child Neurology, University of Colorado and The Children's Hospital, P.O. Box 6507, Mail Stop F-416, Aurora, CO 80045-0507.
E-mail address: timothy.bernard@uchsc.edu (T.J. Bernard).

postnatal. Acute perinatal stroke usually presents with neonatal seizures during the first week of life. This differs from a presumed prenatal stroke, which typically presents at 4 to 8 months of life with an evolving hemiparesis [1]. Because of the difficulty in determining the exact timing of presumed prenatal AIS, some investigators combine the two classifications as presumed prenatal/perinatal AIS. In contrast to neonatal stroke, childhood AIS typically presents with sudden onset of focal neurologic symptoms and signs and (given the broad differential diagnosis) requires an MRI of the brain with diffusion-weighted images to confirm the diagnosis of AIS (AIS presentation discussed later).

Epidemiology

The incidence of neonatal AIS recently is estimated at approximately 1 in 4000 live births annually [2]. Similar estimates are provided by the United States National Hospital Discharge Survey, which recently published an incidence of 18 neonatal strokes per 100,000 births per year [3]. Childhood AIS is less common than neonatal stroke, occurring one third to one tenth as often. The incidence of childhood stroke is approximately 2 to 8 in 100,000 per year in North America [4,5]. Before the advent of MRI techniques, a Mayo Clinic retrospective analysis of cases in Rochester, Minnesota, in the late 1970s yielded an incidence of 2.5 strokes per 100,000 children per year [6]. Although pre-MRI data likely underestimate the incidence of AIS because of the low sensitivity of CT for ischemia, more recent retrospective analyses using medical record review are subject to well-documented inaccuracies engendered by the *International Statistical Classification of Diseases, 9th Revision* coding [7]. In addition, given the low index of suspicion for cerebrovascular events in children, the true incidence of pediatric AIS likely remains underdiagnosed.

Etiology

The etiology of neonatal and childhood AIS is in many instances poorly understood, largely owing to the low incidence of the disease in the pediatric population and the lack of sufficient multicenter data on causal factors. The traditional ischemic stroke risk factors in adults, such as hypertension, atherosclerosis, diabetes, smoking, obesity, and hypercholesterolemia, are infrequent among neonates and older children who have AIS. In some instances of childhood AIS, such as congenital heart disease, sickle cell disease, and arterial dissection, the etiology readily is understood. For instance, with regard to cardiac risk factors, the Canadian Pediatric Stroke Registry found heart disease in 25% of patients who had pediatric AIS [8], whereas the prevalence of patent foramen ovale (PFO) in patients who had cryptogenic stroke was 40% to 50% compared with 10% to 27% in the general population [9,10]. Some additional important risk factors for childhood AIS are identified, including vasculopathy, infection, head and neck trauma, previous transient ischemic attack (TIA) (defined as a focal neurologic deficit lasting less than 24 hours), and prothrombotic disorders [11–21]. Often more than one risk factor is identified. Nevertheless, in the majority of childhood AIS cases, the etiology remains unclear, resulting in a broad subgroup of idiopathic childhood AIS.

Increasingly, arteriopathy (characterized by a disturbance of arterial blood flow within the vessel) is identified as a prevalent risk factor for childhood AIS, occurring in as many as 50% to 80% of cases [13,22]. Often this arteriopathy is secondary to dissection of carotid or vertebral arteries, which accounts for 7% to 20% of all cases of childhood AIS [12,22], and may be caused by neck manipulation or head and neck trauma [23–26] (although this association may be influenced by recall bias) and in rare cases may be related to underlying connective tissues disorders (eg, collagen defects) [27]. Nondissective arteriopathy also is related to certain infections. For example, there is a threefold increased risk for AIS within 1 year of acute varicella zoster virus (VZV) infection in childhood [28]. Postvaricella arteriopathy typically exhibits a characteristic pattern of intracranial narrowing of the internal carotid artery (ICA), middle cerebral artery (MCA), and anterior cerebral artery (ACA), classically causing basal ganglia infarctions [29].

Increasingly, however, angiographic studies in childhood AIS identify MCA, ICA, and ACA arteriopathy without a known infectious or alternative cause; such cases consequently are characterized as idiopathic arteriopathies (Fig. 1) [13]. A minority of these cases represent early moyamoya syndrome (defined as stenosis in the terminal portion of the ICAs bilaterally with the formation of tenuous collateral arteries, producing the classic angiographic "puff of smoke") or possible moyamoya syndrome (recently characterized as unilateral stenosis in the terminal segment of an ICA with collaterals or the presence of bilateral stenosis of the terminal portion of the ICAs without collaterals) (Fig. 2) [12]. Moyamoya, in turn, may be associated with sickle cell anemia, trisomy 21, a history of cranial irradiation for malignancy [30], or fibromuscular dysplasia; in many cases, however, moyamoya is of unclear etiology. In the majority of idiopathic arteriopathies, in which there is no progression to moyamoya, the phenomenon is termed, "transient cerebral arteriopathy," in cases of a monophasic transient lesion that resolves or stabilizes within 6 months, and "chronic cerebral arteriopathy" in progressive cases [12]. An elucidation of the etiology of these currently idiopathic arteriopathies will enhance the understanding of childhood stroke and may have an impact on future therapeutic management and outcomes in these patients.

Thrombophilia may contribute to AIS risk via arterial thrombosis or cerebral embolism of a venous thrombus through a cardiac lesion with right-to-left shunt. Thrombophilia risk factors in pediatric AIS include antiphospholipid antibodies [19,20], anticoagulant deficiencies [21], and hyperhomocysteinemia [31,32]. Protein C is the most commonly associated anticoagulant deficiency, although in cases of AIS (and venous

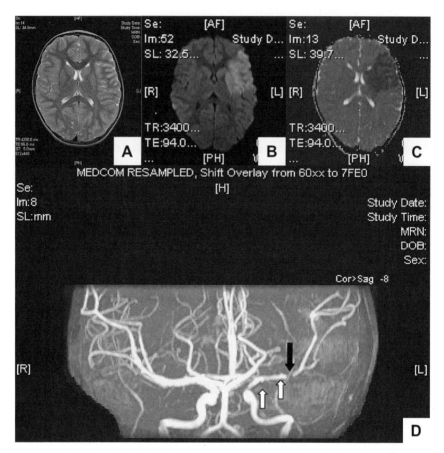

Fig. 1. Idiopathic arteriopathy. A previously healthy 6-year-old boy who had acute-onset right hemiparesis and aphasia. MRI T2 sequences (*A*) are unrevealing 5 hours after onset, but diffusion-weighted imaging (*B*) and ADC mapping (*C*) demonstrate cytotoxic edema, consistent with AIS in the left MCA territory. From the same examination, an anterior-posterior MRA (slightly oblique) image (*D*) demonstrates irregularity of the distal left ICA, extending to the proximal MCA (*white arrows*). There also seems to be an occlusion in the proximal MCA (*black arrow*).

thromboembolism [VTE]) after acute varicella infection, antibody-mediated acquired protein S deficiency seems prevalent [33]. It is likely that anticoagulant deficiencies are acquired most commonly secondary to viral-mediated inflammation, as is the case in varicella. As in VTE, however, severe congenital anticoagulant deficiencies also may be contributory. Although homozygosity for factor V Leiden or prothrombin G20210A polymorphism is a strong risk factor for thrombotic events, it remains unclear whether or not the factor V Leiden or prothrombin G20210A variant in heterozygous form confers a meaningful increase in the risk for pediatric AIS [18–21]. Greatly elevated homocysteine levels classically are associated with

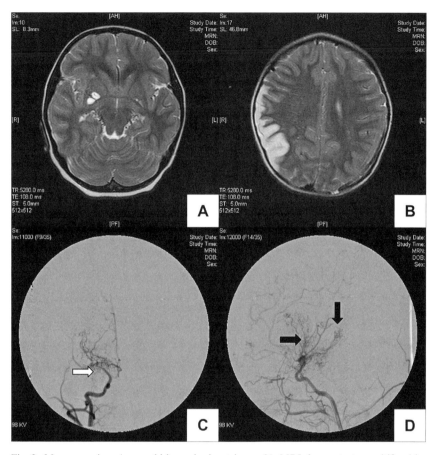

Fig. 2. Moyamoya in a 4-year-old boy who has trisomy 21. MRI demonstrates multifocal infarctions on T2 sequencing; one image reveals an old right-sided basal ganglia infarction (*A*), whereas another illustrates a subacute right parietal infarction (*B*). Follow-up angiogram of the right anterior circulation demonstrates ICA narrowing (*white arrow*) and the classic puff-of-smoke appearance of collateral circulation (*black arrows*) on anterior (*C*) and lateral (*D*) images.

metabolic disorders, such as homocysteinuria (resulting from cystathionine β-synthase deficiency), and mild to moderately elevated levels also occur in homozygous carriers of the methylenetetraydrofolate reductase mutation (MTHFR C677T). Among heterozgyotes, the latter cause of hyperhomocysteinemia is evident particularly in countries where routine folate supplementation of the diet is not undertaken. Another prothrombotic trait, elevated lipoprotein(a) concentration, is associated with increased odds of otherwise idiopathic (ie, apart from thrombophilia) childhood AIS [18]. Other suspected blood-based risk factors for pediatric AIS, supported thus far by evidence from case series or case-control studies, include iron deficiency anemia [34], polycythemia, and thrombocytosis [35].

Given that focal arteriopathy is an uncommon finding in neonatal AIS, stroke etiology is less clear for this group than for childhood AIS. Nevertheless, congenital cardiac anomalies are established risk factors, and thrombophilia investigation has provided additional meaningful contributions. Similar thrombophilic risk factors are identified for neonatal AIS as for childhood stroke, including factor V Leiden, protein C deficiency, and elevated lipoprotein(a) [36]. The possibility of vertical transmission of prothrombotic molecular entities or vasoconstrictive agents (eg, antiphospholipid antibodies or cocaine, respectively) also is important to consider in the etiology of neonatal AIS but has not been studied systematically. In addition, maternal pregestational and gestational factors, such as infertility, placental infection, premature rupture of membranes, and preeclampsia, in the past few years have been found independently associated with neonatal AIS [37]. Recent birth registry data are further suggestive of maternal vascular disease risk factors contributing to neonatal AIS, given the finding of an association with the development of seizures in term neonates (a common manifestation of neonatal AIS) [38]; however, further work is necessary to establish this potential risk factor. In addition, emerging data suggest a combination of maternal- and fetal-specific molecular risk factors in the development of placental pathology may be worthy of additional study regarding perinatal stroke risk [39].

Clinical presentation

The clinical presentation of AIS differs greatly among presumed prenatal, perinatal, postnatal, and childhood stroke. Within each classification, further variance of presentation exists and depends largely on the territory, extent, and timing of ischemia. The most common presentation for presumed prenatal stroke is evolving hemiparesis at 4 to 8 months of life [1]. Typically, the hand is more involved than the arm, because of the high incidence of MCA distribution infarction, and the left hemisphere is affected more commonly than the right [36]. Perinatal AIS has a similar predilection for the left MCA but often presents with focal neonatal seizures during the first week of life. Postnatal stroke may present similarly to perinatal AIS; in other instances, it presentation is like that of childhood stroke (discussed later).

The clinical presentation of childhood AIS is less stereotypical than that of pre- and perinatal AIS and is more dependent on the territory of ischemia. As a general rule, patients who have small- to medium-sized events present with sudden-onset focal neurologic deficits (such as hemiparesis, visual field deficits, aphasia, cranial nerve palsies, dyspahagia, and unilateral ataxia) without major alterations of consciousness. Focal neurologic deficit in the presence of preserved consciousness can aid in the diagnosis, as many more common pediatric illnesses, such as complex partial and generalized seizures or encephalitis, often have alteration of awareness. Larger strokes tend to have multiple deficits and alteration of consciousness. As discussed previously, a history of head or neck trauma, recent varicella infection, and the presence of sickle cell disease or cardiac disease may aid in understanding the underlying etiology. A recent single-center retrospective series of AIS in non-neonatal children found that a nonabrupt pattern of neurologic symptoms or signs (including those in whom the maximum severity of symptoms or signs developed more than 30 minutes from the time of symptom onset, the presentation of symptoms or signs was waxing and waning, or the presentation was preceded by recurrent transient symptoms or signs with intercurrent resolution) often was associated with findings of arteriopathy on diagnostic neuroimaging [40].

Strokes of metabolic etiology frequently manifest a progressive course of stroke-like episodes. Often, there is a family history of early-onset strokes, early-onset dementia, or severe migraines. A classic example of a metabolic stroke occurs in mitochondrial myopathy, encephalopathy, lactic acidosis, and stroke-like episodes (MELAS). MELAS is caused by mitochondrial DNA defects encoding tRNA involved in the generation of ATP and the majority of cases (80%) have the mt3243 mutation [41]. In addition to a maternal history of migraine and stroke, there often is a history of short stature, diabetes, hearing loss, occipital lobe seizures, and optic atrophy [41]. The presentation often is characterized by stroke-like episodes with complete resolution of neurologic function. Over time, however, neurologic deficits persist, often in the form of hemianopia [42]. Acute lesions observed by MRI can be distinguished from typical AIS by virtue of their paradoxic bright appearance on apparent diffusion coefficient (ADC) maps. In cases of a family history of cryptogenic stroke or atypical presentation of stroke, other inherited disorders (eg, non-MELAS mitochondrial DNA defects, organic acidemias, lysosomal diseases, severe congenital thrombophilias, and cerebral autosomal dominant arteriopathy with subcortical infarctions and leukoencephalopathy [CADASIL]), should be considered [41].

Diagnostic evaluation

Diagnostic evaluation of pediatric AIS is more extensive than in adult stroke because of the broad differential diagnosis at presentation and the higher incidence of ateriopathies in childhood AIS. In a child presenting with an acute focal neurologic deficit, multiple alternative etiologies must be considered, including hypoglycemia, prolonged focal seizures, prolonged postictal paresis (Todd's paralysis), acute disseminated encephalomyelitis, meningitis, encephalitis, and brain abscess [43]. For this reason, MRI brain with diffusion-weighted images is becoming the radiographic modality of choice in most cases of childhood AIS. Acutely, CT can rule out hemorrhage, tumor, and abscess and may be an appropriate first-line evaluation in some cases. Typically, this needs to be followed by an MRI with diffusion-weighted images to assess for cytotoxic edema, the hallmark of acute ischemia (see Fig. 1). The use of perfusion-weighted imaging largely is experimental in children [44] but as acute interventions become more available in childhood AIS, this modality likely will be used increasingly as a means by which to identify potentially preservable territories of at-risk functioning brain. Furthermore, the pattern of infarction also may be suggestive of etiology. For example, a case of multiple infarctions in separate arterial distributions likely is thromboembolic, findings of occipital and parietal strokes that cross vascular territories may suggest MELAS, a distribution between vascular territories is consistent with watershed infarction suggestive of a hypotensive etiology, and a pattern of small multifocal lesions at the gray-white junction is suspicious for vasculitis.

Although routine CT and MRI evaluate for ischemia, hemorrhage, mass/mass effect, and other non-AIS pathologies, vascular imaging (magnetic resonance angiography [MRA], CT angiography [CTA], or conventional angiography) can demonstrate arteriopathy, including dissection, stenosis, irregular contour, or intra-arterial thrombosis of the head and neck. Typically, MRA or CTA is the modality used as first-line arterial imaging, unless MRI reveals a pattern consistent with small vessel vasculitis, in which case conventional angiography is indicated. If MRA or CTA suggests moya-moya or atypical vasculature, conventional angiography is warranted, as MRA or CTA may underestimate or overestimate the degree of disease [45].

An additional important component of diagnostic imaging in pediatric AIS is echocardiography with peripheral venous saline injection. In addition to disclosing a septal defect and other congenital cardiac anomalies, echocardiography with saline injection may disclose a small lesion, including a PFO that otherwise may not be detected by conventional transthoracic echocardiography. The prevalence of PFO in patients who have cryptogenic stroke is 40% to 50% compared with 10% to 27% in the general population [9,10]. The use of Doppler imaging during echocardiography assists in determining the direction of shunt through a lesion, although the prognostic significance of the direction of shunt is not well established in pediatric stroke.

At a minimum, diagnostic laboratory evaluation in pediatric acute AIS involves a complete blood count, toxicology screen, complete metabolic panel, erythrocyte sedimentation rate/C-reactive protein (ESR/CRP) to assess for biochemical evidence of systemic inflammation that may suggest vasculitis or infection in the etiology of AIS, β-hCG testing in postmenarchal women, fasting lipid profile, and a comprehensive thrombophilia panel (Box 1). Further investigation into metabolic, genetic, infectious, or rheumatologic diseases should be considered in cases of atypical presentation. In the setting of arteritis, arthritis, or elevated ESR/CRP, rheumatologic evaluation should be considered and include testing of antinuclear antibodies and rheumatoid factor. In childhood AIS with encephalopathy of unclear etiology, nonarterial distribution, or other multisystem disorders of unclear etiology (eg, hearing loss, myopathy, or endocrinopathy), testing should

---

Box 1. Suggested diagnostic laboratory evaluation in children who have acute arterial ischemic stroke

Complete blood count
Comprehensive metabolic panel (including hepatic indices)
ESR
CRP
Antinuclear antibody screen
Disseminated intravascular coagulation screen[a]
Thrombophilia panel[b]
Urine toxicology screen
Urine β-hCG (in postmenarchal woman)
Viral evaluation (if suspected by clinical presentation or if
    cerebral arteriopathy is demonstrated)[c]
Metabolic disease screening (if suspected by clinical
    presentation)[d]
Mitochondrial DNA mutational analyses (if suspected by clinical
    presentation)

---

[a] Includes prothrombin time, activated partial thromboplastin time, fibrinogen, and D-dimer.

[b] Includes protein C activity, free protein S antigen or protein S activity, antithrombin activity, factor VIII activity, factor V Leiden mutation, prothrombin 20,210 mutation, homocysteine concentration (± methylenetetrahydrofolate reductase mutations), antiphospholipid antibody evaluation (lupus anticoagulant testing [eg, dilute Russell's viper venom time or StaClot-LA], anticardiolipin IgG and IgM levels, anti–β2-glycoprotein I IgG and IgM levels), and lipoprotein(a) concentration.

[c] Consider blood titers of VZV, HSV, Epstein-Barr virus (EBV), enterovirus, and parvovirus; blood viral culture; CSF viral culture; CSF VZV, HSV, EBV, enterovirus, and parvovirus testing by polymerase chain reaction (PCR); *Helicobacter pylori* testing; and enteroviral PCR from oral and rectal swabs.

[d] Includes blood lactate concentration, blood pyruvate concentration, serum carnitine concentration, urine organic acids profile, and serum amino acids profile.

---

include lactate and pyruvate to screen for metabolic disorders and mitochondrial DNA testing for MELAS and related disorders. A lumbar puncture is indicated if infectious signs and symptoms are present and in other inflammatory states of unclear etiology. If cerebrospinal fluid (CSF) abnormalities are present, further infectious work-up and routine chemistries and blood counts are warranted. It may be prudent to test routinely for VZV, herpes simplex virus (HSV), enterovirus, and other known viral etiologies in the CSF when a lumbar puncture is performed in addition to performing routine bacterial cultures.

Because the etiology and pathogenesis of childhood AIS often are unclear at the time of diagnosis, thrombophilia testing during the diagnostic evaluation of AIS should be comprehensive (see Box 1). Given the association between recurrence of neonatal AIS and thrombophilia [46], a similar investigation is warranted in neonatal AIS. A particularly important issue of thrombophilia testing specific to neonatal AIS involves antiphospholipid antibody (APA) testing (see Box 1). When APAs are positive in neonates who have AIS, it is informative to evaluate for APA in the mothers, as many case reports have identified vertical (ie, transplacental) transmission of IgG APA in association with neonatal AIS [47].

Treatment

Initial management of childhood stroke should emphasize supportive measures, such as airway stabilization, administration of oxygen, maintenance of euglycemia, and treatment of seizures if they are present. Currently there are no randomized controlled trials on which to base management of medical therapies in childhood or neonatal AIS, with the exception of AIS in the setting of sickle cell disease. Guidelines exist from the American College of Chest Physicians (ACCP) [48] and the Royal College of Physicians [49], with recommendations based on consensus, cohort studies, and extrapolation from adult studies.

Most commonly, childhood AIS is treated with antithrombotic agents, such as aspirin or heparins (unfractionated heparin [UFH] or low-molecular-weight heparin [LMWH]), unless a stroke is a complication of sickle cell anemia. The ACCP recommendations suggest treatment of all nonsickle cell childhood AIS with UFH or LMWH for 5 to 7 days and until cardioembolic stroke and dissection are excluded. For cases of cardioembolic stroke or dissection, the ACCP recommends anticoagulation for 3 to 6 months. After discontinuation of anticoagulation in all patients who have childhood AIS, long-term aspirin therapy is recommended. These ACCP recommendations are based on grade 2C data [48]. In contrast, the Royal College of Physicians recommends initial treatment with aspirin rather than anticoagulation in all childhood AIS. A nonrandomized prospective cohort study of low-dose LMWH versus aspirin in the treatment of AIS (ie, as secondary AIS prophylaxis) in children detected no significant difference in the cumulative incidence of recurrent AIS or significant side effects between these two therapies [50].

Treatment of stroke in sickle cell disease is based largely on clinical experience and retrospective analysis. Recommendations (from ACCP) [48] include exchange transfusion to reduce hemoglobin S to levels less than 30% for acute stroke and maintaining a long-term transfusion program after initial stroke. Based on results from the Stroke Prevention Trial in Sickle Cell Anemia (STOP), which showed that regular transufsions can prevent primary stroke in high-risk children who have sickle cell anemia and whose transcranial Doppler time–averaged maximum velocities exceed 200 cm per second [51], ACCP also recommends primary prevention of AIS through annual transcranial Doppler sceening for arteriopathy in children who have sickle cell disease and are older than 2 years.

Pediatric AIS with moyamoya syndrome usually is treated with surgical intervention. Anticoagulation and antiplatelet agents are considered possible therapies but typically are temporizing measures before surgery. Given heightened risks for recurrent AIS and bleeding, neurosurgical approaches at revascularization (including indirect means, such as encephaloduroarteriomyosyangiosis [EDAMS], and direct means, such as superficial temporal artery branch to MCA branch bypass) generally are preferred as first-line therapy [52,53]. Given the bleeding risk inherent in moyamoya, long-term antithrombotic therapy perhaps best is reserved for children who have appropriately defined "possible moyamoya" in the absence of recurrent symptoms or recurrent AIS/TIA despite appropriate surgical intervention.

Case reports and case series describe the use of systemic intravenous and selective interventional arterial thrombolytic therapy in acute childhood stroke, in many instances used beyond the 3- to 6-hour window from symptom onset for which safety and efficacy is established in adult trials [54–57]. Bleeding risks, efficacy, and outcomes are defined poorly in these studies, making it difficult to assess risk-benefit considerations of this therapy. A multicenter collaborative clinical trial approach with stringent uniform exclusion criteria ultimately will be required to address whether or not adult evidence for a beneficial role of systemic tissue plasminogen activator administration in the immediate period after onset of AIS and the optimal time window for this intervention also apply to children.

In contrast to childhood stroke, neonatal stroke usually is treated acutely with supportive measures only. Antiplatelet therapy and anticoagulation rarely are used, given the low risk for recurrence (cumulative incidence of approximately 3% at a median follow-up duration of 3.5 years) [46]. In the largest follow-up series to date evaluating recurrence in neonatal AIS, all of the recurrent events were associated with an identifiable prothrombotic or cardiac risk factor [46]. Therefore, most neonates who have AIS unlikely benefit from anticoagulation or antiplatelet therapy when these risk factors are evaluated and excluded appropriately. In the event that a potent thrombophilic risk factor is identified, antithrombotic therapy should be considered on a case-by-case basis.

Long-term management of childhood and neonatal AIS ideally should be coordinated by a multidisciplinary team that has pediatric stroke expertise and includes a neurologist, hematologist, rehabilitation physician (along with physical, occupational, and speech therapy services), and neuropsychologist. Children who have hemiparesis should be considered for constraint therapy, a method in which the unaffected arm is restrained, thereby training use of the paretic arm. Recent studies have demonstrated a potential benefit of this therapy [58]. Furthermore, the impact of rehabilitative and neuropsychologic interventions on the neuromotor and academic progress and future needs of patients who have pediatric AIS should be reassessed regularly during extended follow-up. Finally, attention should be given to assessing and monitoring the psychologic impact of AIS on patients and their families.

Outcomes

Recurrent AIS is one of the principal outcomes for which current medical therapies are undertaken (ie, secondary stroke prophylaxis), and the risk for recurrence after non-neonatal AIS varies between approximately 20% and 40% at a fixed follow-up duration of 5 years [17,59]. Certain risk factors in the childhood population are associated with a higher recurrence risk. A recent United States population-based cohort study demonstrated a 66% recurrence risk in children who have abnormal vascular imaging as compared with a neglible recurrence risk in AIS victims who have normal vascular imaging at presentation [60]. Previously, a large multicenter German prospective cohort study of childhood AIS demonstrated a similar increased risk for recurrence in AIS patients who had vasculopathy [61]. It has become clear, therefore, over the past several years that arterial abnormalities impart an increased risk for recurrence. Patients who have moyamoya, in particular, are at greatly increased risk for recurrent AIS and persistent neurologic deficits [17,22,62].

The risk of recurrent AIS also seems to increase with the number of AIS risk factors [59]. In particular, elevated serum levels of lipoprotein(a), congenital protein C deficiency, and vasculopathy are independent risk factors for recurrent AIS [61]. Some studies also suggest a possible relationship between anticardiolipin IgG antibodies and recurrence, although this association has not reached statistical significance [63].

Neuromotor, language, and cognitive outcomes of childhood and neonatal AIS are highly variable and dependent on stroke size, comorbid conditions, and age at diagnosis. Long-term sequelae include residual neurologic deficits (especially hemiparesis), learning disabilities, seizures, and cognitive impairments. The magnitude of these outcomes and their prediction are less clear in childhood AIS than neonatal stroke, perhaps because of the greater heterogeneity in stroke subtypes and distributions (primarily MCA territory) in the former group. A few cohort study analyses indicate that 30% of survivors of childhood AIS have normal motor function at an average follow-up of 6 months to 2.5 years [22,64]. The cumulative incidence of seizure after childhood AIS seems to be 25% to 33% and of behavioral concerns from 29% to 44% at 5 to 7 years of follow-up [65,66].

In neonatal AIS, the risk for recurrence is approximately 0% to 3% at an average follow-up of 3.5 to 6 years [46,59]. As discussed previously, recurrence in neonatal AIS seems confined primarily to patients who have prothrombotic abnormalities and congenital heart disease [46]. Much evidence has emerged recently with regard to prediction of outcomes in neo-natal AIS. An abnormal background on early neonatal encephalography and an ischemia distribution that includes the internal capsule, basal ganglia, and the surrounding cortex are associated with the development of hemiplegia or asymmetry of tone without hemiplegia [67,68]. Acute findings on MRI are predictive of hemiparesis in several series. The presence of signal abnormalities in the posterior limb of the internal capsule or the cerebral peduncles on magnetic resonance with diffusion-weighted imaging and ADC mapping in neonatal acute AIS is associated with the development of unilateral motor deficit [69,70]. Most recently, abnormal signal in the descending corticospinal tract on magnetic resonance with diffusion-weighted imaging in neonates who have AIS has been evaluated; the percentage of cerebral peduncle affected and the total length of descending corticospinal tract involved correlates with the development of hemiparesis [71].

Expressive speech impairments were noted in 12% of perinatal/neonatal and 18% of non-neonatal AIS cases in a single study [53]. As for neuropsychologic outcomes, cognitive or behavioral deficits were discerned in 3% to 14% of children who had neonatal AIS at an average follow-up of 2 to 6 years [68,72].

Despite important work to date in the field, prediction of outcomes and risk stratification in neonatal and childhood stroke remain largely in their infancy. Given the current limited knowledge of prognostic factors in pediatric AIS, it is hoped that within the next few years, large multicenter cohort analyses will permit further risk stratification, laying the foundation for interventional clinical trials.

Acknowledgments

The authors thank Dr. Marilyn Manco-Johnson for helpful comments on the manuscript and Dr. Laura Fenton for expert review of the radiologic imaging studies presented in Figs. 1 and 2.

References

[1] Golomb MR, MacGregor DL, Domi T, et al. Presumed pre- or perinatal arterial ischemic stroke: risk factors and outcomes. Ann Neurol 2001;50(2):163–8.
[2] Nelson K, Lynch JK. Stroke in newborn infants. Lancet Neurol 2004;3:150.
[3] Lynch JK, Hirtz DG, DeVeber G, et al. Report of the National Institute of Neurological Disorders and Stroke workshop on perinatal and childhood stroke. Pediatrics 2002;109: 116–23.
[4] Kittner SJ, Adams RJ. Stroke in children and young adults. Curr Opin Neurol 1996;9:53–6.
[5] Giroud M, Lemesle M, Gouyon JB, et al. Cerebrovascular disease in children under 16 years of age in the city of Dijon, France: a study of incidence and clinical features from 1985 to 1993. J Clin Epidemiol 1995;48:1343–8.
[6] Schoenberg BS, Mellinger JF, Schoenberg DG, et al. Cerebrovascular disease in infants and children: a study of incidence, clinical features, and survival. Neurology 1978;8:763–8.

[7] Golomb MR, Garg BP, Saha C, et al. Accuracy and yield of ICD-9 codes for identifying children with ischemic stroke. Neurology 2006;67:2053–5.

[8] DeVeber G. Risk factors for childhood stroke: little folks have different strokes! Ann Neurol 2003;52(3):167–73.

[9] Wu LA, Malouf JF, Dearani JA, et al. Patent foramen ovale in cryptogenic stroke. Arch Intern Med 2004;164:950–6.

[10] Lechat P, Mas MJ, Lascault P, et al. Prevalence of patent foramen ovule in patients with stroke. N Engl J Med 1988;318:1148–52.

[11] Chabrier S, Lasjaunias P, Husson B, et al. Ischaemic stroke from dissection of the craniofacial arteries in childhood: report of 12 patients. Eur J Paediatr Neurol 2003;7:39–42.

[12] Sebire G, Fullerton H, Riou E, et al. Toward the definition of cerebral arteriopathies in childhood. Curr Opin Pediatr 2004;16:617–22.

[13] Danchaivijitr N, Cox TC, Saunders DE, et al. Evolution of cerebral arteriopathies in childhood arterial ischemic stroke. Ann Neurol 2006;59:620–6.

[14] Shaffer L, Rich PM, Pohl KRE, et al. Can mild head injury cause ischaemic stroke? Arch Dis Child 2003;88:267–9.

[15] Kieslich M, Fiedler A, Heller C, et al. Minor head injury as cause and co-factor in the aetiology of stroke in childhood: a report of eight cases. J Neurol Neurosurg Psychiatry 2002;73: 13–6.

[16] Ganesan V, Prengler M, McShane MA, et al. Investigation of risk factors in children with arterial ischemic stroke. Ann Neurol 2003;53:167–73.

[17] Ganesan V, Prengler M, Wade A, et al. Clinical and radiological recurrence after childhood arterial ischemic stroke. Circulation 2006;114:2170–7.

[18] Nowak-Göttl U, Sträter R, Heinecke A, et al. Lipoprotein (a) and genetic polymorphisms of clotting factor V, prothrombin, and methylenetetrahydrofolate reductase are risk factors of spontaneous ischemic stroke in childhood. Blood 1999;94:3678–82.

[19] Kenet G, Sadetzki S, Murad H, et al. Factor V Leiden and antiphospholipid antibodies are significant risk factors for ischemic stroke in children. Stroke 2000;31:1283–8.

[20] Sträter R, Vielhaber H, Kassenböhmer R, et al. Genetic risk factors of thrombophilia in ischaemic childhood stroke of cardiac origin. A prospective ESPED survey. Eur J Pediatr 1999;158(Suppl 3):S122–5.

[21] Haywood S, Liesner R, Pindora S, et al. Thrombophilia and first arterial ischaemic stroke: a systematic review. Arch Dis Child 2005;90:402–5.

[22] Chabrier S, Husson B, Lasjaunias P, et al. Stroke in childhood: outcome and recurrence risk by mechanism in 59 patients. J Child Neurol 2000;15:290–4.

[23] Rubinstein SM, Peerdeman SM, van Tulder MW, et al. A systematic review of the risk factors for cervical artery dissection. Stroke 2005;36:1575–80.

[24] Patel H, Smith RR, Garg BP. Spontaneous extracranial carotid artery dissection in children. Pediatr Neurol 1995;13:55–60.

[25] Reess J, Pfandl S, Pfeifer T, et al. Traumatic occlusion of the internal carotid artery as an injury sequela of soccer. Sportverletz Sportschaden 1993;2:88–9.

[26] Tekin S, Aykut-Bingol C, Aktan S. Case of intracranial vertebral artery dissection in young age. Pediatr Neurol 1997;16:67–70.

[27] Brandt T, Orberk E, Weber R, et al. Pathogenesis of cervical artery dissections. Association with connective tissue abnormalities. Neurology 2001;57:24–30.

[28] Askalan R, Laughlin S, Mayank S, et al. Chickenpox and stroke in children. Stroke 2002;32: 1257–62.

[29] Lanthier S, Armstron D, Doni T, et al. Post-varicella arteriopathy of childhood. Neurology 2005;64:660–3.

[30] Bowers DC, Liu Y, Leisenring W, et al. Late-occuring stroke among long-term survivors of childhood leukemia and brain tumors: a report form the childhood cancer survivor study. J Clin Oncol 2006;24:5277–82.

[31] van Beynum IM, Smeitink JAM, den Heijer M, et al. Hyperhomocysteinemia. A risk factor for ischemic stroke in children. Circulation 1999;99:2070–2.

[32] Cardo E, Vilaseca MA, Campistol J, et al. Evaluation of hyperhomocysteinemia in children with stroke. Eur J Paediatr Neurol 1999;3:113–7.

[33] Josephson C, Nuss R, Jacobson L, et al. The varicella autoantibody syndrome. Pediatr Res 2001;50:345–52.

[34] Maguire JL, deVeber G, Parkin PC. Association between iron-deficiency anemia and stroke in young children. Pediatrics 2007;120:1053–7.

[35] Alvarez-Larran A, Cervantes F, Bellosillo B, et al. Essential thrombocythemia in young individuals: frequency and risk factors for vascular events and evolution to myelofibrosis in 126 patients. Leukemia 2007;21:1218–23.

[36] Kirton A, deVeber G. Cerebral palsy secondary to perinatal ischemic stroke. Clin Perinatol 2006;33(2):367–86.

[37] Lee J, Croen LA, Backstrand KH, et al. Maternal and infant characteristics associated with perinatal arterial stroke in the infant. JAMA 2005;293:723.

[38] Hall DA, Wadwa RP, Goldenberg NA, et al. Maternal cardiovascular risk factors for term neonatal seizures: a population-based study in Colorado 1989–2003. J Child Neurol 2006;21: 795–8.

[39] Sood R, Zogg M, Westrick RJ, et al. Fetal and maternal thrombophilia genes cooperate to influence pregnancy outcomes. J Exp Med 2007;204:1049–56.

[40] Braun KPJ, Rafay MF, Uiterwaal CSPM, et al. Mode of onset predicts etiological diagnosis of arterial ischemic stroke in children. Stroke 2007;38:298–302.

[41] Pavlakis SG, Kingsley PB, Bialer MG. Stroke in children: genetic and metabolic issues. J Child Neurol 2000;15:308–15.

[42] Hirano M, Pavlakis SG. Mitochondrial myopathy, encephalopathy, lactic acidosis, and stroke-like episodes (MELAS): current concepts. J Child Neurol 1994;9:4–13.

[43] Shellhaas R, Smith SE, O'Tool E, et al. Mimics of childhood stroke: characteristics of a prospective cohort. Pediatrics 2006;118:704.

[44] Gadian DG, Calamante F, Kirkham FJ, et al. Diffusion and perfusion magnetic resonance imaging in childhood stroke. J Child Neurol 2000;15:279–83.

[45] Bernard TJ, Mull BR, Handler MH, et al. An 18-year-old man with fenestrated vertebral arteries, recurrent stroke and successful angiographic coiling. J Neurol Sci 2007;260:279–82.

[46] Kurnik K, Kosch A, Sträter R, et al. Recurrent thromboembolism in infants and children suffering from symptomatic neonatal arterial stroke. A prospective follow-up study. Stroke 2003;34:2887–93.

[47] Boffa MC, Lachassinne E. Review: infant perinatal thrombosis and antiphospholipid antibodies: a review. Lupus 2007;16:634–41.

[48] Monagle P, Chan A, Massicotte P, et al. Antithrombotic therapy in children: the Seventh ACCP Conference on Antithrombotic and Thrombotic Therapy. Chest 2004;126(Suppl 3):645S–87S.

[49] Paediatric Stroke Working Group. Stroke in childhood: Clinical guidelines for diagnosis, management and rehabilitation. Royal College of Physicians, 2004. Available at: http:// www.rcplondon.ac.uk/pubs/books/childstroke/childstroke_guidelines.pdf. Accessed February 25, 2008.

[50] Sträter R, Kurnik K, Heller C, et al. Aspirin versus low-dose molecular-weight heparin: antithrombotic therapy in pediatric ischemic stroke patients. A propsective follow-up study. Stroke 2001;32:2554–8.

[51] Adams R, McKie V, Hsu L, et al. Prevention of a first stroke by transfusion in children with abnormal results of transcranial Doppler ultrasonography. N Engl J Med 1998;339: 5–11.

[52] Ozgur BM, Aryan HE, Levy ML. Indirect revascularization for paediatric moyamoya disease: the EDAMS technique. J Clin Neurosci 2006;13:105–8.

[53] Khan N, Schuknecht B, Boltshauser E, et al. Moyamoya disease and Moyamoya syndrome: experience in Europe; choice of revascularization procedures. Acta Neurochir (Wien) 2003; 145:1061–71.

[54] Amlie-Lefond C, Benedict SL, Benard T, et al. Thrombolysis in children with arterial ischemic stroke: initial results from the International Paediatric Stroke Study [abstract]. Stroke 2007;38:485.

[55] Golomb MR, Rafay M, Armstrong D, et al. Intra-arterial tissue plasminogen activator for thrombosis complicating cerebral angiography in a 17-year-old girl. J Child Neurol 2003;18: 420–3.

[56] Benedict SL, Ni OK, Schloesser P, et al. Intra-arterial thrombolysis in a 2-year-old with cardioembolic stroke. J Child Neurol 2007;22:225–7.

[57] Thirumalai SS, Shubin RA. Successful treatment for stroke in a child using recombinant tissue plasminogen activator. J Child Neurol 2000;15:558.

[58] Taub E, Griffin A, Nick J, et al. Pediatric CI therapy for stroke-induced hemiparesis in young children. Dev Neurorehabil 2007;10:3.

[59] Lanthier S, Carmant L, David M, et al. Stroke in children. The coexistence of multiple risk factors predicts poor outcome. Neurology 2000;54:371–8.

[60] Fullerton HJ, Wu YW, Sidney S, et al. Risk of recurrent childhood arterial ischemic stroke in a population-based cohort: the importance of cerebrovascular imaging. Pediatrics 2007;119: 495–501.

[61] Sträter R, Becker S, von Eckardstein A, et al. Prospective assessment of risk factors for recurrent stroke during childhood—a 5-year follow-up study. Lancet 2002;360:1540–5.

[62] Nagata S, Matsushima T, Morioka T, et al. Unilaterally symptomatic moyamoya disease in children: long-term follow-up of 20 patients. Neurosurgery 2006;59:830–6.

[63] Lanthier S, Kirkham FJ, Mitchell LG, et al. Increased anticardiolipin antibody IgG titers do not predict recurrent stroke or TIA in children. Neurology 2004;62:194–200.

[64] Steinlin M, Pfister I, Pavlovic J, et al. The first three years of the Swiss Neuropaediatric Stroke Registry (SNPSR): a population-based study of incidence, symptoms and risk factors. Neuropediatrics 2005;36:90–7.

[65] DeSchryver EL, Kappelle LJ, Jennekens-Schinkel A, et al. Prognosis of ischemic stroke in childhood: a long term follow up study. Dev Med Child Neurol 2000;42:313–8.

[66] Steinlin M, Roellin K, Schroth G. Long-term follow-up after stroke in childhood. Eur J Pediatr 2004;163:245–50.

[67] Mercuri E, Rutherford M, Cowan F, et al. Early prognostic indicators of outcome in infants with neonatal cerebral infarction: a clinical electroencephalogram, and magnetic resonance imaging study. Pediatrics 1999;103:1–15.

[68] Mercuri E, Barnett A, Rutherford M, et al. Neonatal cerebral infarction and neuromotor outcome at school age. Pediatrics 2004;113:95–100.

[69] De Vries LS, Van der Grond J, Van Haastert IC, et al. Prediction of outcome in new-born infants with arterial ischaemic stroke using diffusion-weighted magnetic resonance imaging. Neuropediatrics 2005;36:12–20.

[70] Boardman JP, Ganesan V, Rutherford MA, et al. Magnetic resonance image correlates of hemiparesis after neonatal and childhood middle cerebral artery stroke. Pediatrics 2005; 115:321–6.

[71] Kirton A, Shroff M, Visvanathan T, et al. Quantified corticospinal tract diffusion restriction predicts neonatal stroke outcome. Stroke 2007;38:974–80.

[72] deVeber GA, MacGregor D, Curtis R, et al. Neurologic outcome in survivors of childhood arterial ischemic stroke and sinovenous thrombosis. J Child Neurol 2000;15:316–24.

PEDIATRIC CLINICS

OF NORTH AMERICA

Pediatr Clin N Am 55 (2008) 339–355

The Role of the Hematologist/Oncologist in the Care of Patients with Vascular Anomalies

Denise M. Adams, MD[a,b,]*, Mary Sue Wentzel, RN[b]

[a]*Division of Hematology/Oncology, Cincinnati Children's Hospital Medical Center, University of Cincinnati, MLC 7015, 3333 Burnet Avenue, Cincinnati, OH 45229, USA*
[b]*Hemangioma and Vascular Malformation Center, Cincinnati Children's Hospital Medical Center, 3333 Burnet Avenue, Cincinnati, OH 45229, USA*

The proper care of children who have vascular anomalies requires the expertise of multiple pediatric specialists. In the past, there was much debate concerning the appropriate treatment of these lesions and which specialists needed to be involved. Many patients were evaluated by specialists who were confused about the diagnosis and the proper medical management. Because of the need for an interdisciplinary approach, several vascular anomalies centers have been developed across the world. These clinics are composed of specialists who have clinical acumen in surgery, radiology, dermatology, hematology, oncology, pathology, neurology, ophthalmology, cardiology, gastroenterology, and basic sciences. This comprehensive multidisciplinary approach offers the best opportunity for children who have vascular anomalies to obtain optimal diagnostic and therapeutic management of these complex lesions.

A classification system for vascular anomalies first was proposed in 1982 by Mulliken and Glowacki [1]. This initial scheme distinguished hemangiomas from vascular malformations based on clinical appearance, histopathologic features, and biologic behavior. Hemangiomas were identified as vascular tumors with an active growth phase, characterized by endothelial proliferation and hypercellularity, followed by an involutional phase. Vascular malformations were described as congenital malformations of the vasculature derived from capillaries, veins, lymphatic vessels, or arteries

* Corresponding author. Division of Hematology/Oncology, Cincinnati Children's Hospital Medical Center, University of Cincinnati, MLC 7015, 3333 Burnet Avenue, Cincinnati, OH 45229.

E-mail address: denise.adams@cchmc.org (D.M. Adams).

0031-3955/08/$ - see front matter. Published by Elsevier Inc.
doi:10.1016/j.pcl.2008.01.007

or a combination of these vessels. In 1996, this classification system was modified to include kaposiform hemangioendothelioma (KHE), tufted angioma (TA), pyogenic granuloma, and hemangiopericytoma. These tumors, once misclassified as hemangiomas, have distinct clinical and histopathologic findings. The revised classification system now has two main categories: vascular tumors and vascular malformations (Fig. 1). Vascular anomaly specialists have identified certain lesions with characteristics of malformations and proliferative lesions, but this system allows diagnosis and classification based primarily on physical examination and medical history. Exceptions may require further imaging studies, biopsy, or observation.

Pediatric hematologist/oncologists play an active role in the care of children who have vascular lesions. In the majority of cases, treatment requires the involvement of medical and surgical specialists. These patients rarely are managed successfully by a surgeon or a pediatrician alone. Often, pediatric hematologist/oncologists provide clinical acumen in establishing a correct diagnosis and guiding the medical management of these patients. Pediatric hematologist/oncologists also can provide insights in the availability and suitability of enrollment into clinical trials or the use of novel, experimental treatments for these complicated conditions.

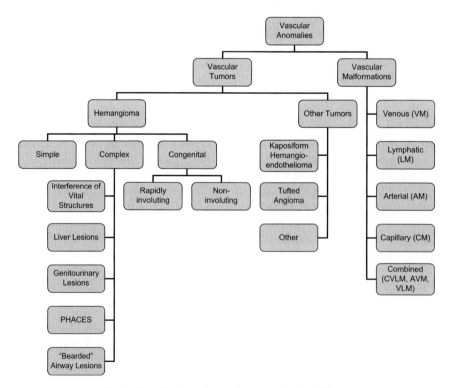

Fig. 1. Classification of vascular anomalies in children.

Vascular tumors

Classification

As illustrated in Fig. 1, vascular tumors represent the first large category of vascular anomalies observed in children. The majority of these vascular tumors are hemangiomas (often called infantile hemangiomas) that appear shortly after birth. Most hemangiomas are simple lesions and require only observation. Some hemangiomas are more complex and cause injury or disfigurement to vital organs, whereas others are associated with other physical abnormalities and syndromes. In contrast, certain lesions are identified as congenital hemangiomas, which are present at birth but are pathologically and clinically different from infantile hemangiomas. Lesions classified as "other" vascular tumors are endothelial cell derived but are not true hemangiomas; these have a more complicated picture (discussed later).

Diagnosis

Hemangiomas are the most common vascular tumor of infancy. Hemangiomas occur more commonly in white newborns, with a higher incidence in female and premature infants [2–5]. They are observed most commonly in the head and neck area followed by the trunk and extremities. The majority occur as single tumors, but as many as 20% of affected infants have multiple lesions [2–5]. Most hemangiomas are not seen at birth but appear during the first several weeks of life. Hemangiomas can be deep or superficial or a combination of the two types. Deep hemangiomas are soft, warm masses with a bluish color. Superficial hemangiomas are red and raised or, rarely, telangiectatic.

Hemangiomas have several phases of growth. The first is the proliferating phase during which they expand rapidly. This phase lasts for 4 to 6 months. In this phase, the hemangioma's superficial component becomes more erythematous or violacious. Expansion can occur superficially and deeply. Deep hemangiomas may proliferate through up to 2 years of age. A stationary phase follows during which the hemangioma grows in proportion to the child. This phase is followed by an involuting phase that can last up to 5 to 6 years. Involuting hemangiomas become more gray in color. Maximum involution occurs in approximately 50% of children by age 5 years and in 90% of children by age 9 [2–5]. The majority of patients do not have sequelae, but 20% to 40 % of patients have residual changes of the skin, such as laxity, discoloration, telangiectasias, fibrofatty masses, or scarring.

Congenital hemangiomas are an entity distinguished from infantile hemangiomas because they are fully developed at birth and even can be diagnosed in utero. There are two subgroups: rapidly involuting congenital hemangiomas (RICH) and noninvoluting congenital hemangiomas (NICH) [6]. The RICH lesions can look very violacious at birth but regress rapidly during the first year of life. In contrast, NICH lesions are fully developed at birth but do not involute. Both lesions are high flow lesions that can be misdiagnosed as arteriovenous malformations [AVMs]. Congenital hemangiomas can cause congestive heart failure that has been reported in utero.

There are distinguishing histochemical endothelial markers (such as GLUT-1), which are present in hemangiomas of infancy but not in the other vascular tumors [7]. Hemangiomas are a mixture of cell types, including endothelial cells (CD31+), pericytes (SMA+), dendritic cells (factor XIIIa+), and mast cells. Continuing research in this area should provide insights into the pathology, pathophysiology, and molecular basis of these benign vascular tumors.

Infantile hemangiomas can be associated with other anomalies or conditions that may require further evaluation or immediate medical management. Hemangiomas in the cervicofacial region that cover the chin, neck, or face in a "bearded" distribution are associated with airway hemangiomas [8]. Any bearded hemangioma should be evaluated by an otolaryngologist whether or not respiratory symptoms are present (Fig. 2). Infants who have hemangiomas in this area should be monitored closely, and medical management should be initiated if airway involvement is suspected.

Hemangiomas in the lumbosacral area can signal underlying occult spinal dysraphism (lipomeningocele, tethered spinal cord, and diastematomyelia). These hemangiomas also can be associated with genital urinary defects [9,10]. Ultrasound (<6 months of age) or MRI (>6 months of age) evaluation of the spine and ultrasound of the genitourinary region is recommended for these patients. Infants who have multiple (>5) cutaneous hemangiomas can have focal visceral tumors involving the liver, spleen, lung, brain, and intestines. Liver hemangiomas (Fig. 3) are the most common of the visceral

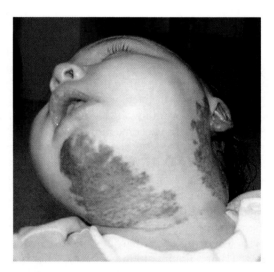

Fig. 2. Bearded hemangioma: high risk for airway lesions; otolaryngolic evaluation is recommended.

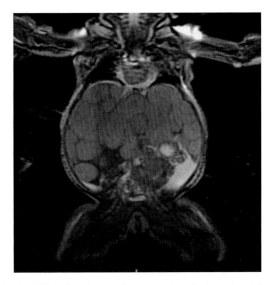

Fig. 3. Diffuse liver hemangioma: monitor for hypothyroidism.

hemangiomas and can lead to serious complications, such as hepatomegaly, leading to compartment syndrome, congestive heart failure, anemia/mild thrombocytopenia, and synthetic hepatic dysfunction [11]. Therefore, infants presenting with multiple cutaneous hemangiomas should undergo further evaluation, including ultrasound evaluation of the abdomen. If liver lesions are found, MRI scanning is indicated to characterize and quantify the lesions better. Liver hemangiomas also can occur without cutaneous lesions, which makes them more difficult to diagnose. Laboratory anomalies can include α-fetoprotein (AFP) elevation but there are no standard values for this population of patients [12]. Recently, a classification system and a registry have been established to gain knowledge about these patients [13]. The differential diagnosis of these lesions includes AVMs, congenital hemangiomas, and other malignant liver tumors, such as hepatoblastoma, angiosarcomas, and epitheloid hemangioendotheliomas [14–16].

Infants who have large hemangiomas, in particular hepatic hemangiomas, should be screened for hypothyroidism. Huang and colleagues [17] reported an association between infantile hemangiomas and severe hypothyroidism. High levels of type 3-iodothyronine deiodinase activity were found in the hemangioma tissue, causing an accelerated uptake of thyroid hormone. Because such patients may require extraordinarily high doses of thyroid replacement, they should be followed by a pediatric endocrinologist [18]. Unidentified, severe hypothyroidism can lead to heart failure and death.

The association of *p*osterior fossa abnormalities, large cervicofacial *h*emangiomas that typically are plaque-like (Fig. 4), *a*rterial anomalies, *c*ardiac anomalies (most commonly coarctation of the aorta), *e*ye anomalies, and *s*ternal cleft or supraumbilical raphe is called PHACES syndrome

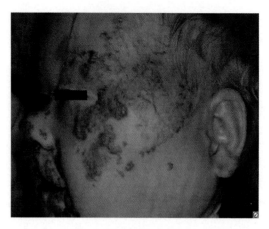

Fig. 4. PHACES syndrome.

[19–21]. Some of these infants are at increased risk for stroke. Because other more complicated hemangiomas also are identified in these patients, the phenotypic spectrum of this syndrome currently is being followed prospectively in an international clinical registry.

Hemangiomas should not be confused with the lesions known as KHE and TA (Fig. 5). These latter lesions first were described in 1940 by Kasabach and Merritt [22], who reported an infant who had thrombocytopenic purpura resulting from what they believed was a giant capillary hemangioma. Subsequently, the association of capillary hemangiomas with thrombocytopenia was referred to as Kasabach-Merritt syndrome.

In 1997, two groups of investigators demonstrated that these lesions were not true hemangiomas, rather, distinct vascular tumors diagnosed

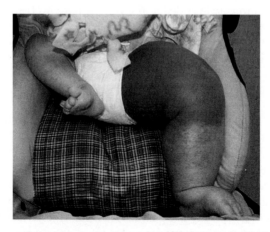

Fig. 5. KHE: aggressive benign vascular tumor with high mortality/morbidity rate associated with KMP.

histologically as KHE or TA [23,24]. KHEs and TAs have a different clinical profile from hemangiomas with a predilection for the upper trunk, extremities, thigh, sacrum, or retroperitoneum. They are warm, firm, indurated purpuric lesions. MRI scans show that these lesions invade the skin and subcutaneous fat and muscle. They usually are focal but some reports describe lymph node spread. These tumors can be associated with what now is called Kasabach-Merritt phenomenon (KMP), which includes an enlarging vascular lesion, profound thrombocytopenia, microangiopathic hemolytic anemia, and a mild consumptive coagulopathy. The phenomenon is associated with a mortality rate as high as 20% to 30%. KHE and TA not always are associated with KMP [25], but it is exactly the coagulopathy seen in KMP that causes morbidity and mortality in patients who have these lesions. The resulting profound thrombocytopenia and hypofibrinogenemia cause the most serious hemorrhagic complications.

Several therapies are reported for the treatment of these lesions but none is uniformly effective. Therapies include the systemic use of corticosteroids, interferon, antifibrinolytic agents, and chemotherapy, including vincristine (VCR), cyclophosphamide, and actinomycin [26–28]. These lesions are challenging to manage as their clinical presentation and response to therapy vary greatly. Clinical response can be subtle and take months to occur. Some lesions remain present for years after resolution of the KMP, leading to other morbidities, such as orthopedic anomalies and chronic pain [29]. Cincinnati Children's Hospital Medical Center has a clinical registry open to prospectively investigate the clinical course of these lesions [30]. As discussed previously, KHEs and TAs should not be confused with hemangiomas and always require supervision by a multidisciplinary team.

Medical management of hemangiomas

The proper management of hemangiomas is based on size, location, presence of complications at the time of diagnosis, patient age, and estimated growth rate [31].

Indications for immediate treatment include interference with vital structures, the possibility of permanent scarring, large facial hemangiomas, and ulcerative hemangiomas. Corticosteroids continue to be first-line therapy for hemangiomas, with response rates varying between 70% and 90% [32,33]. The mechanism of action of corticosteroids remains poorly understood but is believed to include an antiangiogenic effect that decreases endothelial cell proliferation and causes endothelial cell apoptosis. Hasan and colleagues [34] studied the histologic and molecular changes in proliferating hemangioma after steroid therapy and found increased numbers of mast cells, decreased transcriptional expression of cytokines, and enhanced transcription of mitochondrial cytochrome B gene.

Unfortunately, there are limited prospective randomized controlled studies that have looked at steroid dosing or efficacy. Therefore, current data and treatment recommendations are based on retrospective studies and clinical experience. Steroids can be given orally or topically or injected into the lesion. The generally recommended starting dose for systemic steroids is 2 to 5 mg/kg per day of prednisolone as a single morning dose. Typically response is assessed after 2 weeks. If there is good response, the initial dose is maintained for 4 to 6 weeks and then tapered over 4 to 6 months. The use of ranitidine hydrochloride, a histamine H_2-receptor antagonist, or one of the proton pump inhibitors to decrease gastrointestinal irritation is recommended during steroid treatment. In addition, some centers recommend the use of trimethoprim/sulfamethoxazole as prophylactic treatment for *Pneumocytis carinii*, particularly if steroids are used at higher doses or for an excessive period of time [35]. Intralesional corticosteroids are used best for smaller, localized, problematic lesions rather than larger segmental hemangiomas. Topical steroids also are used to treat localized lesions not causing significant impairment, such as on the forehead or cheek.

Short-term side effects of systemic steroids include personality changes, gastric irritation, diminished gain of height and weight, nonsystemic fungal infections, and a cushingoid appearance. Boon and colleagues evaluated 62 patients receiving systemic corticosteroid therapy for problematic infantile hemangiomas and found cushingoid facies in 71% of patients, personality changes in 21%, gastric irritation in 21%, fungal infections in 6%, and reversible myopathy in one patient. Diminished longitudinal growth was seen in 35% and diminished weight in 42%; however, catch-up growth occurred in most patients [36]. Potential long-term side effects of steroid use include immunosuppression, hypertension, significant suppression of the hypothalamic pituitary adrenal function, hyperglycemia, ophthalmologic changes, myositis, osteoporosis, cardiomyopathy, and neurologic changes. Therefore, patients on systemic glucocorticoid therapy should be monitored for the development of potential side effects. Height and weight, blood pressure checks, developmental milestones, and adrenal suppression should be monitored closely. Live vaccines should not be administered while on systemic glucocorticoids. If exposure to varicella occurs, a physician should be called immediately and varicella zoster immune globulin should be administered promptly. Patients should be evaluated for significant febrile events ($> 38.5°C$) and further work-up, including blood cultures and antibiotics, may be needed.

Currently, VCR is the preferred second systemic therapeutic agent for patients who have failed other local medical therapies or cannot tolerate steroids [37–41]. VCR interferes with mitotic spindle microtubules and induces apoptosis in tumor cells in vitro. Its known side-effect profile includes peripheral neuropathy, constipation, jaw pain and irritability, electrolyte disturbances, and neurologic problems. The insertion of a central line is desirable because VCR is a vesicant. The experience with VCR for hemangiomas is described in several retrospective studies with limited numbers of patients [38–41]. Patients included in these studies usually had life-threatening hemangiomas that failed steroid therapy or had significant complications from steroid therapy.

Interferon has been used in the past but has fallen out of favor because of its neurologic side effects. Interferon is an antiangiogenic agent that decreases endothelial cell proliferation by down-regulating basic fibroblast growth factor. Many studies have reported the efficacy of interferon alpha-2a and interferon alpha-2b with a complete response rate of 40% to 50% using doses between 1 and 3 million units/m^2 per day [42,43]. Neurotoxicity, however, consisting of spastic diplegia and other motor developmental disturbances, is reported with all preparations of interferon in approximately 10% to 30% of patients, with several patients experiencing permanent spastic diplegia [44]. There are some data that relate this neurotoxicity to age, with children less than 12 months of age having a higher risk [45]. Interferon also causes flu-like symptoms, anemia, neutropenia, thrombocytopenia, change in the liver enzymes, depression, and hypothyroidism. If used, the recommended dose is 1 million units/m^2 per day for 5 days with a gradual increase to 2 to 3 million units/m^2 per day over 2 months. Total duration of treatment is 4 to 6 months. Some studies report favorable results with interferon on a 3-times-a-week schedule given each Monday, Wednesday, and Friday. Monitoring should include monthly neurologic examinations and laboratory testing twice a month, including complete blood count with differential and liver function tests. Thyroid function should be assessed every 3 months. If any change in neurologic status occurs, interferon should be discontinued immediately.

Novel drugs for hemangiomas

Pediatric hematology/oncology can contribute greatly to the management of hemangiomas by identifying novel therapeutic approaches and subsequently testing these in clinical trials. Targeted therapies for this class of disorders can be based on understanding the pathways involved in angiogenesis, immune regulation, cell cycle inhibition, and gene activation and inhibition (oncongenes and tumor suppressor genes). There are several drugs in development for the management of childhood cancers that may have a role in the treatment of vascular tumors, but more research is required to support this. One such drug is the new thalidomide derivative, lenalidomide (CC5013), used in the treatment of multiple myeloma, solid tumors, Crohn's disease, and congestive heart failure [46]. Thalidomide inhibits secretion of pro-inflammatory cytokines and increases secretion of anti-inflammatory cytokines. Lenalidomide can be taken orally and is a more potent antiangiogenic agent than its parent compound, thalidomide. Other agents of potential interest for the management of vascular tumors include vascular endothelial growth factor (VEGF) inhibitors, such as bevacizumab [47]. The side effects associated with bevacizumab, however, which include serious hemorrhage, thrombotic events, proteinuria, and hypertension, mandate careful evaluation of this drug before its use in benign vascular tumors. Another drug of potential interest is the proangiogenic agent, imiquimod. Topical imiquimod is shown to induce regression of many tumors and to inhibit vascular tumor growth in murine hemangioendothelioma models. Hazen and colleagues [48] showed that the topical application of this drug in children who have hemangiomas can cause resolution in a limited number of patients. Imiquimod stimulates cytokines and causes breakdown and erosion of tissue, which is one of the drug's side effects. Becaplermin, a proangiogenic platelet-derived growth factor gel (Regranex), has been used in a small series of ulcerative hemangiomas, demonstrating some promising responses [49]. Finally, drugs, such as imatinib mesilate, gefitinib, and the retinoids, all used in childhood cancers, also could be studied for managing vascular lesions.

Vascular malformations

Classification

Malformations are congenital abnormalities of the blood vessels and typically are classified according to flow criteria and or the type of vessel involved (see Fig. 1). These malformations can involve the capillaries (capillary malformation [CM]), veins (venous malformation [VM]), arteries (arterial malformation [AM]), or lymphatics (lymphatic malformation [LM]). They commonly are combined lesions involving more than one blood vessel structure (for example, capillary/venous/lymphatic malformations [CVLM], venous/lymphatic malformations [VLM], and arterial venous malformations [AVMs]). Vascular malformations can be associated with other disorders or anomalies and can cause complications to vital structures and organs.

Diagnosis

Unlike vascular tumors, vascular malformations are anomalies in the morphologic development of the vascular system; these lesions are present at birth and grow commensurately with the child. Vascular malformations can be exacerbated by trauma, infection, or hormonal changes. These lesions can result in disfigurement, skeletal abnormalities, infection, venous stasis, and a localized consumptive coagulopathy. They can pose a surgical risk because of hemorrhagic or thrombotic states. The role of pediatric hematologist/oncologists again is to aid in the diagnosis and provide guidance in the medical management.

Coagulopathy and vascular malformations

Hematologists play a key role in management of vascular malformations, because the lesions tend to result in serious coagulopathies. Lesions at high risk for coagulopathies include VMs, VLMs, and CVLMs (Figs. 6 and 7). The risk for coagulopathy is related to the extent of the lesion (diffuse and multiple lesions), but major bleeding or life-threatening thrombotic events rarely occur. The coagulopathy is referred to as localized intravascular coagulopathy (LIC) that is characterized by low plasma levels of fibrinogen, factor V, factor VIII, factor XIII, and antithrombin [50]. D-dimers and fibrin split products also are elevated in LIC. Minor to moderate thrombocytopenia also may be seen. With surgical resection, sclerotherapy, embolization, trauma, infection, or drugs, LIC sometimes progresses to disseminated intravascular coagulopathy that can be life threatening. Furthermore, this chronic consumptive coagulopathy can cause the formation of microthrombi, which calcify (forming phleboliths) and cause pain.

Enjolras and coworkers [51] reviewed 27 cases of extensive pure VMs in the upper and lower limb and found that 88% of these patients had LIC. The coagulopathy was associated with very low levels of plasma fibrinogen and soluble complexes, elevation of fibrin split products, and moderately low platelet counts. This chronic consumptive coagulopathy caused episodes of thrombosis (leading to phlebolith formation) or bleeding (hemarthrosis, hematomas, or intraoperative blood loss). The condition worsened after the cessation of the use of elastic stockings, therapeutic intervention (embolization or surgical procedure), spontaneous fracture of a bone localized in the area of the VM, or during pregnancy or menses in women. This group confirmed their findings in a retrospective evaluation of 24 patients who had extensive VMs [52]. Furthermore, they characterized the difference between LIC caused by these lesions and the coagulopathy that typifies KMP in certain vascular tumors. They also categorized the anomalies based on

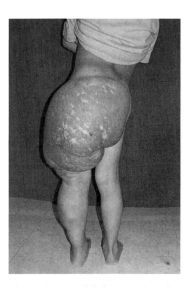

Fig. 6. CVLM: risk for coagulopathy.

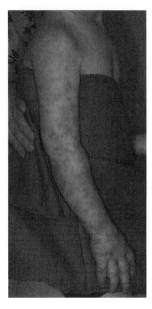

Fig. 7. VM: risk for coagulopathy.

a severity scoring system (a point was given to each involved site) and found that higher VM severity scores were associated with more severe LIC. In this retrospective review, the use of graded permanent elastic compression and low-molecular-weight heparin (LMWH) was effective preventive treatment causing a decrease in pain and phlebolith formation.

At Cincinnati Children's Hospital Medical Center, the authors analyzed 58 patients who had vascular malformations and found a significantly increased risk for coagulopathy in VMs, VLMs, and CVLMs with a diffuse or multifocal presentation. Elevation in the D-dimer was the most common hematologic abnormality. Coagulopathy seemed associated with increased pain in these patients [53].

Finally, there are reports in the literature regarding the risks for coagulopathy during interventional radiologic procedures [54]. Mason and colleagues analyzed coagulation abnormalities in patients undergoing sclerotherapy and embolization for vascular anomalies. An increased incidence of coagulopathy can occur during injection with dehydrated alcohol or sodium tetradecyl sulfate. Coagulopathy consisted of a decrease in platelets and fibrinogen, an increase in prothrombin time, and a conversion from negative to positive D-dimers.

Thrombophilic predisposition

Several congenital or acquired thrombophilic conditions have been identified in the general population as risk factors for venous thromboembolism (see the article by Goldenberg and Bernard elsewhere in this issue for more details). Among these are antithrombin and protein C and S deficiency, factor V Leiden mutation, C677T MTHFR gene mutation, PAI-1 4G/G polymorphism, hyperhomocysteinemia, antiphospholipid antibodies, lupus anticoagulant, and G20210A prothrombin gene mutation [55,56]. There are other situations in which endothelial abnormalities increase the risk for thrombosis, such as sickle cell disease and malignancy [57,58]. In adults, genetic alterations interact with other risk factors, such as the use of oral contraceptives, trauma, immobilization, and surgical procedures, to increase the thrombotic risk for patients. The overall risk in the presence of multiple risk factors can exceed the sum of the separate effects. There is no information about the prevalence of thrombophilic predispositions in patients who have vascular anomalies. It is presumed that patients who have a genetic predisposition toward thrombophilia have an increased risk for thrombosis and coagulopathy if they also have an extensive slow flow vascular malformation, but studies of thrombophilia and vascular anomalies are not published to date.

Management

All patients who have extensive VM, VLM, or CVLM should have a baseline hematologic evaluation. The authors recommend that baseline testing include a complete blood count, prothrombin time, activated partial thromboplastin time, fibrinogen, D-dimer, and prothrombotic assessment (ie, proteins C and S, prothrombin gene mutation, thrombin-antithrombin, factor V Leiden, PAI-1 polymorphism, factor VIII, homocysteine level, lupus anticoagulant, anticardiolipin antibody, and antithrombin III). Patients found to have abnormalities in their initial blood work should have a formal hematology consultation before any surgical or interventional procedure and before or during pregnancy. Those patients at high risk for thrombotic complications should receive LMWH (enoxaparin-LMWH) at 0.5 mg/kg/dose (maximum 60 mg/dose) once or twice a day (adults 30 mg twice daily) for at least 2 weeks before any surgical or invasive radiologic procedure. LWMH should be stopped 12 hours before the procedure and restarted 12 hours after the procedure. Anticoagulant dosing during pregnancy may vary and should be determined and monitored by a hematologist and obstetrician specializing in maternal fetal medicine.

LMWH also can be used daily to alleviate pain caused by inflammation, thrombosis, and formation of phleboliths in patients who have high-risk vascular malformations. Although no prospective studies are available, clinical experience has demonstrated its effectiveness in this setting. While patients are on LMWH, anti-factor Xa levels should be monitored. They normally are drawn 4 to 6 hours after the subcutaneous administration of LMWH. The target anti–factor Xa level should be less than 0.5 units/mL for prophylaxis. A complete blood count and liver function testing should be checked every 4 to 6 months with long-term LMWH dosing.

A dual-energy x-ray absorptiometry scan should be performed when LMWH is used for extensive periods of time because chronic use of LMWH can result in osteopenia.

Patients who have vascular malformations and who develop a serious thrombotic event, such as a pulmonary embolism, require anticoagulation therapy indefinitely [59,60]. In the acute phase, these patients can be treated with LMWH or regular heparin, then converted to an oral vitamin K antagonist, such as warfarin. Some patients who have acute thromboembolic events may require the placement of an inferior or superior vena caval filter in addition to anticoagulation therapy.

Antifibrinolytic agents, such as ∈-aminocaproic acid and tranexamic acid, are used to treat the hemorrhagic coagulopathy that can occur in patients who have vascular lesions [61]. Both agents attach to the lysine-binding sites of plasminogen and plasmin, displacing plasminogen from its fibrin surface. Tranexamic acid is more potent and has a longer half-life than ∈-aminocaproic acid. Widespread use of antifibrinolytic agents is limited secondary to concerns of increased risk for thrombosis, but there are no retrospective or prospective studies concerning the use of these agents in children who have vascular malformations. Furthermore, antiplatelet agents, such as aspirin, ticlopidine, and clopidogrel, have shown little clinical benefit but further, more definitive studies are needed. Compression garments reduce the amount of blood trapping within the vascular lesion and probably decrease LIC. Other nonpharmacologic supportive therapies include massage, physical therapy, and hydrotherapy.

Novel approaches

Vascular malformations are a challenging group of disorders for physicians. Treatment mainly has been surgical or through interventional procedures. Particular attention to new sclerosing agents and embolization techniques will be important in improving the management of these patients. Such agents, however, need to address the pathophysiologic differences in these malformations, because agents effective for arterial malformations may not be effective for lymphatic malformations or VMs.

As with vascular tumors, medical therapy needs to be targeted to the limited knowledge of the pathophysiology of these malformations. One exciting area with great potential is the recent discovery of genetic alterations within these lesions [62]. Some genetic alterations could serve as therapeutic targets and thus aid in treatment options. For example, the PTEN gene mutation has been identified in patients who have extensive AVMs and other anomalies [63]. Rapamycin or other mTOR inhibitors are predicted to be effective agents in disorders in which the PTEN/mTOR/STAT3 pathway is affected [63]. New antithrombotic agents with effectiveness similar to LMWH need to be investigated because life-long anticoagulation is needed after a significant thrombotic event has occurred. At present, clear and agreed-on medical management guidelines are lacking for these complicated patients, highlighting the need for further research.

References

[1] Mulliken JB, Glowacki J. Hemangiomas and vascular malformations in infants and children: a classification based on endothelial characteristics. Plast Reconstr Surg 1982; 69(3):412–22.

[2] Fishman SJ, Mulliken JB. Vascular anomalies. A primer for pediatricians. Pediatr Clin North Am 1998;45(6):1455–77.

[3] Enjolras O, Mulliken JB. Vascular tumors and vascular malformations (new issues). Adv Dermatol 1997;13:375–423.

[4] Drolet B, Esterly N, Frieden IJ. Hemangiomas in children. N Engl J Med 1999;341(3): 173–81.

[5] Haggstrom AN, Drolet BA, Baselga E, et al. Prospective study of infantile hemangiomas: clinical characteristics predicting complications and treatment. Pediatrics 2006;118:882–7.

[6] Mulliken JB, Enjoras O. Congenital hemangiomas and infantile hemangioma: missing links. J Am Acad Dermatol 2004;50(6):875–82.

[7] North PE, Waner M, Mizeracki A, et al. GLUT 1: a newly discovered immunohistochemical marker for juvenile hemangiomas. Human Pathology 2000;31(1):11–22.

[8] Orlow SJ, Isakoff MS, Blei F. Increased risk of symptomatic hemangiomas of the airway in association with cutaneous hemangiomas in a "beard" distribution. J Pediatr 1997;131:643–6.

[9] Stockman A, Boralevi F, Taieb A, et al. SACRAL syndrome: spinal dysraphism, anogenital, cutaneous, renal and urologic anomalies, associated with an angioma of lumbosacral localization. Dermatology 2007;214(1):40–5.

[10] Drolet B, Garzon M. SACRAL syndrome. Dermatology 2007;215(4):360–1.

[11] Isaacs H Jr. Fetal and neonatal hepatic tumors. J Pediatr Surg 2007;42(11):1789–803.

[12] Sari N, Yalcin B, Akuyuz C, et al. Infantile hepatic hemangioendothelioma with elevated serum alpha-fetoprotein. Pediatr Hematol Oncol 2006;23(8):639–47.

[13] Christison-Lagay ER, Burrows PE, Alomari A, et al. Hepatic hemangiomas:subtype classification and development of a clinical algorithm and registry. J Pediatr Surg 2007;42(1):62–7.

[14] Mehrabi A, Kashfi A, Fonauni H, et al. Primary malignant hepatic epithelioid hemangioendothelioma: a comprehensive review of the literature with emphasis on the surgical therapy. Cancer 2006;107(9):2108–21.

[15] Nord KM, Kandel J, Lefkowitch JH, et al. Mulitple cutaneous infantile hemangiomas associated with hepatic angiosarcoma: case report and review of the literature. Pediatrics 2006;118(3):907–13.

[16] Lu M, Greer ML. Hypervascular multifocal hepatoblastoma:dynamic gadolinium-enhanced MRI findings indistinguishable from infantile hemangioendothelioma. Pedriatr Radiol 2007;37(6):587–91.

[17] Huang SA, Tu HM, Harney JW, et al. Severe hypothyroidism caused by type 3 iodothyronine deiodinase in infantile hemangiomas. N Engl J Med 2000;343(3):185–9.

[18] Kalpatthi R, Germak J, Mizelle K, et al. Thyroid abnormalities in infantile hepatic hemangioendothelioma. Pediatr Blood Cancer 2007;49(7):1021–4.

[19] Bronzetti G, Giardini A, Patrizi A, et al. Ipsilateral hemangioma and aortic arch anomalies in posterior fossa malformations, hemangiomas, arterial anomalies, coarctation of the aorta, and cardiac defects and eye abnormalities (PHACE) anomaly: report and review. Pediatrics 2004;113:412–5.

[20] Metry DW, Dowd CF, Barkovich AJ, et al. The many faces of PHACE syndrome. J Pediatr 2001;139:117–23.

[21] Metry DW, Haggstrom AN, Drolet BA, et al. A prospective study of PHACE syndrome in infantile hemangiomas: demographic features, clinical findings, and complications. Am J Med Genet A 2006;140:975–86.

[22] Kasabach H, Merritt K. Capillary hemangioma with extensive purpura: report of a case. Am J Dis Child 1940;59:1063–70.

[23] Sarkar M, Mulliken JB, Kozakewich HP, et al. Thrombocytopenic coagulopathy (Kasabach-Merritt phenomenon) is associated with Kaposiform hemangioendothelioma and not with common infantile hemangioma. Plast Reconstr Surg 1997;100(6):1377–86.

[24] Enjolras O, Wassef M, Mazoyer E, et al. Infants with Kasabach-Merritt syndrome do not have "true" hemangiomas. J Pediatr 1997;130(4):631–40.

[25] Gruman A, Liang MG, Mulliken JB, et al. Kaposiform hemangioendothelioma without Kasabach-Merritt phenomenon. J Am Acad Dermatol 2005;52(4):616–22.

[26] Haisley-Royster C, Enjolras O, Freden JJ, et al. Kasabach-merritt phenomenon: a retrospective study of treatment with vincristine. J Pediatr Hematol Oncol 2002;24(6):459–62.

[27] Mulliken JB, Anupindi S, Ezekowitz RAB, et al. Case 13-2004: a newborn girl with a large cutaneous lesion, thrombocytopenia, and anemia. N Engl J Med 2004;350:1764–75.

[28] Hauer J, Graubner U, Konstantopoulos N, et al. Effective treatment of kaposiform hemangioendotheliomas associated with Kasabach-Merritt phenomenon using four-drug regimen. Pediatr Blood Cancer 2007;49(6):852–4.

[29] Enjolras O, Mulliken JB, Wassef M, et al. Residual lesions after Kasabach-Merritt phenomenon in 41 patients. J Am Acad Dermatol 2000;42:225–35.

[30] Adams D. Hemangioma and vascular malformations center. Available at: http://www.cincinnatichildrens.org/svc/alpha/h/vascular. Accessed March 11, 2008.

[31] Enjolras O, Riche MC, Merland JJ, et al. Management of alarming hemangiomas in infancy: a review of 25 cases. Pediatrics 1990;85(4):491–8.

[32] Bartoshesky LE, Bull M, Ferngold M. Corticosteroid treatment of cutaneous hemangiomas: how effective? A report on 24 children. Clin Pediatr (Phila) 1978;17(8):625, 629–38.

[33] Brown SH Jr, Neerhout RC, Fonkalsrud EW. Prednisone therapy in the management of large hemangiomas in infants and children. Surgery 1972;71(2):168–73.

[34] Hasan Q, Tan ST, Gush J, et al. Steroid therapy of a proliferating hemangioma: histochemical and molecular changes. Pediatrics 2000;105:117–20.

[35] Maronn ML, Corden T, Drolet BA. Pneumocystis carinii pneumonia in infant treated with oral steroids for hemangioma. Arch Dermatol 2007;143(9):1224–5.

[36] Boon LM, MacDonald DM, Mulliken JB. Complications of systemic corticosteroid therapy for problematic hemangioma. Plast Reconstr Surg 1999;104(6):1616–23.

[37] Adams DM. The nonsurgical management of vascular lesions. Facial Plast Surg Clin North Am 2001;9:601–8.

[38] Adams DM, Orme L, Bowers D. Vincristine treatment of complicated hemangiomas. 14th International Workshop on Vascular Anomalies, Netherlands, June 2002.

[39] Enjolras O, Breviere GM, Roger G, et al. Vincristine treatment for function- and life-threatening infantile hemangioma. Arch Pediatr 2004;11:99–107.

[40] Fawcett SL, Grant I, Hall PN, et al. Vincristine as a treatment for a large haemangioma threatening vital functions. Br J Plast Surg 2004;57(2):168–71.

[41] Perez-Valle S, Peinador M, Herraiz P, et al. Vincristine, an efficacious alternative for diffuse neonatal haemangiomatosis. Acta Paediatr 2007; [epub ahead of print].

[42] Ezekowitz R, Mulliken JB, Folkman J. Interferon alfa-2a therapy for life-threatening hemangiomas of infancy. N Engl J Med 1992;326(22):1456–63.

[43] Chang E, Boyd A, Nelson CC, et al. Successful treatment of infantile hemangiomas with interferon-alpha-2b. J Pediatr Hematol Oncol 1997;19(3):237–44.

[44] Barlow CF, Priebe CJ, Mulliken JB, et al. Spastic diplegia as a complication of interferon Alfa-2a treatment of hemangiomas of infancy. J Pediatr 1998;132(3 Pt 1): 527–30.

[45] Michaud AP, Bauman NM, Burke DK, et al. Spastic diplegia and other motor disturbances in infants receiving interferon-alpha. Laryngoscope 2004;114(7):1231–6.

[46] List AF. Lenalidomide—the phoenix rises. N Engl J Med 2007;357(21):2183–6.

[47] Benesch M, Windelberg M, Sauseng W, et al. Compassionate use of bevacizumab (Avastin ®) in children and yound adults with refractory or recurrent solid tumors. Ann Oncol 2007; [epub ahead of print].

[48] Hazen PG, Carney JF, Engstrom CW, et al. Proliferating hemangioma of infancy: successful treatment with topical 5% imiquimod cream. Pediatric Dermatology 2005;22(3):254–6.

[49] Metz BJ, Rubenstein MC, Levy ML, et al. Response of ulcerated perineal hemangiomas of infancy to becaplermin gel, a recombinant human platelet-derived growth factor. Arch Dermatol 2004;140(7):867 70.

[50] Mulliken JB, Young AE, editors. Vascular birthmarks: hemangiomas and malformations. Philadelphia: WB Saunders; 1988.

[51] Enjolras O, Ciabrini D, Mazoyer E, et al. Extensive pure venous malformations in the upper or lower limb: a review of 27 cases. J Am Acad Dermatol 1997;36:219–25.

[52] Mazoyer E, Enjolras O, Laurian C, et al. Coagulation abnormalities associated with extensive venous malformations of the limbs: differentiation from Kasabach-Merritt syndrome. Clin Lab Haematol 2002;24(4):243–51.

[53] Mason KP, Neufeld EJ, Karian VE, et al. Coagulation abnormalities in pediatric and adult patients after sclerotherapy or embolization of vascular anomalies. AJR Am J Roentgenol 2001;177:1359–63.

[54] Nowak-Gottl U, Junker R, Kreuz W, et al. Risk of recurrent venous thrombosis in children with combined prothrombotic risk factors. Blood 2001;97:858–62.

[55] Tormene D, Simioni P, Prandoni P, et al. The incidence of venous thromboembolism in thrombophilic children: a prospective cohort study. Blood 2002;100:2403–5.

[56] Austin H, Key NS, Benson JM, et al. Sickle cell trait and the risk of venous thromboembolism among blacks. Blood 2007;110(3):908–12.

[57] Decousus H, Moulin N, Quenet S, et al. Thrombophilia and risk of venous thrombosis in patients with cancer. Thromb Res 2007;120(Suppl 2):S51–61.

[58] Skourtis G, Lazoura O, Panoussis P, et al. Klippel-Trenaunay syndrom:an unusual cause of pulmonary embolism. Int Angiol 2006;25(3):322–6.

[59] Huiras EE, Barnes CJ, Eichenfield LF, et al. Pulmonary thromboembolism associated with Klippel-Trenaunay syndrome. Pediatrics 2005;116(4):e596–600.

[60] Morad AB, McClain KL, Ogden AK. The role of tranexamic acid in the treatment of giant hemangiomas in newborns. Am J Pediatr Hematol Oncol 1993;15:383–5.

[61] Wang QK. Update on the molecular genetics of vascular anomalies. Lymphat Res Biol 2005; 3(4):226–33.

[62] Tan WH, Baris HN, Burrows PE, et al. The spectrum of vascular anomalies in patients with PTEN mutations: implications for diagnosis and management. J Med Genet 2007;44(9): 594–602.

[63] O'Reilly KE, Rojo F, She QB, et al. mTOR inhibition induces upstream receptor tyrosine kinase signaling and activates Akt. Cancer Res 2006;66(3):1500–8.

PEDIATRIC CLINICS
OF NORTH AMERICA

Pediatr Clin N Am 55 (2008) 357–376

ELSEVIER
SAUNDERS

Advances in Hemophilia: Experimental Aspects and Therapy

Nidra I. Rodriguez, MD[a,b,*], W. Keith Hoots, MD[a,b]

[a]Division of Pediatrics, Hematology Section, The University of Texas
Health Science Center, 6411 Fannin, Houston, TX 77030, USA
[b]Gulf States Hemophilia and Thrombophilia Center, 6655 Travis,
Suite 400 HMC, Houston, TX 77030, USA

Hemophilia A or B is an X-linked recessive disorder that results from the deficiency of blood coagulation factor VIII or IX, respectively (Fig. 1). Hemophilia is classified based on the level of factor VIII or IX activity as severe ($<1\%$), moderate ($1\%–5\%$), or mild ($>5\%–40\%$). The type and frequency of bleeding in hemophilia vary according to its severity. For example, patients who have severe hemophilia present with spontaneous bleeding into the joints or muscles, soft tissue bleeding, and life-threatening hemorrhage in addition to episodes of minor bleeding. Patients who have moderate hemophilia present less commonly with spontaneous bleeding but frequently experience bleeding after minor trauma. Finally, patients who have mild hemophilia typically present bleeding only after surgery or major trauma.

Musculoskeletal bleeding is the most common type of bleeding in hemophilia. Such bleeding can result in arthropathy, a common complication seen in the patient population that has this disease. In general, hemophilia treatment consists of replacing the missing coagulation protein with clotting factor concentrates when bleeding episodes occur (treatment on demand) or by scheduled infusions of clotting factor several times per week (prophylaxis). The development of neutralizing antibodies or inhibitors against factor VIII or IX is another complication encountered as a result of hemophilia treatment.

Multiple factor VIII and IX concentrates are available and categorized based on their source (plasma derived versus recombinant), purity, and viral inactivation methods [1]. Recombinant products are categorized further based on the presence or absence of animal/human protein in the cell culture

* Corresponding author. Gulf States Hemophilia and Thrombophilia Center, 6655 Travis, Suite 400 HMC, Houston, TX 77030.
   E-mail address: nidra.i.rodriguez@uth.tmc.edu (N.I. Rodriguez).

doi:10.1016/j.pcl.2008.01.010

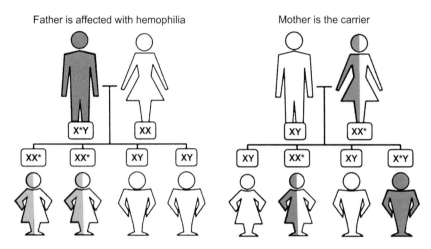

Fig. 1. X-linked recessive inheritance of hemophilia. Asterisk (*) designates affected chromosome. (*From* Pruthi RK. Hemophilia: a practical approach to genetic testing. Mayo Clin Proc 2005;80(11):1485–99; with permission.)

media or in the final stabilized product (Table 1) [1]. Treatment of patients who develop inhibitors against factor VIII or IX is significantly more challenging than treatment of patients who do not have such antibodies. For patients who have high-titer inhibitors, the use of bypassing agents, such as recombinant factor VIIa or activated prothrombin complex concentrates, may be necessary to achieve hemostasis. In these particular patients, however, the ultimate therapeutic goal is to eradicate the inhibitor by means of immune tolerance induction (ITI). With this approach, patients receive repetitive doses of factor VIII or IX, usually once a day, with or without associated immunosuppresion. Typically, there is an initial rise in the antibody titers as a result of anamnestic response. Subsequently, however, a gradual reduction in titer is seen until in the end the inhibitor becomes undetectable. After successful immune tolerance, patients continue on regular factor infusions several times per week.

This article focuses on recent advances. From a clinical standpoint, different prophylactic regimens, including primary, secondary, and tailored prophylaxis, for severe hemophilia are discussed. Some of these regimens may serve as alternatives to primary prophylaxis in developing countries where the high cost of factor concentrates precludes its regular use. Adjuvant treatment options for bleeding management in hemophilia also are discussed along with the role of radionuclide synovectomy with isotopes, such as phosphorus 32 sulfur colloid (P^{32}) to treat joint arthropathy. Current challenges in hemophilia care, including inhibitor development and approaches to achieve ITI, are addressed.

From a research standpoint, some of the mechanisms believed to lead to blood-induced joint disease are discussed. Data suggest that iron deposition in the synovium plays an important role in this process. This article discusses the experimental aspects of synovitis, including the role of iron and cytokines, in inducing an inflammatory response that stimulates angiogenesis and contributes to bone destruction.

Approaches to the medical management of hemophilia

Despite improvements in hemophilia therapy, arthropathy remains a significant clinical problem. The Medical and Scientific Advisory Council of the National Hemophilia Foundation, the World Federation of Hemophilia, and the World Health Organization all recommend that prophylaxis (intravenous factor replacement at least 46 weeks per year through adulthood infused in anticipation of and to prevent bleeding) [2] be considered standard of care to prevent complications, such as arthropathy. Based on this recommendation, a major goal of hemophilia therapy is to prevent any joint disease.

Observational studies support that prophylaxis is superior to on-demand therapy in delaying or preventing the development of hemophilic arthropathy [2]. There are different types of prophylaxis. Primary prophylaxis refers to therapy initiated in young patients who have hemophilia before joint damage (preventive therapy), whereas secondary prophylaxis refers to therapy initiated after joint abnormalities develop.

Since the 1990s, the standard of care for children who have severe hemophilia A or B in developed countries has been long-term prophylaxis, mainly primary, even though there is insufficient data to provide level A evidence of efficacy [3]. Although experience over the past years shows the benefits of such approach, the high cost associated with primary prophylaxis has prevented it from being adopted in developing countries.

Manco-Johnson and colleagues [4] recently published the results of the first prospective, randomized, controlled clinical trial in the United States evaluating the progression of arthropathy in children who have hemophilia treated with prophylaxis versus on-demand therapy. In this multicenter Joint Outcome Study, 65 children who had severe hemophilia (ages 30 months or less) were randomized to receive prophylaxis (25 IU/kg every other day) or an intense, episodic factor replacement (40 IU/kg initially, followed by 20 IU/kg at 24 and 72 hours after a joint bleed). Patients were followed until 6 years of age. Joint damage, the primary outcome of this study, was evaluated by MRI or plain radiographs. An 83% reduction in the risk for joint damage was shown by MRI in the prophylaxis group, supporting that such approach is effective in preventing joint damage. In 14% of cases of MRI changes, there was no evidence of any previous clinical hemarthrosis, suggesting that subclinical bleeding into the joints or the subchondral bone may cause joint damage. Further longitudinal imaging data likely are required to determine whether or not the use of continuous

Table 1
Clotting factor concentrates available in the United States in 2008

Product name (manufacturer)	Viral inactivation procedures	Purity/specific activity (IU factor VIII activity/mg total protein) before addition of stabilizer
Human plasma-derived factor VIII concentrates		
Humate-P (ZLB Behring, Inc.) (contains functional VWF protein)	Pasteurization (heating in solution, 60°C, 10 h)	Intermediate (1–10 IU/mg)
Alphanate SD (Grifols, Inc.) (contains some functional VWF protein)	Solvent detergent (TNBP/polysorbate 80) Affinity chromatography Dry heat (80°C, 72 h)	High (50–100 IU/mg) (>400 IU/mg after correcting for VWF content)
Koate-DVI (Bayer, Inc.) (contains VWF protein)	Solvent detergent (TNBP/polysorbate 80) Dry heat (80°C, 72 h)	High (50–100 IU/mg)
Monoclonal antibody-purified factor VIII concentrates (immunoaffinity purified from human plasma, no intact VWF protein)		
Monarc-M (Baxter/Immuno, Inc., using recovered plasma from the American Red Cross)	Solvent detergent (TNBP/octoxynol 9) Immunoaffinity chromatography	Ultra high (>3000 IU/mg)
Hemofil-M (Baxter/Immuno, Inc.)	Solvent detergent (TNBP/octoxynol 9) Immunoaffinity chromatography	Ultra high (>3000 IU/mg)
Monoclate-P (ZLB Behring, Inc.)	Pasteurization (heated in solution, 60°C, 10 h) Immunoaffinity chromatography	Ultra high (>3000 IU/mg)
Recombinant (genetic-engineered)/first-generation factor VIII concentrates		
Recombinate (Baxter/Immuno, Inc.) (human albumin as a stabilizer)	Immunoaffinity, ion exchange chromatography Bovine serum albumin used in culture medium for Chinese hamster ovary cells	Ultra high (>4000 IU/mg)
Recombinant/second-generation factor VIII concentrates (human albumin-free final formulations)		
Kogenate FS (Bayer, Inc.) Helixate FS (Bayer for ZLB Behring, Inc.) (sucrose as a stabilizer)	Immunoaffinity chromatography ion exchange Solvent detergent (TNBP/polysorbate 80) Ultrafiltration	Ultra high (>4000 IU/mg)

Refacto (Wyeth, Inc.) B-domain deleted (sucrose as a stabilizer)	Ion exchange Solvent detergent (TNBP/Triton X-100) Nanofiltration	Ultra high (>11,200–15,500 IU/mg), measured via chromogenic assay technique
Recombinant/third-generation factor VIII concentrates (no human or animal protein used in the culture medium or manufacturing process; does contain trace amounts of murine monoclonal antibody)		
Advate (Baxter/Immuno, Inc.) (trehalose as a stabilizer)	Immunoaffinity chromatography Ion exchange Solvent detergent (TNBP/polysorbate 80)	Ultra high (>4000–10,000 IU/mg)
Plasma-derived prothrombin complex concentrates/factor IX complex concentrates (nonactivated, also contain factor X and prothrombin but only traces of factor VII)		
Bebulin VH (Baxter/Immuno, Inc.)	Vapor heat (60°C, 10 h at 190 mbar pressure plus 1 h at 80°C, 375 mbar)	Intermediate (<50 IU/mg)
Profilnine SD (Grifols, Inc.)	Solvent detergent (TNBP/polysorbate 80)	Intermediate (<50 IU/mg)
Proplex-T (Baxter/Immuno, Inc.)	Dry heat (60°C, 144 h)	Intermediate (<50 IU/mg)
Plasma-derived prothrombin complex concentrates/factor IX complex concentrates (activated)		
FEIBA (Baxter/Immuno, Inc.)	Vapor heating (60°C, 10 h, 1160 mbar)	Intermediate (<50 U/mg)
Plasma-derived coagulation factor IX (human) concentrates		
AlphaNine SD (Grifols, Inc.)	Dual affinity chromatography Solvent detergent (TNBP/polysorbate 80) Nanofiltration (viral filter)	High (>200 IU/mg)
Mononine (ZLB Behring, Inc.)	Monoclonal antibody immunoaffinity chromatography Sodium thiocyanate Ultrafiltration	High (>160 IU/mg)
Recombinant factor IX concentrates		
BeneFIX (Wyeth, Inc.) (no animal or human-derived protein in cell line; no albumin added to final product)	Affinity chromatography Ultrafiltration	Ultra high (>200 IU/mg)

(continued on next page)

Table 1 (*continued*)

Factor VIII (or factor IX) concentrates useful in treatment of alloantibody and autoantibody inhibitor-related bleeding

Product name (manufacturer)	Viral inactivation method	Dosage
Recombinant factor VIIa (genetic engineered) NovoSeven (Novo Nordisk, Inc.) (stabilized in mannitol; bovine calf serum used in culture medium)	Affinity chromatography Solvent/detergent (TNPB/polysorbate 80)	90-μg/kg intravenous bolus every 2–3 h until bleeding ceases (larger dosing regimens are experimental but may be useful in refractory bleeding). This product is the treatment of choice for individuals who have allofactor IX antibody inhibitors and anaphylaxis or renal disease associated with the use of factor IX containing concentrates.
FEIBA-VH (Baxter Immuno, Inc.) (human plasma derived)	Vapor heated (10 h, 60°C, 190 mbar plus 1 h, 80°C, 375 mbar)	50–100 IU/kg not to exceed 200 IU/kg/24 h (for factor VIII and IX inhibitors)
Porcine plasma-derived factor VIII concentrate Hyate C (Ibsen Biomeasure, Inc.)	No longer available	> 50 IU/mg (for factor VIII inhibitors only)

Adapted from Kessler CM. New perspectives in hemophilia treatment. Hematology Am Soc Hematol Educ Program 2005;429–35; with permission.

prophylaxis can prevent this subclinical bleeding from producing even minimal arthropathy years later.

Timing of prophylaxis

The question of when to start primary prophylaxis has been a subject of controversy among hemophilia caregivers worldwide. To date, there is no consensus. Several studies show that children who have hemophilia and few or no joint bleeds [5–8] who are started on prophylaxis early (mean age of 3 years) exhibit a better musculoskeletal outcome. Progression of joint arthropathy, even after starting prophylaxis, is described in patients who have at least five joint bleeds occurring at the same or different joints [5–8].

In a study published by Astermark and colleagues [5], the only significant predictor for development of hemophilic arthropathy was the age of patients when prophylaxis was started. Using the Pettersson score, a scoring system that allows radiologic evaluation of the joints in patients who have hemophilia, Fischer and colleagues [9] described the Pettersson scores increasing by 8% each year that prophylaxis was postponed after the first occurrence of hemarthrosis. These studies show that irreversible joint damage may follow after a few joint bleeds and that even early prophylaxis may not abrogate that process completely. Therefore, worldwide recommendations to start prophylaxis before joint damage are favored to promote joint integrity, ideally before 3 years of age.

Secondary prophylaxis

Patients who have preexisting joint disease and who experience frequent acute hemarthroses may be treated with periodic use of factor concentrates for a short or long period of time to curtail bleeding recurrence. This approach is known as secondary prophylaxis and is used commonly to minimize bleeding frequency and lessen the progression of joint disease. Even though secondary prophylaxis cannot reverse the changes of chronic arthropathy, it may be beneficial by reducing frequency of bleeding, hospital admissions, and lost days from school or work and by decreasing damage progression.

The use of secondary prophylaxis versus on-demand therapy has been the subject of various studies done in children and adults who have severe hemophilia [10–12]. In summary, the results indicate that patients treated with secondary prophylaxis have decreased number of joint bleeds at the expense of higher clotting factor consumption. A recent study, however, does not confirm the higher cost of this approach.

A long-term outcome study (follow-up of 22 years) published by Fischer and colleagues [13] compared the costs of prophylaxis (primary and secondary) versus secondary prophylaxis alone versus on-demand therapy in patients who had severe hemophilia. In this study, short-term prophylaxis

was administered for 7.5 months (range 3 to 12 months) and long-term prophylaxis was administered over 12 months. Almost half of patients in the
on-demand group occasionally had received short-term prophylaxis for several months to a year. This study showed that clotting factor consumption
per year was similar for both treatment regimens (on-demand group:
median of 1260 IU/kg per /year; prophylaxis group: median 1550 IU/kg
per year). A significant difference, however, was that patients treated on
demand presented a 3.2-fold increase in the frequency of joint bleeds,
a 2.7-fold increase in clinical severity, and a 1.9-fold increase in Pettersson
scores. Not surprisingly, the quality of life for this group of patients was decreased. Hence, these data support that the concept that prophylaxis may
improve clinical outcomes without significantly increasing treatment costs.

Tailored prophylaxis: individualizing therapy to patients' needs

Because the natural history of arthropathy varies in patients who have
hemophilia, even considering those who are classified as having severe
hemophilia, tailoring prophylaxis to a patient's bleeding pattern, joint
involvement, and individual needs seems a reasonable approach.

As discussed previously, data support initiating prophylaxis at an early
age to prevent joint damage. Particularly in young children, however, establishing venous access commonly is a challenge and not surprisingly central
venous catheters (CVCs) often are required in this population for the administration of multiple dosages of factor. The benefit of easy access provided
by such catheters must be balanced by their risks, in particular catheter-
related infection.

Several studies have described different regimens to initiate prophylaxis
early on with a dual goal of preventing joint damage and minimizing the
need for CVC placement in young children. For example, Petrini [14] reported that primary prophylaxis can be started using a weekly infusion of
factor concentrate rather than the standard 3-times-per-week prophylactic
regimen as early as 1 or 2 years of age. This approach reduces the need
for CVC placement in young children without increasing the occurrence
of hemarthrosis. Astermark and colleagues [5] reported in a similar study
that there was no difference in the occurrence of hemarthrosis or arthropathy when comparing children who received factor VIII concentrate infusions
weekly during their first year of prophylaxis versus those who received prophylaxis 3 times a week.

In another study, published by van den Berg and colleagues [15], outcomes of tailored prophylaxis were described for three cohorts according
to the time at which prophylaxis was started in relationship to the number
of joint bleeds. Data from this study also support the use of tailored prophylaxis to prevent hemophilic arthropathy after a first joint bleed has occurred.

A prospective, multicenter Canadian study enrolling children who have
hemophilia is ongoing to evaluate frequency of infusions and dose

escalation [16]. In this study, 25 children who had severe hemophilia A (ages 1 to 2.5 years) and normal joints were enrolled on a dose-escalation protocol defined by breakthrough hemarthroses. With this regimen, the dose of factor VIII concentrate increased from a weekly dose of 50 IU/kg to a twice-a week-dose of 30 IU/kg to an every-other-day dose of 25 IU/kg determined by the frequency of breakthrough musculoskeletal bleeds. An interim report of this cohort has been described after a median follow-up of 4.1 years. Of the 25 patients enrolled, 13 (52%) required a dose escalation to twice-a-week prophylaxis secondary to frequent joint bleeds (median time to escalation 3.42 years). Alternatively, dose escalation had not been required in 12 (48%) of these patients. The occurrence of a target joint, however, one in which recurrent bleeding has occurred on at least four occasions during the previous 6 months or where 20 lifetime bleeding episodes have occurred, was evident in 40% of the patients. This indicates that the long-term effect on joint outcome using this approach warrants further scrutiny.

Adjuvant treatment options for patients who have hemophilia

Desmopressin (DDAVP) has been used to control or prevent bleeding in mild hemophilia A, some cases of moderate hemophilia A, and some types of von Willebrand disease since 1977. Its mechanism of action seems multifactorial, including an increase in plasma levels of factor VIII and von Willebrand factor (VWF), stimulation of platelet adhesion, and increased expression of tissue factor [17,18]. DDAVP is not effective for the treatment of patients who have hemophilia B, as factor IX levels are not influenced by DDAVP.

For mild to moderate hemophilia and von Willebrand disease, the indications for DDAVP use are determined by the type of bleeding episode, baseline, and desired level of factor VIII and VWF. A test dose, also known as DDAVP challenge, should be performed under controlled conditions, such as in a doctor's office, where blood pressure and heart rate can be monitored. A blood sample is obtained before the test dose and approximately 2 hours after administration of the test dose. A twofold to fourfold rise in the levels of factor VIII, von Willebrand antigen, and ristocetin cofactor activity is expected. This expected rise in factor VIII levels explains why patients who have severe hemophilia A are not candidates for this type of therapy to control bleeding. The intranasal route is the administration route of choice for outpatient treatment and commonly is used before dental procedures and oral/nasal mucosal bleeding. The intravenous route also is available and typically used in the inpatient setting. One advantage of intravenous administration is that peak levels tend to be higher and achieved faster. Patients should be advised to limit water intake during DDAVP treatment and to avoid using more than three consecutive daily doses to reduce the risk for developing hyponatremia.

Antifibrinolytic agents, epsilon-aminocaproic acid and tranexamic acid, both lysine derivatives, also are useful adjuvant therapy for patients who have mild to severe hemophilia. They exert their effect by inhibiting the proteolytic activity of plasmin and, therefore, inhibiting fibrinolysis. The use of antifibrinolytic agents is indicated in the presence of mucosal bleeding, primarily oral, nasal, and menstrual blood loss. Its use is contraindicated in presence of hematuria because of increased risk for intrarenal or ureteral thrombosis, in the presence of disseminated intravascular coagulation, or thromboembolic disease. Both drugs are available for use in the United States in an intravenous form (epsilon-aminocaproic acid at 100 mg/kg/dose every 6 hours; tranexamic acid at 10 mg/kg/dose every 6–8 hours). Currently, only epsilon-aminocaproic acid is available for use in the United States in an oral form.

Topical agents, such as fibrin sealant, which is prepared by mixing two plasma-derived protein fractions (fibrinogen-rich concentrate and thrombin concentrate), are used for local bleeding control in hemophilia. There are concerns, however, regarding the use of bovine thrombin in this setting. First, there seems to be a high rate (approximately 20% or higher) of antibody formation [19] against thrombin and factor V, which may inactivate an individual's own endogenous factor V or thrombin production, thereby creating a new bleeding diathesis. Another legitimate concern is the potential risk for transmitting blood-borne pathogens, such as variant Creutzfeldt-Jakob virus [20]. When available commercially, the use of recombinant human thrombin will likely minimize these risks.

A phase 3, prospective, randomized, double-blind, comparative study evaluating the safety and efficacy of topical recombinant human thrombin and bovine thrombin in surgical hemostasis has been published [21]. The primary objective of this study was to evaluate the efficacy of both products whereas the secondary objective was to evaluate safety and antigenicity. This multicenter study enrolled more than 400 patients, who were randomized in a 1:1 ratio. The study showed that both topical agents had a comparable efficacy of 95% with similar adverse events rates. A statistically significant lower incidence of antibodies, however, was identified against recombinant human thrombin (1.5%) compared with antibovine thrombin (21.5%). Based on the results of this study, recombinant human thrombin seems the preferred option to achieve topical hemostasis.

Recombinant factor VIIa is a Food and Drug Administration–approved product used to promote hemostasis in patients who have hemophilia A or B with inhibitors. Its mechanism of action includes binding of activated factor VII to tissue factor, which activates factor X and leads to thrombin generation. Recombinant factor VIIa also binds the surface of activated platelets independent of tissue factor, activating factor X and leading to thrombin generation. The standard dose in hemophilia with inhibitors is 90 to 120 µg/kg every 2 to 3 hours until hemostasis is achieved. Subsequent dosing and interval is based on clinical judgment. At the present time, there is no validated laboratory test to monitor recombinant factor VIIa therapy. Clinical experience shows an excellent or effective response in more than 90% of patients who have hemophilia and low risk for thrombosis [22,23].

Experimental aspects of synovitis and alternative methods for intervention

In hemophilia, the joints are the most common site of serious bleeding [10]. Synovitis occurs after repeated episodes of bleeding into the joints and is characterized by a highly vascular synovial membrane with prominent proliferation of synovial fibroblasts and infiltration by inflammatory cells [24]. Ultimately, destruction of the cartilage and bone leads to crippling arthritis if adequate treatment is not administered in a timely manner. The exact mechanisms leading to the characteristic changes seen in synovitis are not understood fully. It is hypothesized, however, that synovial cell proliferation, immune system activation, and angiogenesis (the formation of new blood vessels from preexisting ones) occur secondary to the presence of blood components, especially iron, in the joint space. These events self-amplify each other, ultimately leading to cartilage and bone destruction (Fig. 2). Different therapeutic options for synovial control in hemophilia are available. For example, the synovium can be removed surgically by means of an open or arthroscopic synovectomy. Another alternative, synoviorthesis, allows for the destruction of the synovial tissue by intra-articular injection of a chemical or radioactive agent. The main indications for synoviorthesis are chronic synovitis and recurrent hemarthroses. The procedure is performed by an orthopedic surgeon or invasive radiologist/nuclear medicine specialist who has expertise in hemophilia. The majority of patients require a single injection, although a few patients may require more than one injection to the same joint at different time periods. Synoviorthesis offers several advantages over surgical synovectomy. It is less invasive and costly, requires minimal factor coverage, is associated with fewer

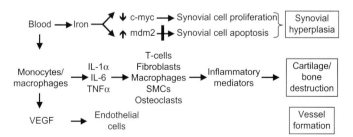

Fig. 2. Proposed mechanism in the pathogenesis of hemophilic synovitis. IL-6, interleukin 6; IL-1α, interleukin 1α; SMC, synovial mesenchymal cell; TNFα, tumor necrosis factor alpha; VEGF, vascular endothelial growth factor. (*Adapted from* Valentino LA, Hakobyan N, Rodriguez N, et al. Pathogenesis of haemophilic synovitis: experimental studies on blood-induced joint damage. Haemophilia 2007;13(3):10–3; with permission.)

infections and minimal pain, and does not require extensive rehabilitation. Even though this procedure may not halt joint degeneration, it may effectively reduce the frequency of joint bleeding along with a reduction in arthropathic pain.

Radioactive synovectomy (RS) using P^{32} has been used for chronic synovitis in the United States since 1988. Initial comprehensive review of its use suggested that this technique was efficient, safe, and not associated with malignancies [25]. Subsequently, however, two cases of acute lymphoblastic leukemia (ALL) after RS were reported in children who had hemophilia. The first patient was a 9-year-old boy who had severe hemophilia A who developed pre–B-cell ALL. The second was a 14-year-old boy who had severe hemophilia A who developed T-cell ALL. Both patients developed their ALL less than 1 year after treatment with RS [26], which raises the question as to whether or not this may be too early for radiation-induced malignancy. Both patients had a history of exaggerated immunologic response or autoimmune disease.

There have been no further reports of cancer after RS in hemophilia or rheumatoid arthritis in the United States. Data from a retrospective, long-term, Canadian study evaluating the incidence of cancer in more than 2400 patients who had chronic synovitis from multiple diseases, including rheumatoid arthritis and hemophilia, and who underwent RS were presented at World Federation of Hemophilia (Georges Rivard, MD, Montreal, Canada, unpublished data, 2007). In this study, Infante-Rivard and colleagues [27] compared the incidence rates of cancer in a cohort of patients treated with RS to the incidence rates of cancer in the general Quebec population, as documented in the Quebec Province Cancer Registry. The majority of the patients (80%) received one or two treatments using radioactive isotopes, whereas the remaining underwent three or more procedures. Most patients received yttrium^{90} (70%) whereas close to 30% of the patients received P^{32}. Data analysis using a Cox regression model showed no evidence of increased risk for cancer with the use of RS [27].

Currently, the use of RS is based on defined risks versus benefits. Therefore, this approach may be recommended for patients who have no known risk factors for malignancy who have developed a target joint and continue to present recurrent hemarthrosis despite prophylactic therapy or in whom prophylaxis is not an option. Nevertheless, informed consent should describe the risks (discussed previously) clearly to parents and, when applicable, to patients.

Current challenges in hemophilia management

Inhibitor development

There is no question that the development of inhibitory antibodies in hemophilia is one of the most challenging aspects of current management. The incidence of inhibitors in patients who have hemophilia A is estimated at 30%, whereas the incidence in hemophilia B is much lower, at approximately 3%. Genetic and environmental risk factors for inhibitor development are described [28,29]. These antibodies, usually of the IgG4 subtype, occur early within the first 50 exposure days and are classified as low- or high-titer inhibitor according to measurement by the Bethesda unit (BU) laboratory assay (<5 BU is referred to as low titer, >5 BU as high titer) and the propensity of the antibody to anamnese after re-exposure to the antigen (factor VIII or IX). Patients who have low-titer inhibitors may be treated successfully with high doses of factor VIII or IX. Alternatively, patients who have high-titer inhibitors require bypassing agents, such as recombinant factor VIIa or activated prothrombin complex concentrates, for bleeding control. Ultimately, ITI to eradicate the inhibitor is desired. This intervention is effective at eradicating all inhibitors in approximately 70% of patients.

An ongoing international multicenter trial, International Immune Tolerance Study , investigates the impact of factor VIII dose on the rate of ITI success along with the time to ITI success. Patients who have severe hemophilia are randomized to receive either a high-dose factor VIII (200 U/kg daily) or a low-dose factor VIII (50 U/kg 3 times per week for 33 months). The primary endpoints of this study are to compare the success rate, time to achieve tolerance, complications, and cost of both regimens.

Whether or not the type of factor VIII concentrate to treat hemophilia A influences inhibitor development has been a subject of debate since the introduction of recombinant products in the 1990s. Although some studies suggest an increased risk for inhibitor development with the use of recombinant products compared with the experience with plasma-derived products, other studies have not confirmed such findings [29–31]. Now, with almost 2 decades of experience with the use of recombinant products, it is clear that the incidence of inhibitor development has remained stable when compared with historical data.

More recently, a possible therapeutic advantage of using VWF-containing products to achieve ITI has been proposed. Inhibitory antibodies against the factor VIII molecule are directed primarily against epitopes located at the A2, A3, and C2 domains [28]. VWF is known to bind the A3 and C2 domains of factor VIII [32], which may result in a blockade to inhibitor binding (Fig. 3). Another proposed mechanism is that VWF may protect the infused factor VIII from rapid degradation by plasma proteases [33]. In vitro studies show that VWF protects factor VIII from neutralizing antibodies [34,35]. In vivo confirmation of these findings in an animal model showed that VWF-C2 binding confers protection against inhibitor development [36].

In 2006, Gringeri and colleagues [37] reported a low incidence of inhibitors (9.8%) in patients who had severe hemophilia A who previously were untreated and received a VWF-containing factor VIII concentrate. More

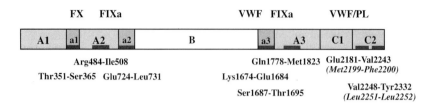

Fig. 3. Schematic model showing the domain structure of factor VIII (FVIII) and the localization of the main binding epitopes of FVIII antibodies. (*From* Astermark J. Basic aspects of inhibitors to factors VIII and IX and the influence of non-genetic risk factors. Haemophilia 2006;12(Suppl 6):8–13; with permission.)

recently, Gringeri and colleagues [38] reported the results of the first prospective ITI study using a VWF-containing factor VIII concentrate in patients who had hemophilia A considered at high risk for a poor response to ITI. This study showed successful inhibitor eradication in 9 of the 16 (53%) patients who completed this study. The median time to inhibitor eradication was 24 months (range 4–30 months). The remaining seven patients showed partial success documented by a decreased inhibitor titer (median of 1.5 BU, range 1.1–2.8 BU), without complete disappearance. One patient was withdrawn 12 months after enrollment as a result of persistent high-titer inhibitor (70 BU). Overall, this study demonstrated a relatively high success rate of inhibitor eradication, taking into consideration that this group of patients was at high risk for a poor response and two of them previously had failed ITI.

Rituximab experience in hemophilia with inhibitors

Rituximab, a human-mouse chimeric monoclonal antibody directed against the CD20 antigen, has demonstrated a therapeutic benefit in the treatment of B-cell–mediated malignancies and immune-mediated disorders, such as immune thrombocytopenic purpura and autoimmune hemolytic anemia [39–41]. The use of rituximab in acquired hemophilia versus congenital hemophilia is reported more extensively [42,43]. The standard dose for rituximab use in hemophilia has been 375 mg/m^2/dose, administered weekly for 4 weeks and then monthly (up to 5 months) until the inhibitor disappears.

Rituximab has been used in congenital hemophilia with inhibitors in only 18 documented patients (12 who had severe hemophilia A, four who had mild or moderate hemophilia A, and two who had severe hemophilia B). Thirteen of them responded favorably to rituximab, three with a complete response and 10 with a partial response, whereas the remaining five patients had no response [42,43]. The data suggest that the efficacy of rituximab may be enhanced by concomitant administration of factor VIII. The long-term success of such an approach is not clear, however, as further follow-up is needed.

Carrier state and genetic testing in hemophilia

Carrier status in women cannot be established based solely on factor VIII or IX levels because there is a significant overlap between factor levels in carrier and noncarrier women. For this reason, genetic testing is recommended. Women who are obligate carriers (daughter of a man who has hemophilia or the mother of more than one son who has hemophilia) do not need carrier testing as it is evident that they have inherited an affected X chromosome from a father who has hemophilia (see Fig. 1).

In approximately 30% of patients who have hemophilia, there is no family history of the disease and it seems to occur as a result of spontaneous novel mutations [44]. In such cases, molecular testing can identify mutations in 95% to 98% of patients who have hemophilia A or B [45].

Candidates for genetic testing include patients who have a diagnosis of hemophilia A or B, at-risk women who are related to an affected man (proband) who has a known mutation, and female carriers of hemophilia A or B seeking prenatal diagnosis.

Although in many cases the whole gene needs to be sequenced, this is not necessarily the case for patients who have severe hemophilia A, in whom intron 22 inversion is found in approximately 45%. In hemophilia A, therefore, it is recommended initially to perform intron 22 gene inversion analysis and, if not present, to proceed with full sequencing of the factor VIII gene. For patients who have mild or moderate hemophilia A, full sequencing of the factor VIII gene is recommended unless a mutation already is identified in another family member. To identify a mutation in patients who have hemophilia B, full sequencing of the factor IX gene is performed. After a mutation is identified in a proband with hemophilia A or B, carrier testing and prenatal diagnosis can be offered to at-risk family members. If a proband is not available for testing, genetic analysis can be performed on a blood sample from an obligate carrier.

Potential new therapies in the horizon

Gene therapy

Gene therapy involves the transfer of genes that express a particular gene product into human cells resulting in a therapeutic advantage. Particularly for hemophilia, the goal of gene transfer is aimed at the secretion of a functional factor VIII or IX protein. Different strategies for hemophilia using animal models or humans include retroviral, lentiviral, adenoviral, and adeno-associated viral vectors.

There have been several gene therapy phase I clinical trials using direct in vivo gene delivery or ex vivo plasmid transfections with hepatic reimplantation of gene-engineered cells [46,47]. Even though a therapeutic effect has been seen in some of these studies, stable production of the coagulation protein is not yet demonstrated in human subjects. These trials have failed to show long-term gene expression observed in preclinical animal models [1].

The only active human clinical trial is in patients who have severe hemophilia B, evaluating the safety of adeno-associated viral vector in delivering human factor IX gene into the liver using immunomodulation at the time of gene transfer. Hence, gene therapy in hemophilia continues to be a topic of intense investigation and holds promise as an enduring therapy for hemophilia A and B.

Novel bioengineering technologies

Another novel approach aims to improve recombinant factor VIII synthesis and secretion by targeting modifications, such as increased mRNA expression, reduced interaction with endoplasmic reticulum chaperones, or increased endoplasmic reticulum–Golgi transport [48]. Strategies to improve factor VIII functional activity may be achieved by increasing molecular activation or by inducing resistance to inactivation. Targets to reduce factor VIII immunogenicity also are foci of current research. Similar strategies are being evaluated in hemophilia B, in particular modifications to increase factor IX synthesis, secretion, and activity [49].

Another promising approach is the development of strategies that result in a longer plasma half-life for factor VIII, thereby reducing the frequency of factor infusions. Three of these strategies are described.

Polyethylene glycol conjugation

Pegylation, the modification of proteins by conjugation with polyethylene glycol (PEG) polymers, initially was described in the 1970s [50]. These polymers incorporate water molecules within their hydrophilic structure. As a result, pegylation increases the size of the conjugated protein above the renal threshold for filtration, resulting in an extended half-life. Pegylation also may result in antigenic shielding for the factor VIII molecule [51]. Animal studies show an increased half-life of pegylated factor VIII, resulting in improved hemostasis [52].

Pegylated liposomes

Liposomes are able to encapsulate drugs within their lipid bilayer or within their aqueous phase [53]. As they may be cleared rapidly, however, structural modifications are incorporated to reduce clearance and extend half-life. Animal studies using pegylated liposomal factor VIII (PEGLip-FVIII) have shown an increased half-life and hemostatic efficacy for PEGLip-FVIII compared with standard factor VIII. Spira and colleagues [54] recently published the results of a clinical pilot study showing prolongation in the mean number of days without bleeding episodes in patients receiving PEGLip-FVIII compared with nonpegylated factor VIII. Although these early results are encouraging, concerns regarding its clearance mechanism have been raised. A phase I clinical trial using this PEGLip formulation of Kogenate has demonstrated similar pharmacokinetics as native Kogenate. Further studies are required to ascertain whether or not this is the case.

Polysialic acid polymers

Polysialic acids are polymers of N-acetylneuraminic acid. Similarly to pegylation, the hydrophilic properties of polysialic acids allow the formation of a "watery cloud" that protects the target molecule from degradation and rapid clearance. In contrast to pegylation, however, these polymers are biodegradable. Hence, concerns regarding long-term product accumulation in the body should not apply to this strategy.

Summary

From a clinical perspective, the use of prophylaxis in patients who have hemophilia is strongly recommended to prevent arthropathy. Different prophylactic regimens are used to achieve this goal. The use of radionuclide synovectomy with radioisotopes, such as P^{32}, seems a safe and efficacious approach to treat arthropathy, a major complication of chronic joint bleedings. The management of patients who have inhibitory antibodies against factor VIII or IX remains challenging. Further clinical studies are necessary in this field.

Understanding the pathogenesis of hemophilic arthropathy likely begins with deciphering the biochemical and cellular response after blood-induced joint damage. Information gleaned from early in vitro models indicates a role for oxidative iron in inducing genetic alteration in proximal synovial cells of the joint that lead to their enhanced proliferation. In addition, the cytokine response to the initial iron injury creates an inflammatory milieu that incites chondrocyte dysfunction, resulting in dysfunctional cartilage matrix, and the initiation of osteoclastogenesis. When this process is repetitive, as seen in hemophilic arthropathy, accentuation of these destructive and inflammatory processes is accompanied by significant angiogenesis. In addition, the fragility of the blood vessels in these neovascularized tissues may predispose to renewed hemorrhage, a process that spirals out of control gradually until end-stage hemarthropathy is the outcome.

Much experimental work is yet to be done to demonstrate definitively each step along this evolutionary process. Some may mimic other joint disease states, such as rheumatoid arthritis. Others may be unique to hemophilic arthropathy. New investigative capacities in genomics and proteomics may provide the tools to elucidate the pathogenesis and to point to new avenues of prevention and therapy.

References

[1] Kessler CM. New perspectives in hemophilia treatment. Hematology Am Soc Hematol Educ Program 2005;429–35.

 [2] Berntorp E, Astermark J, Bjorkman S, et al. Consensus perspectives on prophylactic therapy
     for haemophilia: summary statement. Haemophilia 2003;9(Suppl 1):1–4.
 [3] Galiè N, Seeger W, Naeije R, et al. Comparative analysis of clinical trials and evidence-based
     treatment algorithm in pulmonary arterial hypertension. J Am Coll Cardiol 2004;43:81–8.
 [4] Manco-Johnson MJ, Abshire TC, Shapiro AD, et al. Prophylaxis versus episodic treat-
     ment to prevent joint disease in boys with severe hemophilia. N Engl J Med 2007;
     357(6):535–44.
 [5] Astermark J, Petrini P, Tengborn L, et al. Primary prophylaxis in severe haemophilia should
     be started at an early age but can be individualized. Br J Haematol 1999;105(4):1109–13.
 [6] Funk M, Schmidt H, Escuriola-Ettingshausen C, et al. Radiological and orthopedic score in
     pediatric hemophilic patients with early and late prophylaxis. Ann Hematol 1998;77(4):
     171–4.
 [7] Kreuz W, Escuriola-Ettingshausen C, Funk M, et al. When should prophylactic treatment in
     patients with haemophilia A and B start?–The German experience. Haemophilia 1998;4(4):
     413–7.
 [8] Petrini P, Lindvall N, Egberg N, et al. Prophylaxis with factor concentrates in preventing
     hemophilic arthropathy. Am J Pediatr Hematol Oncol 1991;13(3):280–7.
 [9] Fischer K, van der Bom JG, Mauser-Bunschoten EP, et al. The effects of postponing prophy-
     lactic treatment on long-term outcome in patients with severe hemophilia. Blood 2002;99(7):
     2337–41.
[10] Aledort LM, Haschmeyer RH, Pettersson H. A longitudinal study of orthopaedic outcomes
     for severe factor-VIII-deficient haemophiliacs. The Orthopaedic Outcome Study Group.
     J Intern Med 1994;236(4):391–9.
[11] Smith PS, Teutsch SM, Shaffer PA, et al. Episodic versus prophylactic infusions for hemo-
     philia A: a cost-effectiveness analysis. J Pediatr 1996;129(3):424–31.
[12] Szucs TD, Offner A, Kroner B, et al. Resource utilisation in haemophiliacs treated in
     Europe: results from the European Study on Socioeconomic Aspects of Haemophilia
     Care. The European Socioeconomic Study Group. Haemophilia 1998;4(4):498–501.
[13] Fischer K, van der Bom JG, Molho P, et al. Prophylactic versus on-demand treatment strat-
     egies for severe haemophilia: a comparison of costs and long-term outcome. Haemophilia
     2002;8(6):745–52.
[14] Petrini P. What factors should influence the dosage and interval of prophylactic treatment in
     patients with severe haemophilia A and B? Haemophilia 2001;7(1):99–102.
[15] van den Berg HM, Fischer K, Mauser-Bunschoten EP, et al. Long-term outcome of individ-
     ualized prophylactic treatment of children with severe haemophilia. Br J Haematol 2001;
     112(3):561–5.
[16] Feldman BM, Pai M, Rivard GE, et al. Tailored prophylaxis in severe hemophilia A: interim
     results from the first 5 years of the Canadian Hemophilia Primary Prophylaxis Study.
     J Thromb Haemost 2006;4(6):1228–36.
[17] Villar A, Jimenez-Yuste V, Quintana M, et al. The use of haemostatic drugs in haemophilia:
     desmopressin and antifibrinolytic agents. Haemophilia 2002;8:189–93.
[18] Galves A, Gomez-Ortiz G, Diaz-Ricart M, et al. Desmopressin (DDAVP) enhances platelet
     adhesion to the extracellular matrix of cultured human endothelial cells through increased
     expression of tissue factor. Thromb Haemost 1997;77:975–80.
[19] Winterbottom N, Kuo JM, Nguyen K, et al. Antigenic responses to bovine thrombin expo-
     sure during surgery: a prospective study of 309 patients. Journal of Applied Research 2002;2:
     1–11.
[20] Bruce ME, Will RG, Ironside JW, et al. Transmissions to mice indicate that 'new variant'
     CJD is caused by the BSE agent. Nature 1997;389(6650):498–501.
[21] Chapman WC, Singla N, Genyk Y, et al. A phase 3, randomized, double-blind comparative
     study of the efficacy and safety of topical recombinant human thrombin and bovine throm-
     bin in surgical hemostasis. J Am Coll Surg 2007 Aug;205(2):256–65.

[22] O'Connell N, Mc Mahon C, Smith J, et al. Recombinant factor VIIa in the management of surgery and acute bleeding episodes in children with haemophilia and high responding inhibitors. Br J Haematol 2002;116(3):632–5.

[23] Hedner U. Treatment of patients with factor VIII and IX inhibitors with special focus on the use of recombinant factor VIIa. Thromb Haemost 1999;82(2):531–9.

[24] Rodriguez-Merchan EC. Effects of hemophilia on articulations of children and adults. Clin Orthop Relat Res 1996;(328):7–13.

[25] Dunn AL, Busch MT, Wyly JB, et al. Radionuclide synovectomy for hemophilic arthropathy: a comprehensive review of safety and efficacy and recommendation for a standarized treatment protocol. Thromb Haemost 2002;87:383–93.

[26] Manco-Johnson MJ, Nuss R, Lear J, et al. 32P radiosynoviorthesis in children with hemophilia. J Pediatr Hematol Oncol 2002;24:534–9.

[27] Infante-Rivard C, Rivard G, Winikoff R, et al. Is there an increased risk of cancer associated with radiosynoviorthesis? Haemophilia 2006;12(2):[abstract 18FP539].

[28] Astermark J. Basic aspects of inhibitors to factors VIII and IX and the influence of non-genetic risk factors. Haemophilia 2006;12(6):8–14.

[29] Scharrer I, Bray GL, Neutzling O. Incidence of inhibitors in haemophilia A patients—a review of recent studies of recombinant and plasma-derived factor VIII concentrates. Haemophilia 1999;5:145–54.

[30] Goudemand J, Rothschild C, Demiguel V, et al. Influence of the type of factor VIII concentrate on the incidence of factor VIII inhibitors in previously untreated patients with severe hemophilia A. Blood 2006;107(1):46–51.

[31] Gouw SC, van der Bom JG, Auerswald G, et al. Recombinant versus plasma-derived factor VIII products and the development of inhibitors in previously untreated patients with severe hemophilia A: the CANAL cohort study. Blood 2007;109(11):4693–7.

[32] Scandella D, de Graaf Mahoney S, Mattingly M, et al. Epitope mapping of human FVIII inhibitor antibodies by deletion analysis of FVIII fragments expressed in Escherichia coli. Proc Natl Acad Sci U S A 1988;85:6152–6.

[33] Auerswald G, Spranger T, Brackmann HH. The role of plasma-derived factor VIII/von Willebrand factor concentrates in the treatment of hemophilia A patients. Haematologica 2003;88(9):16–20.

[34] Suzuki T, Arai M, Amano K, et al. Factor VIII inhibitor antibodies with C2 domain specificity are less inhibitory to factor VIII complexed with von Willebrand factor. Thromb Haemost 1996;76:749–54.

[35] Gensana M, Altisent C, Aznar JA, et al. Influence of von Willebrand factor on the reactivity of human factor VIII inhibitors with factor VIII. Haemophilia 2001;7:369–74.

[36] Behrmann M, Pasi J, Saint-Remy JM, et al. von Willebrand factor modulates factor VIII immunogenicity: comparative study of different factor VIII concentrates in a haemophilia A mouse model. Thromb Haemost 2002;88:221–9.

[37] Gringeri A, Monzini M, Tagariello G, et al. Occurrence of inhibitors in previously untreated or minimally treated patients with haemophilia A after exposure to a plasma-derived solvent-detergent factor VIII concentrate. Haemophilia 2006;12:128–32.

[38] Gringeri A, Musso R, Mazzucconi G, et al. Immune tolerance induction with a high purity von Willebrand factor/VIII complex concentrate in haemophilia A patients with inhibitors at high risk of a poor response. Haemophilia 2007;13:373–9.

[39] Gopal AK, Press OW. Clinical applications of anti CD 20 antibodies. J Lab Clin Med 1999; 134:445–50.

[40] Stasi R, Pagano A, Stipa E, et al. Rituximab chimeric anti-CD 20 monoclonal antibody treatment for adults with chronic idiopathic thrombocytopenic purpura. Blood 2001;98: 952–7.

[41] Zecca M, Nobili B, Ramenghi U, et al. Rituximab for the treatment of refractory autoimmune hemolytic anemia in children. Blood 2003;101:3857–61.

[42] Carcao M, St. Louis J, Poon MC, et al. Rituximab for congenital haemophiliacs with inhibitors: a Canadian experience. Haemophilia 2006;12:7–18.

[43] Fox RA, Neufeld EJ, Bennett CM. Rituximab for adolescents with haemophilia and high titre inhibitors. Haemophilia 2006;12:218–22.

[44] Lawn RM. The molecular genetics of hemophilia: blood clotting factors VIII and IX. Cell 1985;42:405–6.

[45] Goodeve AC, Peake IR. The molecular basis of hemophilia A: genotype-phenotype relationships and inhibitor development. Semin Thromb Hemost 2003;29(1):23–30.

[46] Pierce GF, Lillicrap D, Pipe SW, et al. Gene therapy, bioengineered clotting factors and novel technologies for hemophilia treatment. J Thromb Haemost 2007;5:901–6.

[47] Ponder KP. Gene therapy for hemophilia. Curr Opin Hematol 2006;13(5):301–7.

[48] Miao HZ, Sirachainan N, Palmer L, et al. Bioengineering of coagulation factor VIII for improved secretion. Blood 2004;103:3412–9.

[49] Pipe SW. The promise and challenges of bioengineered recombinant clotting factors. J Thromb Haemost 2005;3:1692–701.

[50] Abuchowski A, van Es T, Palczuk NC, et al. Alteration of immunological properties of bovine serum albumin by covalent attachment of polyethylene glycol. J Biol Chem 1977; 252:3578–81.

[51] Molineaux G. Pegylation: engineering improved biopharmaceuticals for oncology. Pharmacotherapy 2003;23:3S–8S.

[52] Baru M, Carmel-Goren L, Barenholz Y, et al. Factor VIII efficient and specific non-covalent binding to PEGylated liposomes enables prolongation of its circulation time and haemostatic efficacy. Thromb Haemost 2005;93:1061–8.

[53] Goyal P, Goyal K, Vijaya Kumar SG, et al. Liposomal drug delivery systems—clinical applications. Acta Pharm 2005;55:1–25.

[54] Spira J, Ply Ushch OP, Andreeva TA, et al. Prolonged bleeding-free period following prophylactic infusion of recombinant factor VIII (Kogenate (R) FS) reconstituted with pegylated liposomes. Blood 2006;108:3668–73.

ELSEVIER
SAUNDERS

PEDIATRIC CLINICS
OF NORTH AMERICA

Pediatr Clin N Am 55 (2008) 377–392

von Willebrand Disease

Jeremy Robertson, MD[a], David Lillicrap, MD[b],
Paula D. James, MD[c],*

[a]Division of Hematology/Oncology, Hospital for Sick Children, 555 University Avenue,
Toronto, ON M5G 1X8, Canada
[b]Department of Pathology and Molecular Medicine, Richardson Labs, Queen's University,
108 Stuart Street, Kingston, ON K7L 3N6, Canada
[c]Department of Medicine, Queen's University, Room 2025, Etherington Hall,
94 Stuart Street, Kingston, ON K7l 2V6, Canada

History

von Willebrand disease (VWD) first was described in 1926 by a Finnish physician named Dr. Erik von Willebrand. In the original publication [1] he described a severe mucocutaneous bleeding problem in a family living on the Åland archipelago in the Baltic Sea. The index case in this family, a young woman named Hjördis, bled to death during her fourth menstrual period. At least four other family members died from severe bleeding and, although the condition originally was referred to as "pseudohemophilia," Dr. von Willebrand noted that in contrast to hemophilia, both genders were affected. He also noted that affected individuals exhibited prolonged bleeding times despite normal platelet counts.

In the mid-1950s, it was recognized that the condition usually was accompanied by a reduced level of factor VIII (FVIII) activity and that the bleeding phenotype could be corrected by the infusion of normal plasma. In the early 1970s, the critical immunologic distinction between FVIII and von Willebrand factor (VWF) was made and since that time significant progress has been made in understanding the molecular pathophysiology of this condition.

JR is the 2007/2008 recipient of the Baxter BioScience Pediatric Thrombosis and Hemostasis Fellowship in the Division of Hematology/Oncology at the Hospital for Sick Children. DL holds a Canada Research Chair in Molecular Hemostasis and is a Career Investigator of the Heart and Stroke Foundation of Ontario.

* Corresponding author.

E-mail address: jamesp@queensu.ca (P.D. James).

doi:10.1016/j.pcl.2008.01.008
pediatric.theclinics.com

von Willebrand factor

Cloning and characterization of the *VWF* gene, by four groups simultaneously in 1985 [2–5], has facilitated understanding of the molecular biology of VWD. Located on the short arm of chromosome 12 at p13.3, the *VWF* gene spans 178 kilobases (kb) and comprises 52 exons that range in size from 1.3 kb (exon 28) to 40 base pairs (bp) (exon 50) [6]. The encoded VWF mRNA is 9 kb in length and the translated pre-pro-VWF molecule contains 2813 amino acids (AA), comprising a 22 AA signal peptide, a 741 AA propolypeptide, and a 2050 AA-secreted mature subunit that possesses all the adhesive sites required for VWF's hemostatic function [7]. There is a partial, unprocessed pseudogene located on chromosome 22, which duplicates the *VWF* gene sequence for exons 23–34 with 97% sequence homology [8]. Also, the *VWF* gene is highly polymorphic, and to date, 140 polymorphisms are reported, including promoter polymorphisms, a highly variable tetranucleotide repeat in intron 40, two insertion/deletion polymorphisms, and 132 distinct single nucleotide polymorphisms involving exon and intron sequences [9].

VWF is synthesized in endothelial cells [10] and megakaryocytes [11] as a protein subunit that undergoes a complex series of post-translational modifications, including dimerization, glycosylation, sulfation, and ultimately multimerization. The fully processed protein then is released into the circulation or stored in specialized organelles: the Weibel-Palade bodies of endothelial cells or the α-granules of platelets. VWF is secreted into the plasma, where it circulates as a very large protein that has a molecular weight ranging from 500 to 20,000 kd depending on the extent of subunit multimerization [12]. After secretion, under the influence of shear flow, high-molecular-weight (HMW) VWF, multimers undergo partial proteolysis mediated by the ADAMTS-13 plasma protease (*A D*isintegrin *A*nd *M*etalloprotease with *Thromb S*opondin type 1 motif, member 13), with cleavage occurring between AA residues tyrosine 1605 and methionine 1606 in the A2 domain of the VWF protein [13].

VWF is a multifunctional adhesive protein that plays major hemostatic roles, including:

     A critical role in the initial cellular stages of the hemostatic process. VWF binds to the platelet glycoprotein (GP)Ib/IX receptor complex to initiate platelet adhesion to the subendothelium [14]. After adhesion, platelet activation results in the exposure of the GPIIb/IIIa integrin receptor through which VWF and fibrinogen mediate platelet aggregation (Fig. 1) [15].

     As a carrier protein for the procoagulant cofactor FVIII. VWF binds to and stabilizes FVIII; therefore, low levels of VWF or defective binding of VWF to FVIII results in correspondingly low levels of FVIII because of its accelerated proteolytic degradation by activated protein C [16].

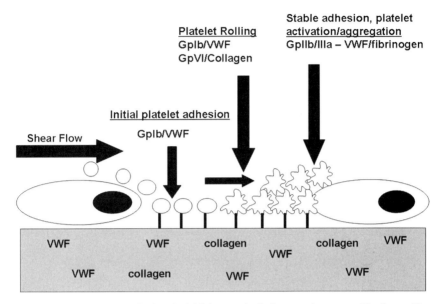

Fig. 1. Role of VWF in mediating the initial events in the hemostatic process. Platelets, rolling along the endothelial cell surface, are tethered to the site of endothelial cell injury through the binding of subendothelial VWF to the GpIb protein of the Ib/IX receptor. The platelets subsequently are activated and the GpIIb/IIIa complex is exposed on the platelet surface. Interaction of fibrinogen and VWF with GpIIb/IIIa then consolidates the platelet adhesive event and initiates platelet aggregation.

Clinical features of von Willebrand disease

VWD is stated as the most common inherited bleeding disorder known in humans. This is based on two large epidemiologic studies that reported the prevalence of VWD in healthy school-aged children to be approximately 1% [17,18]. More recent studies, however, suggest that the prevalence of individuals who have VWD who present to primary care physicians with symptomatic bleeding or bruising is closer to 1 in 1000 [19]. The number of individuals referred to a tertiary care center for management of VWD is much lower, at approximately 1 in 10,000 [20].

VWD is characterized by three key features: a personal history of excessive mucocutaneous bleeding, abnormal VWF laboratory studies, and evidence of a family history of the condition. A diagnostic algorithm for possible VWD cases is presented in Fig. 2.

Bleeding histories

The clinical hallmark of VWD is the presence of excessive and prolonged mucocutaneous bleeding. Most often, this involves bruising, epistaxis, bleeding from the gums and trivial wounds, and menorrhagia and postpartum hemorrhage in women. Prolonged and excessive bleeding also occurs

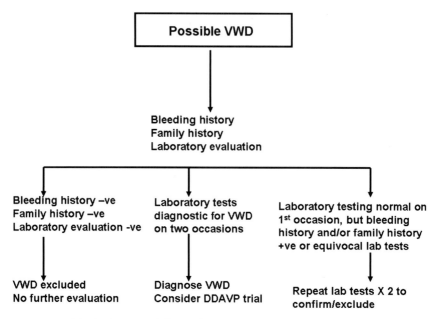

Fig. 2. A proposed diagnostic algorithm for possible VWD cases.

after surgical and dental procedures. Children who have VWD also may experience bruising after routine immunizations and gum bleeding after the loss of primary teeth. Typically, only patients who have type 3 VWD (characterized by an absence of VWF, accompanied by low FVIII levels, less than 0.10 IU/mL [10%]) experience spontaneous musculoskeletal bleeding, such as that seen in patients who have severe hemophilia. An accurate assessment of hemorrhagic symptoms is a key component in diagnosing VWD but often presents a significant challenge, particularly in the pediatric population.

Although bruising and epistaxis are common among children who have VWD, these symptoms also are reported in normal children. An additional consideration is that bleeding symptoms manifest in children in distinctly different ways compared with adults. Some of the classical symptoms of VWD in adults (eg, menorrhagia and postsurgical bleeding) are not prevalent in the pediatric population. Children who have a bleeding disorder may not have had surgery or (in the case of girls) reached the age of menarche; however, they may have symptoms that cause difficulty and merit treatment. To address these issues, there has been significant recent interest in developing new clinical tools for quantifying bleeding, and although much of this work has focused on adult populations, tools have been developed that are specific to pediatrics [21]. The Epistaxis Scoring System is a semiquantitative system, in which children with recurrent epistaxis are either categorized as "mild" or "severe," and represents one such tool [22].

Abnormal von Willebrand factor laboratory studies

The laboratory evaluation for VWD involves qualitative and quantitative measurements of VWF and FVIII. The results from affected individuals are highly variable, ranging from the near complete absence of VWF in type 3 VWD to modest quantitative reductions in VWF and FVIII levels as seen in type 1 VWD. The type 2 variants are characterized by qualitative abnormalities in VWF and include four subtypes, 2A, 2B, 2M, and 2N (see classification later). It is critical that the laboratory investigations for VWD be interpreted by physicians who have experience in this area, given the heterogeneity of possible results.

Although it is important to perform screening tests in the diagnostic work-up of patients who have possible VWD, it also is important to recognize the limitations of these tests. The complete blood count can be completely normal in individuals who have VWD but may show evidence of an iron deficiency anemia resulting from chronic blood loss; type 2B VWD often is associated with mild thrombocytopenia. If the VWF level is reduced to levels less than approximately 0.35 IU/mL (35%), the commensurate low level of FVIII may result in the prolongation of the activated partial thromboplastin time (aPTT); however a normal aPTT does not rule out VWD, particularly in milder cases. The bleeding time may be prolonged [23]; however, this test lacks sensitivity and specificity and patients who have known VWD may have normal bleeding times. Parenthetically, the bleeding time is poorly reproducible and invasive and no longer should be a routine component of the investigation of children who have possible VWD. Recently, a newer analyzer, known as the PFA-100, has been evaluated in the diagnostic work-up of VWD. Its reported sensitivity for VWD is high (ranging from 71%–97%); however, given that it is a test of global hemostasis, the specificity is lower. As a result, the PFA-100 may have a role as a screening test; however, its precise clinical usefulness remains unresolved [21,24,25].

Laboratory tests specific for VWD include a measurement of the amount of circulating plasma VWF antigen, a measurement of the VWF function (a ristocetin-based platelet aggregation test, known as the VWF ristocetin cofactor assay [VWF:RCo] [26], or the VWF collagen-binding assay) [27] and a measurement of FVIII coagulant activity. One other VWF test also uses ristocetin, the ristocetin-induced platelet agglutination (RIPA) assay. In contrast to the VWF:RCo (which evaluates the interaction between patients' VWF and formalin-fixed platelets), the RIPA assay evaluates the sensitivity of patients' platelets to low-dose ristocetin and is useful particularly in identifying individuals who have type 2B VWD. In these cases, the platelet membrane is "overloaded" with high-affinity mutant VWF, resulting in platelet agglutination at low ristocetin concentrations, less than 0.6 mg/mL [27]. The final laboratory test performed to characterize VWD involves the assessment of the molecular-weight profile of circulating plasma VWF [28]. As discussed previously, VWF circulates in the plasma as a heterogenous mixture of multimers. HMW multimers are the most hemostatically active, as they contain the most active binding sites for platelets, and characteristically are absent in some type 2 forms of VWD. The molecular-weight profile of VWF is evaluated most often using sodium dodecyl sulfate polyacrylamide gel electrophoresis (SDS-PAGE), which is technically challenging and available only in a few laboratories (Fig. 3). Recent efforts have been made to simplify and enhance the objectivity of this assay by combining nonradioactive, chemiluminescent detection methods with densitometric analysis of the multimer bands.

Normal plasma levels of VWF are approximately 1 U/mL (100%, correlating to approximately10 µg/mL) with a wide population range of 0.50 to 2.0 U/mL (50%–200%). These variations are influenced by several genetic and environmental factors. ABO blood group is the genetic influence characterized best; VWF and FVIII levels in individuals who have blood group O are approximately 25% lower than individuals who have blood group A, B, or AB [29]. This difference is believed a result of the lack of glycosylation (and therefore stabilization) of VWF in individuals who are in blood group O. Two major environmental factors affecting VWF levels are stress and hormones. The plasma levels of VWF and FVIII increase approximately twofold to fivefold during physiologic stress, such as fainting [30] or exercise [31]. VWF and FVIII levels also fluctuate over the course of a menstrual cycle and under the influence of oral contraceptive pills and pregnancy [32]. Additionally, VWF levels vary with age, with neonatal levels higher than adult levels [33,34], although many laboratories do not report age-specific normal ranges. These factors all must be considered when interpreting VWF laboratory results and, as a result, most clinicians support at least two sets of tests to confirm or refute a diagnosis of VWD.

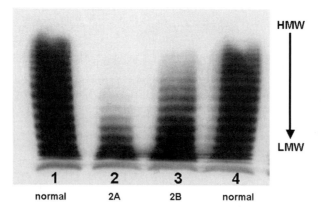

Fig. 3. VMF multimer analysis. Multimer analysis in two patients who have type 2 VWD. Lanes 1 and 4 represent normal plasma multimer patterns. Lane 2 shows the plasma VWF multimers for a patient who had type 2A and lane 3 the plasma multimers for a patient who has type 2B VWD. LMW, low molecular weight.

Family history

Most cases of VWD are inherited, and often there is evidence of a family history of excessive bleeding. This issue is complicated, however, by some forms of the disease showing incomplete penetrance of bleeding symptoms. As a result, many clinicians do not consider the lack of a positive family history (especially in type 1 VWD) an exclusion criterion. The disease is inherited as a dominant trait in type 1 and in the qualitative variants types 2A, 2B, and 2M. In contrast, the rare type 2N and severe type 3 forms of the disease show a recessive pattern of inheritance.

Classification of von Willebrand disease

The current International Society on Thrombosis and Haemostasis established classification of VWD comprises three types: type 1 VWD, a partial quantitative deficiency of qualitatively normal VWF; type 2 VWD, a qualitative deficiency caused by functionally abnormal VWF; and type 3 VWD, which represents a virtual absence of the VWF protein (Table 1) [35].

Type 1 von Willebrand disease

Type 1 VWD, which represents approximately 80% of VWD cases unfortunately is the most difficult subtype of VWD to diagnose. As discussed previously, circulating VWF levels are influenced by several factors, and there is overlap between normal individuals who have VWF levels at the lower end of the normal range and those who have mild type 1 VWD. Additionally, mucocutaneous bleeding symptoms in individuals who have type 1 VWD can be mild and potentially overlooked by patients and physicians. Convincing family histories may be absent, given the incomplete penetrance of this subtype. Consideration of all of these factors has led to much recent debate about the proper definition of this disorder [36]. The suggestion has been made that a diagnosis of type 1 VWD be reserved for individuals who have significant reductions in VWF to less than 0.15 IU/mL (15%); although this may not have become a widely accepted clinical definition, it highlights the importance

Table 1
Characteristic laboratory findings in von Willebrand disease by subtype

von Willebrand disease subtype	VWF:Ag	VWF:RCo	FVIII:C	RCo:Ag ratio	Multimer pattern	RIPA
1	↓	↓	↓ or ↔	>0.60	Normal	—
2A	↓	↓↓	↓ or ↔	<0.60	Abnormal	↓
2B	↓	↓↓	↓ or ↔	<0.60	Abnormal	↑
2M	↓	↓↓	↓ or ↔	<0.60	Normal	—
2N	↓ or ↔	↓ or ↔	0.10–0.40	>0.60	Normal	—
3	↓↓↓	↓↓↓	<0.10	—	—	—

Abbreviations: FVIII:C, Factor VIII coagulant activity; RCo:Ag Ratio, VWF, ristocetin cofactor/VWF antigen ratio.

of considering a diagnosis carefully. Assigning an incorrect diagnostic label of VWD to patients can be difficult to revise subsequently and may lead to confusion and inappropriate management. In addition, the wider implications of this diagnosis, including the potential social stigma and health insurance implications, should be considered carefully before making a diagnosis. In contrast, underdiagnosis of type 1 VWD can be a concern in young children who may not have been subjected to a sufficient hemostatic challenge to manifest a bleeding tendency that would lead to consideration of a diagnosis of VWD. Taking all of these factors into consideration, a suggested definition of type 1 VWD in children could include both definite (for children with excessive mucocutaneous bleeding and low VWF levels) and possible (for children with low VWF levels but no history of excessive mucocutaneous bleeding potentially because of the lack of opportunity).

The genetic basis of type 1 VWD has been the focus of much recent investigation, and two large multicenter trials have reported consistent results [37,38]. Mutations throughout the *VWF* gene were identified in approximately 65% of index cases and the majority of these were missense mutations. Mutations were identified more frequently in cases of lower VWF levels and more highly penetrant in those cases. The genetic variation reported most frequently identified in both studies was a missense mutation resulting in an AA substitution of tyrosine to cysteine at codon 1584 (Y1584C), identified in 10% to 20% of patients who had type 1 VWD [39]. In both studies, however, some patients who had type 1 VWD had no obvious VWF mutation identified, and in these (often milder) cases, the genetic determinants likely are more complex and could involve other genetic loci. At this time, genetic testing for type 1 VWD generally is neither available nor required for establishing the diagnosis.

Type 2 von Willebrand disease

Type 2 VWD is characterized by a qualitative deficiency of VWF activity and is classified further into the qualitative variants that affect VWF-platelet interactions (2A, 2B, and 2M) and the rare type 2N characterized by defective VWF binding to FVIII. The clinical presentation of type 2 VWD is similar to type 1 VWD in that patients present with excessive mucocutaneous bleeding; however, in contrast to the variably positive family histories in type 1 VWD, patients who have type 2 VWD usually present with a clearly positive family history.

Type 2A

Type 2A VWD accounts for approximately 10% of all VWD cases and is characterized by the loss of HMW and intermediate-molecular-weight multimers. This is the result of a defect in the synthesis of the higher-molecular-weight multimers (group 1 mutations) or the synthesis of multimers that are more susceptible to cleavage by ADAMTS-13 (group 2 mutations) [40]. Type 2A can be suspected because of disproportionately low functional activity compared with von Willebrand factor antigen level (VWF:Ag) (ie, VWF:RCo to VWF:Ag ratio of <0.60). The FVIII level may be low or normal. RIPA is reduced and the multimer profile shows a loss of HMW and sometimes intermediate-molecular-weight multimers. The molecular genetic basis of type 2A VWD is well characterized, with missense mutations in the VWF A2 domain predominating. Other type 2A cases are caused by mutations that disrupt dimerization or multimerization; these mutations are located outside of the A2 domain (Fig. 4).

Type 2B

Type 2B VWD is the result of gain-of-function mutations within the GpIb-binding site on VWF. This leads to an increase in VWF-platelet interactions that result in the selective depletion of HMW multimers [27,41]. The increased binding of mutant VWF to platelets also results in the formation of circulating platelet aggregates and subsequent thrombocytopenia. As in type 2A VWD, the laboratory profile shows a decrease in VWF:RCo to VWF:Ag ratio; however, in contrast to 2A, there is increased sensitivity to low doses of ristocetin in the RIPA. HMW multimers are absent in the plasma. Type 2B mutations are well characterized and represent a variety of different missense mutations in the region of the *VWF* gene encoding the GpIb-binding site in the A1 protein domain. A disorder known as platelet-type VWD (PT-VWD) exhibits identical clinical and laboratory features to those of type 2B VWD [42]. This condition is caused by mutations within the platelet *GPIB* gene that affect the region of the GPIb/IX receptor that binds to VWF [43]. It can be distinguished from type 2B VWD using platelet aggregation tests that identify enhanced ristocetin-induced binding of VWF, by mixing combinations of patient and normal plasma with patient and normal washed platelets. In rare cases, genetic analysis of the A1 domain of the *VWF* gene and the *GPIB* gene can be performed. It is assumed that PT-VWD is less prevalent than type 2B VWD although the level of misdiagnosis is not known. The distinction is important, however, because the treatment is plasma based in type 2B VWD and platelet based in PT-VWD.

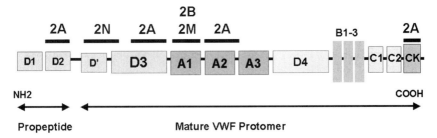

Fig. 4. Type 2 VWD mutations. Repeating multidomain structure of the VWF protein. The regions of the protein comprising the prepropolypeptide and mature VWF subunits are indicated at the bottom of the diagram. Regions of the protein in which the causative mutations for types 2A, 2B, 2M, and 2N VWD are shown above the protein diagram.

Type 2M

Type 2M VWD (the "M" refers to multimer) is characterized by decreased VWF-platelet interactions. The laboratory work-up shows a reduced ratio of VWF:RCo to VWF:Ag but a normal multimer pattern. RIPA also is reduced. Causative mutations are localized to the platelet GPIB-binding site in the A1 domain of VWF [44].

Type 2N

Type 2N VWD (the "N" refers to Normandy, where the first cases were reported) is described as an autosomal form of hemophilia A [45] and is an important differential in the investigation of all individuals (male and female) presenting with a low FVIII level. The characteristic laboratory feature is a significant reduction in FVIII level when compared with VWF level (which may be low or normal). The VWF multimer pattern in 2N is normal. The definitive diagnosis requires the demonstration of reduced FVIII binding in a microtiter plate-based assay or the identification of causative mutations in the FVIII-binding region of the *VWF* gene [46].

Type 3 von Willebrand disease

Patients who have type 3 VWD typically manifest a severe bleeding phenotype from early childhood, although clinical heterogeneity exists. In addition to more significant presentations of the cardinal mucocutaneous bleeding symptoms seen in the other subtypes, individuals who have type 3 VWD experience joint and soft tissue bleeds frequently, similar to patients who have hemophilia A, because of the commensurate reduction in plasma FVIII levels. In the laboratory, this condition is characterized by prolongation of the aPTT and bleeding time, undetectable levels of VWF:Ag, and VWF:Rco, and FVIII levels less than 0.10 IU/mL (10%). The inheritance of type 3 VWD is autosomal recessive and although parents of affected individuals often are unaffected, there is a growing realization that some obligate carriers of type 3 VWD mutations manifest an increase in mucocutaneous bleeding symptoms compared with normal individuals [47]. Molecular genetic studies of individuals who have type 3 VWD reveal that the phenotype is the result of a variety of genetic defects, including large gene deletions and frameshift and nonsense mutations within the VWF gene, all of which result in a premature stop codon [48]. As a result of the lack of circulating VWF, these mutations in some cases are associated with the development of alloantibodies to VWF, which represent a serious complication of treatment [49,50].

Clinical management of von Willebrand disease

In general, the management of VWD can be divided into three main categories: (1) localized measures to stop or minimize bleeding; (2)

pharmacologic agents that provide indirect hemostatic benefit; and (3) treatments that increase plasma VWF and FVIII levels directly.

Localized measures

The importance of localized measures to control bleeding in VWD, such as the application of direct pressure to a site of bleeding or injury, should not be understated. Biting down on a piece of gauze may halt bleeding from a tooth socket, and application of a compression bandage and cold pack to an injured limb may reduce subsequent hematoma formation. Management of nosebleeds can be problematic particularly for some affected children, however, and patients may benefit from a stepwise action plan that escalates from initial direct pressure to packing after a certain time period and that includes guidelines regarding how long to wait before seeking medical attention. In selected cases, nasal cautery may be required for prolonged or excessive epistaxis.

Adjunctive therapies

Several adjunctive therapies can be used with significant benefit in VWD, particularly at the time of minor surgical and dental procedures and to treat menorrhagia. These interventions include the use of antifibrinolytic agents, such as tranexamic acid and epsilon aminocaproic acid, and the application of topical hemostatic preparations, such as fibrin glue, to exposed sites of bleeding. In women who have menorrhagia, the administration of estrogens (that work, at least in part, by elevating plasma VWF and FVIII levels) often results in significant clinical benefit. Topical estrogen creams applied to the nasal mucosa also are used in children to reduce epistaxis with variable efficacy.

Desmopressin

Desmopressin (1-deamino-8-D-arginine vasopressin) is a synthetic analog of the antidiuretic hormone vasopressin [51]. Its administration increases plasma VWF and FVIII levels by approximately twofold to eightfold within 1to 2 hours of administration [52]. The effect is presumed to be the result of the release of stored VWF from endothelial cell Weibel-Palade bodies, with the secondary stabilization of additional FVIII. Desmopressin can be administered by the intravenous, subcutaneous, or intranasal route [53]. Its peak effect is achieved within 30 and 90 minutes with the intravenous and intranasal routes, respectively. The usual parenteral dose is 0.3 μg/kg (maximum dose 20 μg) infused in approximately 50 mL of normal saline over approximately 30 minutes. The dose of the highly concentrated intranasal preparation is 150 μg for children under 50 kg and 300 μg for larger children. Highly concentrated products (eg, Stimate) deliver 150 μg per spray, a much higher concentration than found in the nasal sprays used to treat enuresis.

Desmopressin is safe and generally well tolerated; however, its use in pediatric patients must be undertaken cautiously. Common mild side effects include facial flushing and headache. Tachycardia and mild reductions in blood pressure can occur and, given that patients sometimes feel lightheaded during the infusion, it is best to administer it with patients lying down. The most serious side effects that can develop are severe hyponatremia and seizures [54,55] because of the antidiuretic effect of the medication. Reduction of fluid intake for 24 hours after administration to maintenance levels is an important precaution to prevent water intoxication. Children under 3 years of age are especially prone to this complication and extra attention must be paid in these cases. With repeated desmopressin administrations, serial monitoring of serum sodium levels should be performed.

An important limitation in the use of desmopressin is the development of tachyphylaxis with repeated administration. The magnitude of the VWF and FVIII increments often falls to approximately 70% of that documented with the initial dose when given at repeated intervals of less than 24 hours [56]. Presumably, a greater period of time is required for the Weibel-Palade body VWF stores to be replenished. For practical purposes, a single dose of desmopressin before dental procedures or at the onset of menses usually is sufficient. Doses can be repeated at 12 or 24 hours; however, the potential decrease in efficacy (described previously) must be considered. Additionally, in situations where repeat dosing is considered, the duration of fluid restriction must be increased. Generally, more than three doses of desmopressin (preprocedure, at 12 hours, and at 24 hours) are not recommended.

Most patients who have type 1 VWD respond to desmopressin; however, patients who have severe type 1 and many who have type 2 VWD do not respond adequately [57]. Therefore, it is critical to perform a therapeutic trial of the agent before any clinical use. VWF and FVIII levels should be checked before desmopressin administration and at several time points after (eg, at 1, 2, and 4 hours). Although the repeated phlebotomies can present a significant challenge, particularly for young patients, documentation of an adequate response is recommended strongly. An increment of VWF and FVIII to threefold over baseline and to at least 0.30 IU/mL (30%) usually is considered adequate for situations, such as dental procedures, minor surgery, or the treatment of epistaxis or menorrhagia; however, major surgery and significant bleeding episodes should be treated with factor replacement therapy. Desmopressin responsiveness may be suboptimal in young children (<3 years), and repeat assessment at an older age may be warranted. In addition, certain VWF mutants that show increased clearance are described, limiting the clinical usefullness of desmopressin in this setting [58].

Most patients who have type 1 VWD respond adequately to desmopressin and, for these patients, the concomitant use of desmopressin and an antifibrinolytic agent is sufficient for most clinical situations. Patients who have type 3 VWD typically do not respond to desmopressin, however, given the lack of stored VWF in this condition. Patients who have type 2 VWD respond variably to desmopressin. Patients who have type 2A often exhibit adequate responses and, therefore, may benefit from a therapeutic trial. Patients who have type 2M typically do not respond well to desmopressin. Desmopressin long has been considered contraindicated in type 2B VWD because of the transient thrombocytopenia that follows the release of the mutant VWF; however, its hemostatic efficacy is documented, allowing its use on an individualized basis [59,60]. Finally, desmopressin has been used in patients who have type 2N, with a twofold to ninefold increase in the VWF and FVIII levels [61]; however, the duration of the FVIII increment usually is only approximately 3 hours. This suggests that for patients who have type 2N, desmopressin should be considered only in clinical situations where a brief, transient rise in FVIII is required.

Blood component therapy

Situations, such as major surgery, trauma, and life-threatening bleeding, require intravenous treatment with plasma-derived concentrates of VWF and FVIII. Cryoprecipitate was used commonly in these settings in the 1970s and 1980s, but it no longer is the treatment of choice because of the lack of an effective viral inactivation process for this product. The blood components currently used are plasma-derived, intermediate purity concentrates that have undergone several viral inactivation steps to prevent viral transmission [62–64] (eg, Humate-P and Alphanate). Dosing recommendations currently are made in VWF:RCo units and are weight based; repeat infusions can be given every 12 to 24 hours depending on the clinical situation. It is recommended to measure VWF:RCo and FVIII levels in patients receiving repeat infusions not only to ensure adequate hemostasis but also to monitor for supraphysiologic levels of FVIII. High FVIII levels associated with treatment with these concentrates can contribute to venous thrombosis [65]. In the rare event that infusion of an intermediate purity concentrate is ineffective at stopping bleeding, transfusion of a platelet concentrate is beneficial [66], presumably because it facilitates the delivery of a small amount of VWF (contained in normal platelets) to the site of vascular injury. The role of prophylactic factor infusions in patients who are affected severely currently is the subject of an international randomized trial.

Summary

VWD is a common inherited bleeding disorder and many cases are diagnosed in childhood. VWD has a negative impact on the quality of life of affected individuals; therefore, it is important that the condition be recognized and diagnosed. This article reviews the pathophysiology of the condition, the current classification scheme, and the available treatments, highlighting issues specific to the pediatric population.

References

[1] von Willebrand EA. Hereditar pseudohemofili. Fin Lakaresallsk Handl 1926;67:7–112.
[2] Sadler JE, Shelton-Inloes BB, Sorace JM, et al. Cloning and characterization of two cDNAs coding for human von Willebrand factor. Proc Natl Acad Sci U S A 1985;82:6394–8.
[3] Ginsburg D, Handin RI, Bonthron DT, et al. Human von Willebrand factor (vWF): isolation of complementary DNA (cDNA) clones and chromosomal localization. Science 1985;228:1401–3.
[4] Verweij CL, Diergaarde PJ, Hart M, et al. Full-length von Willebrand factor (vWF) cDNA encodes a highly repetitive protein considerably larger than the mature vWF subunit. EMBO J 1986;5:1839–47.
[5] Lynch DC, Zimmerman TS, Collins CJ, et al. Molecular cloning of cDNA for human von Willebrand factor: authentication by a new method. Cell 1985;41:49–56.
[6] Mancuso DJ, Tuley EA, Westfield LA, et al. Structure of the gene for human von Willebrand factor. J Biol Chem 1989;264(33):19514–27.
[7] Titani K, Kumar S, Takio K, et al. Amino acid sequence of human von Willebrand factor. Biochemistry 1986;25:3171–84.
[8] Hampshire D. The University of Sheffield ISTH SSC VWF database. Available at: http://www.vwf.group.shef.ac.uk/. Accessed on January 3, 2008.
[9] Mancuso DJ, Tuley EA, Westfield LA, et al. Human von Willebrand factor gene and pseudogene: structural analysis and differentiation by polymerase chain reaction. Biochemistry 1991;30:253–69.
[10] Wagner DD, Marder VJ. Biosynthesis of von Willebrand protein by human endothelial cells: processing steps and their intracellular localization. J Cell Biol 1984;99:2123–30.
[11] Sporn LA, Chavin SI, Marder VJ, et al. Biosynthesis of von Willebrand protein by human megakaryocytes. J Clin Invest 1985;76:1102–6.
[12] Ruggeri Z, Zimmerman T. The complex multimeric composition of factor VIII/von Willebrand factor. Blood 1981;57:1140–3.
[13] Dong JF, Moake JL, Nolasco L, et al. ADAMTS-13 rapidly cleaves newly secreted ultralarge von Willebrand factor multimers on the endothelial surface under flowing conditions. Blood 2002;100:4033–9.
[14] Savage B, Saldivar E, Ruggeri ZM. Initiation of platelet adhesion by arrest onto fibrinogen or translocation on von Willebrand factor. Cell 1996;84:289–97.
[15] Ruggeri ZM. Mechanisms of shear-induced platelet adhesion and aggregation. Thromb Haemost 1993;70:119–23.
[16] Koedam JA, Meijers JC, Sixma JJ, et al. Inactivation of human factor VIII by activated protein C. Cofactor activity of protein S and protective effect of von Willebrand factor. J Clin Invest 1988;82:1236–43.
[17] Rodeghiero F, Castaman G, Dini E. Epidemiological investigation of the prevalence of von Willebrand's disease. Blood 1987;69:454–9.
[18] Werner EJ, Broxson EH, Tucker EL, et al. Prevalence of von Willebrand disease in children: a multiethnic study. J Pediatr 1993;123:893–8.
[19] Bowman M, James P, Godwin M, et al. The prevalence of VWD in the primary care setting. Blood 2007;106:1780 [(ASH Annual Meeting abstracts)].
[20] Sadler JE, Mannucci PM, Berntorp E, et al. Impact, diagnosis and treatment of von Willebrand disease. Thromb Haemost 2000;84:160–74.
[21] Dean JA, Blanchette VS, Carcao MD, et al. von Willebrand disease in a pediatric-based population–comparison of type 1 diagnostic criteria and use of the PFA-100 and a von Willebrand factor/collagen-binding assay. Thromb Haemost 2000;84:401–9.
[22] Katsanis E, Luke KH, Hsu E, et al. Prevalence and significance of mild bleeding disorders in children with recurrent epistaxis. J Pediatr 1988;113:73–6.
[23] Mannucci PM, Pareti FI, Holmberg L, et al. Studies on the prolonged bleeding time in von Willebrand's disease. J Lab Clin Med 1976;88:662–73.

[24] Fressinaud E, Veyradier A, Truchaud F, et al. Screening for von Willebrand disease with a new analyzer using high shear stress: a study of 60 cases. Blood 1998;91:1325–31.

[25] Favaloro EJ. The utility of the PFA-100 in the identification of von Willebrand disease: a concise review. Semin Thromb Hemost 2006;32:537–45.

[26] Howard MA, Firkin BG. Ristocetin—a new tool in the investigation of platelet aggregation. Thromb Diath Haemorrh 1971;26:362–9.

[27] Cooney KA, Lyons SE, Ginsburg D. Functional analysis of a type IIB von Willebrand disease missense mutation: increased binding of large von Willebrand factor multimers to platelets. Proc Natl Acad Sci U S A 1992;89:2869–72.

[28] Hoyer LW, Rizza CR, Tuddenham EGD, et al. Von Willebrand factor multimer patterns in von Willebrand's disease. Br J Haematol 1983;55:493–507.

[29] Gill JC, Endres-Brooks J, Bauer PJ, et al. The effect of ABO blood group on the diagnosis of von Willebrand disease. Blood 1987;69:1691–5.

[30] Casonato A, Pontara E, Bertomoro A, et al. Fainting induces an acute increase in the concentration of plasma factor VIII and von Willebrand factor. Haematologica 2003;88: 688–93.

[31] Stakiw J, Bowman M, Hegadorn C, et al. The effect of exercise on von Willebrand factor and ADAMTS-13 in individuals with type 1 and type 2B von Willebrand disease. J Thromb Haemost 2008;6:90–6.

[32] Kadir RA, Chi C. Women and von Willebrand disease: controversies in diagnosis and management. Semin Thromb Hemost 2006;32:605–15.

[33] Andrew M, Vegh P, Johnston M, et al. Maturation of the hemostatic system during childhood. Blood 1992;80:1998–2005.

[34] Sosothikul D, Seksarn P, Lusher JM. Pediatric reference values for molecular markers in hemostasis. J Pediatr Hematol Oncol 2007;29:19–22.

[35] Sadler JE, Budde U, Eikenboom JC, et al. Update on the pathophysiology and classification of von Willebrand disease: a report of the Subcommittee on von Willebrand Factor. J Thromb Haemost 2006;4:2103–14.

[36] Sadler JE. Von Willebrand disease type 1: a diagnosis in search of a disease. Blood 2003;101: 2089–93.

[37] James PD, Notley C, Hegadorn C, et al. The mutational spectrum of type 1 von Willebrand disease: results from a Canadian cohort study. Blood 2007;109:145–54.

[38] Goodeve A, Eikenboom J, Castaman G, et al. Phenotype and genotype of a cohort of families historically diagnosed with type 1 von Willebrand disease in the European study, molecular and clinical markers for the diagnosis and management of Type 1 von Willebrand disease (MCMDM-1VWD). Blood 2007;109:112–21.

[39] O'Brien LA, James PD, Othman M, et al. Founder von Willebrand factor haplotype associated with type 1 von Willebrand disease. Blood 2003;102:549–57.

[40] Lyons SE, Bruck ME, Bowie EJW, et al. Impaired intracellular transport produced by a subset of type IIA von Willebrand disease mutations. J Biol Chem 1992;267:4424–30.

[41] Ruggeri ZM, Pareti FI, Mannucci PM, et al. Heightened interaction between platelets and factor VIII/von Willebrand factor in a new subtype of von Willebrand's disease. N Engl J Med 1980;302:1047–51.

[42] Miller JL, Castella A. Platelet-type von Willebrand's disease: characterization of a new bleeding disorder. Blood 1982;60:790–4.

[43] Brychaert MC, Pietu G, Ruan C, et al. Abnormality of glycoprotein Ib in two cases of "pseudo" von Willebrand's disease. J Lab Clin Med 1985;106:393–400.

[44] Mancuso DJ, Kroner PA, Christopherson PA, et al. Type 2M:Milwaukee-1 von Willebrand disease: an in-frame deletion in the Cys509-Cys695 loop of the von Willebrand factor A1 domain causes deficient binding of von Willebrand factor to platelets. Blood 1996;88:2559–68.

[45] Mazurier C. von Willebrand disease masquerading as haemophilia A. Thromb Haemost 1992;67:391–6.

[46] Nesbitt IM, Goodeve AC, Guilliatt AM, et al. Characterisation of type 2N von Willebrand disease using phenotypic and molecular techniques. Thromb Haemost 1996;75:959–64.

[47] Castaman G, Rodeghiero F, Tosetto A, et al. Hemorrhagic symptoms and bleeding risk in obligatory carriers of type 3 von Willebrand disease: an international, multicenter study. J Thromb Haemost 2006;4:2164–9.

[48] Baronciani L, Cozzi G, Canciani MT, et al. Molecular defects in type 3 von Willebrand disease: updated results from 40 multiethnic patients. Blood Cells Mol Dis 2003;30:264–70.

[49] Shelton-Inloes B, Chehab F, Mannucci P, et al. Gene deletions correlate with the development of alloantibodies in von Willebrand's disease. J Clin Invest 1987;79:1459–65.

[50] Ngo K, Glotz Trifard V, Koziol J, et al. Homozygous and heterozygous deletions of the von Willebrand factor gene in patients and carriers of severe von Willebrand disease. Proc Natl Acad Sci U S A 1988;85:2753–7.

[51] Mannucci PM. Desmopressin: a nontransfusional form of treatment for congenital and acquired bleeding disorders. Blood 1988;72:1449–55.

[52] Rodeghiero F, Castaman G, Di Bona E, et al. Consistency of responses to repeated DDAVP infusions in patients with von Willebrand's disease and hemophilia A. Blood 1989;74:1997–2000.

[53] Rose EH, Aledort LM. Nasal spray desmopressin (DDAVP) for mild hemophilia A and von Willebrand disease. Ann Intern Med 1991;114:563–8.

[54] Humphries JE, Siragy H. Significant hyponatremia following DDAVP administration in a healthy adult. Am J Hematol 1993;44:12–5.

[55] Weinstein RE, Bona RD, Altman AJ, et al. Severe hyponatremia after repeated intravenous administration of desmopressin. Am J Hematol 1989;32:258–61.

[56] Mannucci PM, Bettega D, Cattaneo M. Patterns of development of tachyphylaxis in patients with haemophilia and von Willebrand disease after repeated doses of desmopressin (DDAVP). Br J Haematol 1992;82:87–93.

[57] Federici AB, Mazurier C, Berntorp E, et al. Biologic response to desmopressin in patients with severe type 1 and type 2 von Willebrand disease: results of a multicenter European study. Blood 2004;103:2032–8.

[58] Haberichter SL, Balistreri M, Christopherson P, et al. Assay of the von Willebrand factor (VWF) propeptide to identify patients with type 1 von Willebrand disease with decreased VWF survival. Blood 2006;108:3344–51.

[59] Fowler WE, Berkowitz LR, Roberts HR. DDAVP for type IIB von Willebrand disease. Blood 1989;74:1859–60.

[60] Casonato A, Sartori MT, De Marco L, et al. 1-Desamino-8-D-arginine vasopressin (DDAVP) infusion in type IIB von Willebrand's disease: shortening of bleeding time and induction of a variable pseudothrombocytopenia. Thromb Haemost 1990;64:117–20.

[61] Mazurier C, Gaucher C, Jorieux S, et al. Biological effect of desmopressin in eight patients with type 2N (Normandy) von Willebrand disease. Br J Haematol 1994;88:849–54.

[62] Rodeghiero F, Castaman G, Meyer D, et al. Replacement therapy with virus-inactivated plasma concentrates in von Willebrand disease. Vox Sang 1992;62:193–9.

[63] Mannucci PM, Chediak J, Hanna W, et al. Treatment of von Willebrand disease with a high-purity factor VIII/von Willebrand factor concentrate: a prospective, multicenter study. Blood 2002;99:450–6.

[64] Lillicrap D, Poon MC, Walker I, et al. Efficacy and safety of the factor VIII/von Willebrand factor concentrate, haemate-P/humate-P: ristocetin cofactor unit dosing in patients with von Willebrand disease. Thromb Haemost 2002;87:224–30.

[65] Mannucci PM. Venous thromboembolism in von Willebrand disease. Thromb Haemost 2002;88:378–9.

[66] Castillo R, Monteagudo J, Escolar G, et al. Hemostatic effect of normal platelet transfusion in severe von Willebrand disease patients. Blood 1991;77:1901–5.

ELSEVIER
SAUNDERS

PEDIATRIC CLINICS
OF NORTH AMERICA

Pediatr Clin N Am 55 (2008) 393–420

Childhood Immune Thrombocytopenic Purpura: Diagnosis and Management

Victor Blanchette, FRCP[a],*,
Paula Bolton-Maggs, DM, FRCP[b]

[a]Division of Hematology/Oncology, The Hospital for Sick Children, Department of Pediatrics,
University of Toronto, 555 University Avenue, Toronto, Ontario M5G 1X8, Canada
[b]University Department of Haematology, Manchester Royal Infirmary,
Oxford Road, Manchester M13 9WL, United Kingdom

Immune thrombocytopenic purpura (ITP) is an autoimmune disorder characterized by a low circulating platelet count caused by destruction of antibody-sensitized platelets in the reticuloendothelial system [1]. ITP can be classified based on patient age (childhood versus adult), duration of illness (acute versus chronic), and presence of an underlying disorder (primary versus secondary). Persistence of thrombocytopenia, generally defined as a platelet count of less than $150 \times 10^9/L$ for longer than 6 months, defines the chronic form of the disorder. Secondary causes of ITP include collagen vascular disorders, such as systemic lupus erythematosus (SLE); immune deficiencies, such as common variable immunodeficiency (CVID); and some chronic infections (eg, HIV and hepatitis C).

This article focuses on the diagnosis and management of children (under 18 years of age) who have acute and chronic ITP. Emphasis is placed on areas of controversy and new therapies.

Pathophysiology

The pathophysiology of ITP increasingly is understood better (reviewed by Cines and Blanchette [1]). Not surprisingly, it is complex with involvement of many players in the human immune orchestra, including antibodies, cytokines, antigen-presenting cells, costimulatory molecules, and T and B lymphocytes (including T-helper, T-cytotoxic, and T-regulatory lymphocytes). Current knowledge is summarized later.

---

* Corresponding author.
E-mail address: victor.blanchette@sickkids.ca (V. Blanchette).

A key element in the pathophysiology of ITP is loss of self tolerance leading to the production of autoantibodies directed against platelet antigens. Evidence for an "antiplatelet factor" in the plasma of subjects who have ITP was provided in a seminal report from Harrington and coworkers [2] in 1951. The investigators demonstrated that the infusion of plasma from subjects who had ITP into volunteers induced a rapid fall in platelet count and a clinical picture that mimics ITP. The "antiplatelet factor" subsequently was confirmed as an immunoglobulin [3]. Now it is known that the autoantibodies in patients who have ITP mostly are of the IgG class with specificity against platelet-specific antigens, in particular, glycoproteins IIb/IIIa and Ib/IX. Unfortunately, accurate detection of platelet autoantibodies is difficult and not available routinely in most clinical hematology laboratories; clinicians should be aware that indirect platelet autoantibody tests (tests that detect free autoantibodies in the plasma) are inferior to direct tests (tests that detect platelet-bound autoantibodies) and that even with the best direct tests performed in expert immunohematology laboratories, the positivity rate in patients who have well-characterized ITP does not exceed 80% [4]. A negative platelet antibody test, therefore, does not exclude a diagnosis of ITP. For this reason, platelet antibody testing is not recommended as part of the routine diagnostic strategy [5].

It is increasingly clear that cellular immune mechanisms play a pivotal role in ITP [1]. The production of antiplatelet antibodies by B cells requires antigen-specific, CD4-postive, T-cell help (Fig. 1). It also is possible that in some ITP cases, cytotoxic T cells play a role in the destruction of platelets. A possible sequence of events in ITP is as follows. A trigger, possibly an infection or toxin, leads to the formation of antibodies/immune complexes that attach to platelets. Antibody-coated platelets then bind to antigen-presenting cells (macrophages or dendritic cells) through low-affinity Fcγ receptors (Fcγ RIIA/Fcγ RIIIA) and are internalized and degraded. Activated antigen-presenting cells then expose novel peptides on the cell surface and with costimulatory help facilitate the proliferation of platelet antigen-specific, CD4-positive, T-cell clones. These T-cell clones drive autoantibody production by platelet antigen-specific B-cell clones. As part of the platelet destructive process in ITP, cryptic epitopes from platelet antigens are exposed, leading to the formation of secondary platelet antigen-specific T-cell clones, with stimulation of new platelet antigen-specific B-cell clones and broadening of the immune response. The autoantibody profile of individual patients who have ITP reflects activity of polyclonal autoreactive B-cell clones derived by antigen-driven affinity selection and somatic mutation.

Although increased platelet destruction clearly plays a key role in the pathogenesis of ITP, it is now recognized that impaired platelet production also is important in many cases. In adults, as many as 40% of ITP cases may have reduced platelet turnover, reflecting the inhibitory effect of platelet autoantibodies on megakaryopoiesis [6]. Studies of platelet kinetics in

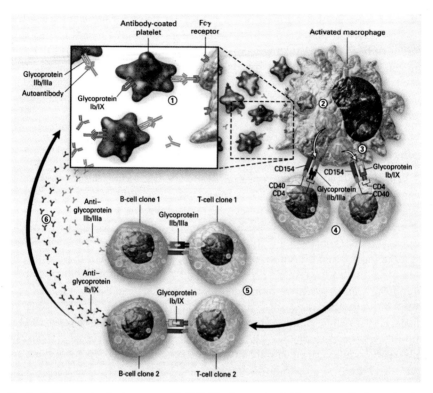

Fig. 1. Pathogenesis of epitope spread in ITP. The factors that initiate autoantibody production are unknown. Most patients have antibodies against several platelet-surface glycoproteins at the time the disease becomes clinically evident. Here, glycoprotein IIb/IIIa is recognized by auto-antibody (orange, inset), whereas antibodies that recognize the glycoprotein Ib/IX complex have not been generated at this stage (1). Antibody-coated platelets bind to antigen-presenting cells (macrophages or dendritic cells) through Fcγ receptors and then are internalized and degraded (2). Antigen-presenting cells not only degrade glycoprotein IIb/IIIa (light blue oval), thereby amplifying the initial immune response, but also may generate cryptic epitopes from other platelet glycoproteins (light blue cylinder) (3). Activated antigen-presenting cells (4) express these novel peptides on the cell surface along with costimulatory help (represented in part by the interaction between CD154 and CD40) and the relevant cytokines that facilitate the proliferation of the initiating CD4-positive T-cell clones (T-cell clone 1) and those with additional specificities (T-cell clone 2) (5). B-cell immunoglobulin receptors that recognize additional platelet antigens (B-cell clone 2) thereby also are induced to proliferate and synthesize antiglycoprotein Ib/IX antibodies (green) in addition to amplifying the production of anti-glycoprotein IIb/IIIa antibodies (orange) by B-cell clone 1 (6). (*From* Cines DB, Blanchette VS. Immune thrombocytopenic purpura. N Engl J Med 2002;346:995–1008; with permission. Copyright © 2002, Massachusetts Medical Society. All rights reserved.)

children who have ITP are limited but it is possible that a similar situation exists. There also is evidence that platelet autoantibodies may induce thrombocytopenia by inhibiting proplatelet formation [7]. Circulating thrombopoietin (TPO) levels in patients who have ITP typically are normal or increased only slightly, reflecting the normal or only slightly reduced TPO receptor mass in this acquired platelet disorder. In contrast, TPO levels are high in inherited platelet production disorders, such as thrombocytopenia-absent radii or congenital amegakaryocytic thrombocytopenia [8]. TPO testing generally is not available, but these observations have led to the question of whether or not TPO or molecules mimicking TPO may increase platelet production and be a new treatment strategy in ITP. Several such agents currently are in clinical trials.

Differential diagnosis

Primary ITP is a diagnosis of exclusion. The question, "When does a low platelet count not mean ITP?" is important, especially for atypical cases. When an unexpected low platelet count in a child is obtained, artifact or laboratory error should be considered first and excluded. Pseudothrombocytopenia is an example of spurious thrombocytopenia that is caused by platelet aggregation and clumping in the presence of ethylenediamine tetraacetic acid (EDTA) anticoagulant [9]. Examination of well-stained blood smears prepared from a venous blood sample collected separately into EDTA and 3.8% sodium citrate anticoagulant usually confirms or excludes pseudothrombocytopenia. A smear prepared from the collection tube with EDTA should demonstrate platelet clumping, whereas a smear prepared from the tube with sodium citrate should not. Some patients, however, have platelets that also clump in citrate anticoagulant.

A detailed history, careful physical examination, and results of selected tests confirm or eliminate common causes of secondary thrombocytopenia, such as SLE. A positive antinuclear antibody is common in children who have ITP and, as an isolated finding, does not confirm or exclude SLE [10]; more specific tests, such as an anti–double-stranded DNA test, should be ordered if a diagnosis of SLE-associated ITP is suspected. A transfusion history should be obtained in all cases and, depending on the age of the child, the history should include questioning about drug use (prescription and nonprescription) and sexual activity. If relevant, testing for antibodies to hepatitis C and HIV should be performed.

A detailed family history should be obtained in all cases. Especially in children who have apparent "chronic" ITP and isolated moderate thrombocytopenia, the possibility of an inherited thrombocytopenia should be considered. The topic, "inherited thrombocytopenia: when a low platelet count does not mean ITP," is the focus of an excellent review [11]. The inherited thrombocytopenias can be classified based on platelet size (large, normal, and small) and gene mutations. They include conditions, such as the MYH9-related macrothrombocytopenias, Wiskott-Aldrich syndrome (WAS), and rare conditions, such as gray platelet syndrome (Box 1). The pattern of inheritance (eg, X-linked in boys who have WAS) and abnormalities on peripheral blood smear (eg, Döhle-like inclusions in neutrophils of patients who have MYH9 disorders or pale agranular platelets in gray platelet syndrome) may provide

---

Box 1. Inherited thrombocytopenias classified by platelet size

Small platelets [MPV < 7 fL]
WAS
X-linked thrombocytopenia

Normal-sized platelets [MPV 7–11 fL]
Thrombocytopenia-absent radii
Congenital amegakaryocytic thrombocytopenia
Radioulnar synostosis and amegakaryocytic thrombocytopenia
Familial platelet disorder with associated myeloid malignancy

Large/giant platelets [MPV > 11 fL]
MYH9[a] syndromes
  • May-Hegglin anomaly
  • Fechtner syndrome
  • Epstein syndrome
  • Sebastian syndrome
Mediterranean thrombocytopenia
Bernard-Soulier syndrome
Velocardiofacial/DiGeorge syndrome
Paris-Trousseau thrombocytopenia/Jacobsen syndrome
Gray platelet syndrome

Abbreviation: MPV, mean platelet volume.
[a] MYH9 gene encodes for the nonmuscle myosin heavy-chain IIA.
Data from Drachman JG. Inherited thrombocytopenia: when a low platelet count does not mean ITP. Blood 2004;103:390–8.

---

important clues to the underlying disorder. Failure of patients who have apparent "chronic ITP" and moderate thrombocytopenia to respond to front-line platelet-enhancing therapies, such as high-dose intravenous (IV) immunoglobulin G (IVIG) or IV anti-D, should prompt consideration of an alternate diagnosis. Additional investigation in such cases should include screening for type 2B von Willebrand disease, pseudo–von Willebrand disease, and Bernard-Soulier syndrome. In males who have small platelets, WAS or X-linked thrombocytopenia should be considered. These latter conditions can be confirmed by screening for mutations in the WASP gene. Boys who have WASP gene mutations may have significant immunologic abnormalities.

Childhood acute immune thrombocytopenic purpura

Clinical and laboratory features

Thrombocytopenia for less than 6 months defines the entity acute ITP. Typically, children who have acute ITP are young, of previous good health, and present with sudden onset of bruising or a petechial rash. In a series of 2031 children who had newly diagnosed ITP, reported by Kühne and colleagues [12] in 2001 for the Intercontinental Childhood ITP Study Group (ICIS), the mean age at presentation was 5.7 years. Approximately 70% of the cohort were children ages 1 to 10 years with 10% of the cohort infants (older than 3 and less than 12 months old) and the remainder 20% older children (ages 10 to 16 years) [13]. Male and female children were affected approximately equally with the caveat that boys outnumbered girls in young children, especially those less than 1 year of age (Fig. 2) [12]. The predominance of boys who had ITP in children under 10 years of age is reported in several other studies [14–16]. In approximately two thirds of cases, the onset of acute ITP is preceded by an infectious illness, most often an upper respiratory tract infection; in a minority of cases, ITP follows a specific viral illness (rubella, varicella, mumps, rubeola, or infectious mononucleosis) or immunization with a live virus vaccine [17,18]. The risk for ITP after mumps-measles-rubella vaccine is estimated at approximately 1 in 25,000 doses [19]. In children who have acute ITP, the interval between the preceding infection and the onset of purpura varies from a few days to several weeks, with the most frequent interval approximately 2 weeks [20]. Physical examination at presentation is remarkable only for the cutaneous manifestations of severe thrombocytopenia with bruising or a petechial rash present in almost all cases (Table 1). Clinically significant lymphadenopathy or marked hepatosplenomegaly are atypical features; however, shotty cervical adenopathy is common in young children and a spleen tip may be palpable in 5% to 10% of cases [20,21]. Epistaxis (often minor, sometimes severe) is a presenting symptom in approximately one quarter of affected children; hematuria occurs less frequently [20].

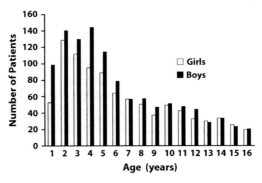

Fig. 2. Age (years) of children who had newly diagnosed ITP entered into the Intercontinental Childhood ITP Registry. (*From* Kühne T, Imbach P, Bolton-Maggs PHB, et al. Newly diagnosed idiopathic thrombocytopenic purpura in childhood: an observational study. Lancet 2001;358:2122–25; with permission.)

Table 1
Presenting features in children who have acute immune thrombocytopenic purpura

Investigator	Number of cases	Male:female ratio	Preceding infectious illness	Hemorrhagic manifestations		
				Purpura/ petechiae	Epistaxis	Hematuria
Choi (1950–1964)[a] [20]	239	117:122	119/239	235/239	76/239	20/239
Lusher (1956–1964) [21]	152	69:83	122/146	—	46/152	8/152
Blanchette (1974–1982) [22]	80	37:43	58/80	75/80	20/80	3/80
Bolton-Maggs (1995–1996) [14]	427	213:214	245/427	310/427	85/427	6/427
Total	898	436:462	544/892 (60.9%)	620/746 (83.1%)	227/898 (25.3%)	37/898 (4.1%)

[a] Years in parenthesis represent the period of observation.

The key laboratory finding in children who have acute ITP is isolated, and often severe, thrombocytopenia. In more than half of cases, platelet counts at presentation are less than $20 \times 10^9/L$ (Fig. 3). Other hematologic abnormalities are consistent with a diagnosis of childhood acute ITP only if they can be explained easily (eg, anemia secondary to epistaxis/

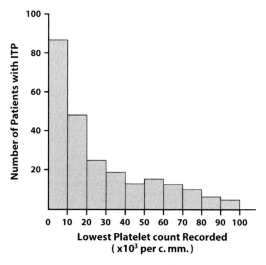

Fig. 3. Lowest platelet count observed in children who had ITP. (*From* Choi SI, McClure PD. Idiopathic thrombocytopenic purpura in childhood. Can Med Assoc J 1967;97:562–8; with permission. Copyright © 1967, Canadian Medical Association.)

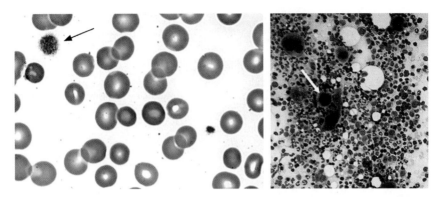

Fig. 4. Blood smear and bone marrow aspirate from a child who had ITP showing large plate-lets (blood smear [*left*]) and increased numbers of megakaryocytes, many of which appear im-mature (bone marrow aspirate [*right*]).

menorrhagia) or atypical lymphocytosis in cases of infectious mononucleo-sis. The one exception is mild eosinophilia, which is a common finding [21]. The blood smear shows a marked decrease in platelets with some platelets that are large (megathrombocytes) (Fig. 4). A bone marrow aspirate, if per-formed, typically shows normal to increased numbers of megakaryocytes, many of which are immature (see Fig. 4). An increase in the number of bone marrow eosinophil precursors is present in some cases.

Natural history of childhood acute immune thrombocytopenic purpura

The natural history of childhood acute ITP is well documented (reviewed by Blanchette and Carcao [22]). Complete remission, defined as a platelet count greater than $150 \times 10^9/L$ within 6 months of initial diagnosis and without the need for ongoing platelet-enhancing therapy, occurs in at least two thirds of cases. This excellent outcome seems independent of any man-agement strategy. As an example, in the prospective study reported by Kühne and colleagues [12], complete remission rates of 68%, 73%, and 66% were reported in children who received no treatment, IVIG, or cortico-steroids, respectively. These data are similar to the 76% complete remission rate reported by George and colleagues [5] on the basis of a review of 12 case series involving 1597 cases. A recent study of children from five Nordic stud-ies described a simple clinical score that predicts early remission [23]. If con-firmed, this could identify those children who might be left without active therapy for low platelet counts. Predictors of early remission were abrupt onset of illness, preceding infection, male gender, age under 10 years, wet purpura, and a platelet count less than $5 \times 10^9/L$.

The outcome for children who have acute ITP who continue to manifest thrombocytopenia beyond 6 months from initial presentation generally is good. Published reports suggest that as many as one third of such children have spontaneous remission of their illness from a few months to several years after initial diagnosis [5,24]. In one study, 61% was predicted at 15 years of follow-up [25]. Most spontaneous remissions occur early, and the number of children who have severe thrombocytopenia (platelet counts $<20 \times 10^9/L$) and who are symptomatic with bleeding symptoms and, therefore, are therapy dependent more than 1 year after initial diagnosis is small. In a Swiss-Canadian retrospective analysis of 554 children who had newly diagnosed ITP and platelet counts less than $20 \times 10^9/L$, the percentages of children who had platelet counts less than $20 \times 10^9/L$ at 6, 12, 18, and 24 months after diagnosis were 9%, 6%, 4%, and 3%, respectively (Fig. 5) [26]. This is the small subgroup of children for whom splenectomy ultimately may need to be considered.

The case for treatment of children who have acute ITP relates to those who have significant bleeding and consideration of the very small, but finite, risk for intracranial hemorrhage (ICH). The risk of this feared complication was 0.9% in a series of 1693 children reviewed by George and colleagues [5]. This figure, however, probably is an overestimate reflecting that reports in the literature mainly are from academic centers that likely are referred the most severe cases. Based on data in the United Kingdom, Lilleyman has estimated an incidence of 0.2% of ICH in children who have newly diagnosed ITP [27], a figure consistent with the 0.17% incidence rate (3 of 1742 children who had newly diagnosed acute ITP) reported by Kühne and colleagues [13] on behalf of the ICIS.

Whatever the true incidence of ICH in children who have acute ITP, there is no doubt that this event is a devastating and sometimes fatal complication in this generally benign childhood disorder. The percent of cases of ICH occurring within 4 weeks of initial diagnosis varied from 19% to 50%

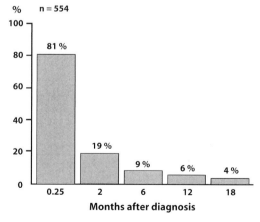

Fig. 5. Percentage of children (n = 554) who had ITP and platelet counts below $20 \times 10^9/L$ at 1 week, 2, 6, 12, and 18 months after diagnosis of acute ITP. Swiss-Canadian retrospective analysis. (*From* Imbach P, Akatsuka J, Blanchette V, et al. Immunthrombocytopenic purpura as a model for pathogenesis and treatment of autoimmunity. Eur J Pediatr 1995;154(Suppl 3): S60–4; with permission.)

in different reports [5,27,28]; in one retrospective review, 10% (7/69) of cases of ICH occurred within 3 days of diagnosis of ITP [29]. Trauma to the head and use of antiplatelet drugs, such as aspirin, were identified as risk factors for ICH in children who had ITP and very low platelet counts [30].

Unfortunately, a prospective randomized controlled trial to determine definitively whether or not therapeutic intervention can decrease the incidence of ICH significantly in children who have newly diagnosed ITP and platelet counts below $20 \times 10^9/L$ is not feasible, because of the large numbers of cases required to ensure a statistically significant outcome. Physicians who care for children who have acute ITP, therefore, must act in the best interest of each child without the benefit of definitive data. Because of the significant morbidity and mortality associated with ICH and the availability of highly effective platelet-enhancing therapies, some recommend that families of young children who have newly diagnosed acute ITP at risk for ICH (who have platelet counts $<10 \times 10^9/L$) be offered the option of treatment using the minimum therapy necessary to increase the platelet count rapidly to a safe, hemostatic level. There is no current evidence, however, that such a management strategy significantly reduces the incidence of ICH in children who have ITP, although intuitively this seems probable.

In addition, there is evidence to suggest that the rate of platelet response to frontline therapies (corticosteroids or IVIG) in the subset of children who have ITP and clinically significant hemorrhage is suboptimal [31]. Discussion with parents and children, if of appropriate age, should include consideration of best available evidence with regard to the three key issues: (1) to treat or not to treat (2) to perform a bone marrow aspirate or not and (3) to hospitalize or not.

To treat or not to treat

Observation

The case for observation of children who have acute ITP rests with the knowledge that acute ITP is, for the majority of affected children, a benign self-limiting disorder, usually with mild clinical symptoms and has a low risk for serious bleeding (approximately 3% with ICH being rare) and the fact that there are no prospective studies that clearly indicate a decrease in the incidence of ICH associated with treatment [32]. Several children who had ITP-associated ICH were receiving platelet-enhancing therapy at the time of the hemorrhage [28]. In addition, all treatments suffer from the disadvantage of side effects, which can be severe.

Guidelines for initial management of children who have acute ITP have been published and reflect the ongoing debate, "to treat or not to treat" [5,33–36]. Recommendations from the Working Party of the British Committee for Standards in Haematology General Haematology Task Force state that treatment of children who have acute ITP should be decided on the basis of clinical symptoms in addition to cutaneous signs, not the platelet count alone [36]. The Working Party considered it appropriate to manage children who have acute ITP and mild clinical disease expectantly, with supportive advice, and a 24-hour contact point irrespective of the platelet count. Based on these guidelines, intervention is reserved for the few children who have overt hemorrhage and platelet counts below $20 \times 10^9/L$ or those who have organ- or life-threatening bleeding irrespective of the circulating platelet count [34,36]. Many clinicians in Europe manage children who have ITP expectantly (ie, without medication to increase the platelet count) because of the rapid remissions in most cases, the low risk for bleeding, and toxicities of currently available medical therapies. Data are reported from the United Kingdom and Germany promoting the use of advice and support to children and their families during the usually short duration of the illness [15,32,37].

Corticosteroids

The corticosteroid treatment regimen used to treat children who have newly diagnosed ITP in most reported studies, and worldwide, is oral prednisone at a dose of 1 to 2 mg/kg per day given in divided doses and continued for a few weeks. Two randomized studies support the benefit of corticosteroid therapy in children who have ITP. In the first study, conducted by Sartorius [38] and reported in 1984, 73 children ages 10 months to 14 years who had newly diagnosed ITP were randomized to receive oral prednisolone (60 mg/m^2 per day for 21 days) or a placebo. Platelet responses were significantly faster in the corticosteroid-treated group, with 90% of children achieving a platelet count of $30 \times 10^9/L$ within the first 10 days of treatment compared with 45% of children in the placebo no-treatment group. The Rumpel-Leede test, which measures capillary resistance (blood vessel integrity), became negative sooner in the corticosteroid-treated group. In the second study, reported by Buchanan and Holtkamp [39] in 1984, 27 children who had acute ITP were randomized to receive oral prednisone (2 mg/kg per day for 14 days, with tapering and discontinuation of corticosteroids by day 21) or placebo. Although there was a definite trend in favor of corticosteroids, only on day 7 of therapy did the prednisone-treated patients have significantly higher platelet counts, lower bleeding scores, and shorter bleeding times than children receiving placebo. Taken together, these two studies suggest limited early benefit from conventional dose oral corticosteroid therapy in children who have acute ITP.

The risks and benefits of high-dose corticosteroid therapy administered orally or IV to children who have acute ITP merit discussion. In a study of 20 children randomized to receive oral megadose methylprednisolone (30 mg/kg for 3 days followed by 20 mg/kg for 4 days) or IVIG (0.4 g/kg $\times$ 5 days), Özsoylu and colleagues [40] reported that 80% of children in both groups had platelet counts greater than $50 \times 10^9/L$ by 72 hours after the start of treatment. Corticosteroids were given before 9:00 AM and adverse effects were not observed. In contrast, Suarez and colleagues [41] reported that hyperactivity and behavioral problems occurred in 5 of 9 children who had acute ITP given 6 to 8 mg/kg per day of oral prednisone for 3 days or until platelet counts had increased to $20 \times 10^9/L$. Immediate platelet responses with this regimen were impressive: the mean time to achieve a platelet count of $20 \times 10^9/L$ was 1.9 ± 0.6 days (range 1–3 days).

A commonly used high-dose corticosteroid regimen is that reported by van Hoff and Ritchey [42]. The investigators treated 21 consecutive children who had ITP using IV methylprednisolone (30 mg/kg, maximum dose 1 g) given daily for 3 days. The median time to achieving a platelet count greater than $20 \times 10^9/L$ was 24 hours. Ten children (48%) had transient glycosuria but no cases of hyperglycemia were observed. Similar results were reported by Jayabose and colleagues [43], who treated 20 children who had acute ITP with IV methylprednisolone (5 mg/kg per day in four divided doses). By 48 hours from start of treatment, 90% of children had platelet counts greater than $20 \times 10^9/L$, and all children achieved this hemostatic threshold by 72 hours from the start of treatment. No patients developed symptomatic hyperglycemia or hypertension; the investigators did not comment about weight gain or mood/behavioral changes. The authors' experience with short-course oral prednisone (4 mg/kg per day $\times$ 4 days without tapering) is complementary. Eighty-three percent of children who had acute ITP and platelet counts less than $20 \times 10^9/L$ achieved a platelet count above $20 \times 10^9/L$ within 48 hours of starting corticosteroid therapy (Fig. 6) [44].

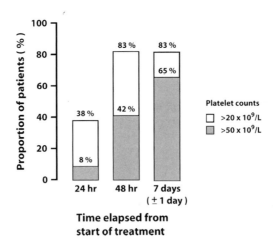

Fig. 6. Platelet response to short-course oral prednisone (4 mg kg^{-1} d^{-1} for 4 d) among 25 children who had acute ITP. (*From* Carcao MD, Zipursky A, Butchart S, et al. Short-course oral prednisone therapy in children presenting with acute immune thrombocytopenic purpura (ITP). Acta Paediatr Suppl 1998;424:71–4; with permission.)

On the basis of these studies, it can be concluded that a clinically significant increment in platelet count can be achieved rapidly in the majority of children who have acute ITP after the administration of high-doses of corticosteroids (approximately 4 mg/kg per day of prednisone or an equivalent corticosteroid preparation) administered orally or parenterally. The frequency and severity of corticosteroid toxicity relates to dose and duration of therapy and merits further study. If a decision is made to use corticosteroid therapy for children who have acute ITP, it seems wise to use high-dose corticosteroid regimens for as short a period of time as is necessary to achieve a clinically meaningful endpoint (eg, cessation of bleeding or achievement of a platelet count $>20 \times 10^9/L$). This approach minimizes the predictable, and sometimes serious, adverse effects of long-term corticosteroid therapy (reviewed by Beck and colleagues [45]). A fall in platelet count often occurs during the period of tapering corticosteroids but not usually to clinically significant levels.

Intravenous immunoglobulin G

Imbach and colleagues [46] first reported that IV infusion of a pooled, largely monomeric IgG preparation produced a rapid reversal of thrombocytopenia in children who had acute and chronic ITP. This landmark observation was confirmed subsequently by several investigators (reviewed by Blanchette and Carcao [22]). Transient blockade of Fc receptors on macrophages in the reticuloendothelial system, especially the spleen, is believed to play a major role in the immediate, and often dramatic, platelet responses observed after treatment of children who have ITP using a high dose of IVIG (1–2 g/kg). Two Canadian prospective randomized clinical trials are instructive in the context of IVIG treatment of children who have acute ITP. In the first study, reported by Blanchette and colleagues [47] in 1993, 53 children who had acute ITP and platelet counts less than $20 \times 10^9/L$ were randomized to receive IVIG (1 g/kg on 2 consecutive days), oral prednisone (4 mg/kg per day $\times$ 7 days with tapering and discontinuation by day 21), or expectant management (no treatment). The rate of platelet response was significantly faster in children who received treatment compared with those managed expectantly; for the endpoint of time (days) taken to achieve a platelet count greater than or equal to $20 \times 10^9/L$, IVIG and corticosteroids were equivalent, whereas IVIG was superior to oral corticosteroid therapy for the endpoint of time (days) taken to achieve a platelet count greater than $50 \times 10^9/L$. Bleeding symptoms were not recorded in this study, however; the platelet count alone was used as a surrogate marker for response. The follow-up Canadian randomized trial compared two IVIG treatment regimens (1 g/kg on 2 consecutive days and 0.8 g/kg once), oral prednisone (4 mg/kg per day for 7 days with tapering and discontinuation by day 21), and for the subset of children who were blood group rhesus (D) positive, IV anti-D (25 µg/kg on 2 consecutive days) [48]. The key

findings from this second randomized trial in children who had newly diagnosed ITP and platelet counts less than $20 \times 10^9/L$ were (1) a single dose of
IVIG (0.8 g/kg) was as effective as the larger dose of IVIG 1 g/kg for 2 days
in raising the platelet count and (2) both IVIG regimens were superior to IV
anti-D administered as 25 μg/kg for 2 days for the clinically important
endpoint of time (number of days) to achieve a platelet count greater than
or equal to $20 \times 10^9/L$. Bleeding symptoms were not recorded in the study.
The choice of the 0.8 g/kg dose as a single infusion reflected the early observation by Imbach and colleagues [49] that in children who had acute ITP
treated with 0.4 g/kg of IVIG daily for 5 consecutive days, platelet responses
often were observed after the first two infusions. These studies show that
treatment with corticosteroids or IVIG can produce a rapid rise in the platelet count of children who have ITP with the caveat that the effect on bleeding symptoms was not assessed. As a result of these observations, the
authors recommend that if a decision is made to treat children who have
newly diagnosed ITP with IVIG, the initial dose should be 0.8 to 1.0 g/kg
administered as a single infusion with subsequent IVIG doses given based
on the clinical situation and follow-up platelet counts. Reflex administration
of a second dose of IVIG (ie, a total dose of 2 g/kg) generally is not necessary and for the majority of children only leads to an increased frequency of
adverse side effects (eg, headache, nausea, or vomiting) and higher costs.

It generally is accepted that IVIG therapy in children who have ITP,
although expensive, is safe. High doses (2 g/kg), however, frequently are
associated with side effects, principally fever and headache [47]. Other uncommon but clinically significant treatment-associated adverse effects include
neutropenia and hemolytic anemia caused by alloantibodies in the IVIG preparations and self-limiting aseptic meningitis that generally occurs a few days
after IVIG therapy. This latter complication is characterized by severe headache and, for the subset of children who still are significantly thrombocytopenic, often prompts investigation with a CT scan to rule out an ICH. On
a reassuring note, although IVIG is a human plasma–derived product, current commercially available IVIG preparations are treated with highly effective measures to inactivate lipid-coated viruses, such as HIV and hepatitis C.

Intravenous anti-D

In 1983, Salama and colleagues [50] reported that the IV infusion of anti-D
resulted in the reversal of thrombocytopenia in patients who had ITP and
were rhesus (D) positive. The investigators speculated that the beneficial
effect of anti-D was due to the competitive inhibition of reticuloendothelial
function by preferential sequestration of immunoglobulin-coated autologous
red blood cells (RBCs). These observations subsequently were confirmed by
several investigators. In a report that detailed experience with IV anti-D treatment in 272 subjects who had ITP, Scaradavou and colleagues [51] documented several important findings, including (1) anti-D at conventional

doses is ineffective in splenectomized subjects; (2) platelet responses are significantly better in children compared with adults; and (3) responders to IV anti-D generally respond on retreatment. There was a trend toward a higher platelet count after therapy in patients who received 40 to 60 μg/kg of IV anti-D compared with those who received less than or equal to 40 μg/kg. The dose response to IV anti-D is of importance. A recent report by Tarantino and colleagues [52], describing the results of a prospective randomized clinical trial of IV anti-D (50 μg/kg and 75 μg/kg) and IVIG (0.8 g/kg) in 101 children who had acute ITP and platelet counts less than $20 \times 10^9/L$, clearly established that IV anti-D (75 μg/kg) is superior to IV anti-D (50 μg/kg) and equivalent to IVIG (0.8 g/kg) with respect to the numbers of cases with platelet counts greater than $20 \times 10^9/L$ at 24 hours after therapy.

Short-term adverse effects, such as fever, chills, and nausea/vomiting, are more frequent with a 75-μg/kg than a 50-μg/kg dose and are likely related to release of pro-inflammatory cytokines/chemokines after IV anti-D [53]. These side effects can be ameliorated/prevented by premedication of patients with acetaminophen/corticosteroids. The most predictable adverse effect of anti-D therapy in subjects who are rhesus (D) positive is a fall in hemoglobin level due to RBC destruction by infused RBC alloantibodies. The fall in hemoglobin occurs within 1 week of the anti-D therapy with recovery generally evident by day 21. In the Scaradavou study, the mean hemoglobin decrease was 0.8 g/dL at 7 days post IV anti-D treatment, and only 16% of cases had a hemoglobin decrease greater than 2.1 g/dL [51]. In occasional cases, abrupt severe intravascular hemolysis is reported after therapy; the majority of these cases were in adults, some of whom had comorbid diseases [54]. This complication also is reported in rare cases after IVIG therapy. Physicians who treat children who have ITP using anti-D should be aware of this complication and advise parents and children to report symptoms and signs, such as excessive tiredness or pallor or passage of dark (tea-colored) urine, promptly. No clinically significant increase in treatment-related hemolysis has been reported with 75 versus 50 μg/kg of IV anti-D, and a single dose of 75 μg/kg of anti-D now can be recommended as standard dosing for the treatment of children who have acute ITP and are rhesus (D) positive.

To perform a bone marrow aspirate or not

There is consensus that bone marrow aspiration is not necessary for children who have newly diagnosed typical acute ITP if management involves observation or plasma based therapies, such as IVIG or anti-D. The contentious issue is whether or not a bone marrow aspirate should be performed in children who have typical acute ITP before starting corticosteroids to avoid missing, and therefore treating inappropriately, an underlying leukemia. The results of a retrospective study of bone marrow aspirates performed in children who have suspected acute ITP are instructive in this regard [55]. No children who had typical laboratory features, defined as a normal hemoglobin level and total white blood cell and neutrophil count for age, had underlying leukemia; cases of leukemia, however, were observed in children who had atypical laboratory features. A bone marrow examination, therefore, should be considered mandatory in atypical cases of childhood acute ITP, defined as those who have lassitude, protracted fever, bone or joint pain, and unexplained anemia, neutropenia, or macrocytosis. The diagnosis should be questioned, particularly in those children who fail to remit. The most common diagnosis to emerge after isolated thrombocytopenia in a well child is aplastic anemia.

To hospitalize or not

The majority of children who have newly diagnosed acute ITP and platelet counts less than $20 \times 10^9/L$ are hospitalized. The figure was 83% in the first United Kingdom National Survey [14] and 78% of 1995 children who had newly diagnosed ITP reported by Kühne and colleagues [12] on behalf of the ICIS. This high hospitalization rate is driven by the decision to treat and the perceived need for a bone marrow aspirate before starting corticosteroid therapy. If a conservative management approach is used, with bone marrow aspiration and treatment reserved for selected cases only (eg, those with atypical features or clinically significant bleeding), a low rate of hospitalization can be achieved [37]. Outpatient infusion of IVIG or anti-D also is an option in selected cases.

Chronic immune thrombocytopenic purpura

Conventionally, chronic ITP is defined as thrombocytopenia (platelet count less than $150 \times 10^9/L$) persisting for longer than 6 months from the onset of illness. Using this definition, approximately 20% to 25% of children manifest chronic ITP at 6 months after the initial diagnosis of ITP. Many children who have platelet counts in the range of 30 to $150 \times 10^9/L$, however, require no platelet-enhancing therapy and some enter a spontaneous complete remission in the 6 to 24 months after initial presentation [24]. The clinically important subgroup of children is those who have platelet counts less than or equal to $20 \times 10^9/L$ at 6 months from initial diagnosis and who require ongoing platelet-enhancing therapy because of bleeding symptoms. This is the small group of children for whom second-line therapies (eg, rituximab) or splenectomy may need to be considered, approximately 5% of children who have acute ITP at the time point of 18 months after initial presentation [26].

Management

Presplenectomy management

Medical management is preferred over splenectomy for children who have chronic ITP for less than 12 months. Treatment options include oral corticosteroids (including pulse oral dexamethasone), IVIG, and IV anti-D (reviewed by Blanchette and Price [56]). Avoidance of medications known to affect platelet function adversely, especially aspirin, should be stressed and high-risk competitive or contact activities should be avoided during periods of severe thrombocytopenia. The goal should be to maintain a hemostatically "safe" platelet count while avoiding the potential toxicities and cost of overtreatment, in particular the well-known adverse effects of protracted corticosteroid therapy. If treatment is recommended, the authors' preference is to use short courses of relatively high-dose oral prednisone (4 mg/kg per day for 4 days, maximum daily dose 180 mg), IVIG (0.8 to 1.0 g/kg once), or, for children who are rhesus (D) positive, IV anti-D (75 µg/kg once), with all treatments given intermittently based on clinical need. Treatment is, in the main, outpatient based and parents and children (if of an appropriate age) should be informed about the risk, benefits, and alternatives to treatment, including the remote risk for transfusion-transmitted infections with virus-inactivated plasma-based therapies, such as IVIG and IV anti-D. The advantage of anti-D over IVIG in this clinical setting relates to the ease of administration (anti-D can be infused over 5–10 minutes compared with several hours for IVIG), significantly lower cost in some countries, and a comparable platelet-enhancing effect.

Splenectomy

Guidelines for splenectomy in children who have ITP are conservative, reflecting the significant spontaneous remissions that occur in children who have early chronic ITP and the small but finite risk of overwhelming postsplenectomy sepsis, a complication especially worrisome in children under 6 years of age. A group of United Kingdom pediatric hematologists recommended in 1992 that in children who have ITP, "splenectomy should not be considered before at least six months and preferably 12 months from the time of diagnosis, unless there are very major problems" [33]. New guidelines published in 2003 state that splenectomy rarely is indicated in children who have ITP but comment that "severe lifestyle restrictions, crippling menorrhagia and life-threatening hemorrhage may give good reason for the procedure" [36]. Practice guidelines developed for the American Society of Hematology (ASH) advocate that elective splenectomy be considered in children who have persistence of ITP for at least 12 months and who manifest bleeding symptoms and a platelet count below 10×10^9/L (children ages 3 to 12) or 10 to 30×10^9/L (children ages 8 to 12 years) [5]. Only a few scenarios were considered, however. The efficacy and relative safety of splenectomy led Mantadakis and Buchanan [57] to recommend splenectomy for children older than 5 years who have had symptomatic ITP longer than 6 months' duration and whose quality of life is affected adversely by hemorrhagic manifestations, constant fear of bleeding, or complication of medical therapies. In contrast, the Israeli ITP Study Group recommends early splenectomy in children not responding rapidly to corticosteroid therapy [58]. This seems premature as many children likely remit spontaneously given time.

If elective splenectomy is performed, the laparoscopic technique is preferred; accessory spleens often are present and should be removed at the time of surgical intervention. Preoperative treatment with corticosteroids, IVIG, or anti-D is considered appropriate for children who have platelet counts less than $30 \times 10^9/L$. The outcome after splenectomy in children who have primary ITP is good, and a complete remission rate of approximately 70% can be expected after the procedure (Table 2). Some of the children reported in these series, however, may have entered a spontaneous remission over time without splenectomy. In adults, potential predictors of success after splenectomy include imaging studies to document the sites of platelet destruction and the historical response to medical therapies, such as IVIG and IV anti-D [63–65]. The results of imaging studies are insufficiently specific, however, and reports of the predictive value of prior responses to medical therapies too conflicting to recommend that this information be used to determine reliably whether or not a splenectomy should be performed in children who have chronic ITP.

Protection against overwhelming postsplenectomy infection

Before elective splenectomy, children who have ITP should be immunized with the hemophilus influenza type b and pneumococcal vaccines; depending on their age and immunization history, meningococcal vaccine also is recommended [66]. Because the protection provided after immunization is incomplete (not all pneumococcal serotypes are included in the currently available vaccines), daily prophylaxis with penicillin, or an equivalent antibiotic if the child is allergic to penicillin, is recommended for children up to 5 years of age and for at least 1 year after splenectomy to prevent pneumococcal sepsis, in particular. Some physicians recommend continuing antibiotic prophylaxis into adulthood. All febrile episodes should be assessed carefully and the use of parenteral antibiotics considered because overwhelming postsplenectomy

Table 2
Complete remission rates after splenectomy in children who had immune thrombocytopenic purpura

	Number of cases	Complete remission (%)
ASH review [5]	271	72
Blanchette (1992) [59]	21	81
Ben Yehuda (1994) [58]	27	67
Mantadakis (2000) [57]	38	76
Aronis (2004) [60]	33	79
Kühne (2006) [61]	134	67
Wang (2006) [62]	65	89
	589	74

infection can occur despite immunization and use of antibiotic prophylaxis. Children should wear a medical alert bracelet indicating that they have had a splenectomy and when traveling abroad should carry an explanatory letter and a supply of antibiotics to be started in the event of a febrile episode while arranging for medical assessment. In the United Kingdom, patients are issued with a card stating that they are asplenic.

Emergency treatment

On rare occasions, children who have acute ITP and severe thrombocytopenia may manifest symptoms or signs suggestive of organ- or life-threatening hemorrhage (eg, ICH). Management of such cases is challenging and should involve measures that have the potential to increase the circulating platelet count rapidly. An approach commonly used involves the immediate IV administration of methylprednisolone (30 mg/kg, maximum dose 1 g) over 20 to 30 minutes plus a larger than usual (two- to threefold) infusion of donor platelets in an attempt to boost the circulating platelet count temporarily. After administration of IV methylprednisolone and platelets, an infusion of IVIG (1 g/kg) should be started with IVIG and methylprednisolone repeated daily as indicated clinically, generally for at least 1 to 2 days. Survival of transfused donor platelets may be improved after IVIG therapy [67]. Depending on the specific clinical circumstances, an emergency splenectomy may need to be considered. Continuous infusion of platelets may be beneficial in selected cases. Experience with recombinant factor VIIa is limited but this hemostatic agent can be administered rapidly and should be considered in critical situations [68].

Combined cytopenias

The combination of ITP and clinically significant autoimmune hemolytic anemia (Evans's syndrome) or autoimmune neutropenia occurs in a minority of cases [69–73]. Affected children often are older than those who present with typical acute ITP. The clinical course is variable and often prolonged

Table 3
Retrospective reviews of patients who had Evans's syndrome

Investigator	Number of cases	Median age at onset (y)	Male:female ratio	Associated neutropenia	Number of deaths
Wang (1988) [69]	10	7.5	6:4	50%	3/10
Savaşan (1997) [70]	11	5.5	10:1	55%	4/11
Matthew (1997) [71]	42	7.7	22:20	38%	3/42
Blouin (2005) [72]	36	4.0	20:16	27%	3/36
	99		58:41	37%	13/99 (13.1%)

with significant morbidity and mortality reported in retrospective series (Table 3). Response to single-agent therapy or splenectomy often is poor [74]; combination immunosuppressive therapy may yield improved results [74–77]. Underlying causes for the combined cytopenias include SLE, CVID, and the autoimmune lymphoproliferative syndrome (ALPS). Malignancies (eg, Hodgkin's disease and lymphomas) and chronic infections (eg, HIV and hepatitis C) also need to be considered. The possibility of these conditions should be kept in mind in children who have combined immune cytopenias and appropriate investigations performed.

Features of CVID include recurrent bacterial infections (especially sinopulmonary), gastrointestinal disturbances similar to those seen in children who have inflammatory bowel disease, and granulomatous disease, especially affecting the lungs [78–82]. Laboratory features include low serum IgG levels and in some cases low serum IgA and IgM levels, absent or impaired specific antibody responses to infection or vaccination, and variable abnormalities of the immune system (eg, decreased numbers or function of T and B cells). Approximately 10% to 20% of subjects who have CVID manifest autoimmune cytopenias [79]. Treatment consists of regular IVIG replacement therapy [82]. Caution should be exercised about performing splenectomy in cases of CVID-associated ITP because of the risk for overwhelming postsplenectomy infection.

ALPS is a rare but important disorder because of defects in programmed cell death of lymphocytes [83–87]. Mutations in the Fas receptor, Fas ligand, and caspase genes are identified in approximately 70% of cases. Clinical features of the disorder include massive lymphadenopathy, most often in the cervical and axillary areas, and hepatosplenomegaly. The laboratory hallmark of ALPS is an increased number of double-negative (CD4-negative and CD8-negative) T cells that express the α/β T-cell receptor. Defective in vitro antigen-induced apoptosis in cultured lymphocytes can be demonstrated in affected cases. For accurate diagnosis of ALPS, these tests should be performed by laboratories familiar with the test methods and in which local normal values are established [88]. The best frontline treatment of patients who have ALPS is with mycophenolate mofetil (MMF); in the largest series of ALPS reported to date of treatment with this immunosuppressive agent, a response rate of 92% was observed [89]. Splenectomy should be avoided in ALPS cases because of the high risk for overwhelming postsplenectomy sepsis.

New therapies

First-line therapies in children include corticosteroids, high-dose IVIG, and, for children who are rhesus positive, IV anti-D. Splenectomy is the traditional second-line treatment of those children who have well-established, symptomatic chronic ITP who have failed or are intolerant of first-line therapies. An array of third-line therapies is available for children in whom splenectomy is refused or contraindicated. Agents include azathioprine, cyclophosphamide, danazol, vinca alkaloids, dapsone, cyclosporine, MMF, or combination therapy. As with adults, current evidence supporting effectiveness and safety of these therapies in children who have severe chronic refractory ITP is minimal [5,90]. The decision to choose one of these agents or combinations usually is based on physician preferences and experience. A major difficulty with many of these third-line therapies is modest response rates and frequently a slow onset of action. In addition, bone marrow suppression and an increased incidence of infection complicate treatment with many of the immunosuppressive agents. Before physicians can confidently know the best management for their patients, these treatments, and perhaps combinations of agents and new approaches to treatment, must be evaluated for effectiveness and safety in prospective cohort studies of consecutive patients or randomized controlled trials. Such trials should include measurement of relevant clinical outcomes (eg, bleeding manifestations and quality of life) other than the platelet count alone [90].

Rituximab is a human murine (chimeric) monoclonal antibody directed against the CD20 antigen expressed on pre-B and mature B lymphocytes. Rituximab eliminates most circulating B cells with recovery of B-cell counts 6 to 12 months after therapy. Rituximab currently is indicated for the treatment of lymphoma in adults. Because of its ability to deplete autoantibody-producing lymphocytes, it is used off-label to treat patients who have a variety of autoimmune diseases. Experience with rituximab therapy for patients who have ITP is greatest for adults. In a recent systematic review that involved 313 patients from 19 studies, Arnold and colleagues [91] reported a complete response rate, defined as a platelet count greater than 150×10^9/L, in 43.6% of cases (95% CI, 29.5% to 57.7%); 62.5% of cases (95% CI, 52.6% to 72.5%) achieved platelet counts greater than 50×10^9/L. The treatment regimen used most frequently was 375 mg/m^2 administered weekly for 4 weeks. The median time to response was 5.5 weeks and the median response duration 10.5 months. Durable responses were more frequent in patients who achieved complete remission. The largest pediatric series reported data including 36 patients, ages 2.6 to 18.3 years, six of whom had Evans's syndrome [92]. Responses, defined as a platelet count greater than 50×10^9/L during 4 consecutive weeks starting in weeks 9 to 12 after 4 weekly doses of rituximab (375 mg/m^2 per dose), were observed in 31% of cases (CI, 16% to 48%). In adults who had chronic ITP, durable responses lasting longer than 1 year were more likely in complete responders, and these patients also were more likely to respond to retreatment after relapse [93,94]. Although these results are promising, there is an urgent need for randomized control trials to define the role of rituximab as a splenectomy-sparing strategy or as treatment of patients who fail splenectomy and who have severe, symptomatic ITP. Clinically severe, short- and medium-term adverse effects after rituximab therapy for patients who have ITP fortunately are rare. They include therapy-associated serum sickness, immediate and delayed neutropenia, and reactivation of coexisting chronic infections (eg, hepatitis B) [95,96]. The recent report of two patients who had SLE who developed progressive multifocal leukoencephalopathy after rituximab therapy prompted an alert from the Food and Drug Administration's MedWatch Program [96]. Although changes in circulating immunoglobulin levels are observed in some children after rituximab therapy, it seems that IVIG replacement therapy for otherwise healthy pediatric patients who have ITP and who do not have underlying immunodeficiency treated with rituximab is unnecessary [92].

TPO is the primary growth factor in regulation of platelet production [97]. Megakaryopoiesis is controlled by signaling through the c-Mpl receptor present on megakaryocytes and platelets. On the basis that platelet production is impaired in some patients who have ITP, studies evaluated the use of a pegylated, truncated form of human TPO (PEG-megakaryocyte growth and development factor [MGDF]) with encouraging results. PEG-MGDF was immunogenic and induced production of neutralizing anti-TPO antibodies in some recipients, resulting in thrombocytopenia [98]. It was withdrawn, therefore, from further clinical investigation. Recently, nonimmunogenic thrombopoietic peptides (AMG 531) and small nonpeptide molecules (eltrombopag and AKR-501) have been developed [99] (reviewed by Kuter [100]). AMG 531 consists of a peptide-binding domain, which stimulates megakaryopoiesis in the same way as TPO, and a carrier Fc domain. AMG 531 activates c-Mpl receptors to stimulate the growth and maturation of megakaryocytes and this effect ultimately results in increased production of platelets. Preliminary studies with AMG 531 in adults who have ITP are encouraging [101,102]. A prospective pediatric study is underway. Eltrombopag and AKR-501 are small-molecule thrombopoietic receptor agonists administered orally [99]. Early results with eltrombopag in adults who have ITP also are encouraging [103]. Apart from reversible marrow fibrosis in some adult patients treated with AMG 531, these novel platelet-enhancing therapies seem remarkably nontoxic. Their true place in the management of children who have ITP remains to be determined through prospective clinical trials. It should be borne in mind that, based on experience in adults, recurrence of thrombocytopenia in cases of chronic, refractory ITP is likely in most cases once these novel thrombopoiesis-stimulating agents are discontinued.

Future directions

Although much has been learned about the pathogenesis and treatment of ITP over the past 3 decades, many questions remain unanswered. Optimal management of children who have newly diagnosed acute ITP and platelet counts less than 20×10^9/L remains the subject of debate and there is an urgent need for a well-designed large trial to address the issues of to treat or not, to perform a bone marrow aspirate or not, and whether or not to hospitalize such children. Experience from the United Kingdom suggests that promotion of conservative guidelines for management of childhood acute ITP can result in a decrease in the frequency of treatment and invasive procedures, such as bone marrow aspirates [104]. The role of new therapies, such as rituximab and thrombopoietic agents, remains to be defined by well-designed, prospective clinical trials. All future clinical trials for childhood ITP should include outcome measures more than the platelet count alone (eg, bleeding scores, health-related quality-of-life assessments, and economic analyses) [105–111]. Finally, exchange of information between adult and pediatric hematologists who care for patients who have ITP must be encouraged, especially with regard to guidelines for investigation and management [112].

References

[1] Cines DB, Blanchette VS. Immune thrombocytopenic purpura. N Engl J Med 2002;346: 995–1008.

[2] Harrington WJ, Minnich V, Hollingsworth JW, et al. Demonstration of a thrombocytopenic factor in the blood of patients with thrombocytopenic purpura. J Lab Clin Med 1951;38: 1–10.

[3] Shulman NR, Marder VJ, Weinrach RS. Similarities between known antiplatelet antibodies and the factor responsible for thrombocytopenia in idiopathic purpura. Physiologic, serologic and isotopic studies. Ann N Y Acad Sci 1965;124:499–542.

[4] Berchtold P, Muller D, Beardsley D, et al. International study to compare antigen-specific methods used for the measurement of antiplatelet autoantibodies. Br J Haematol 1997;96: 477–83.

[5] George JN, Woolf SH, Raskob GE, et al. Idiopathic thrombocytopenic purpura: a practice guideline developed by explicit methods for the American Society of Hematology. Blood 1996;88:3–40.

[6] Louwes H, Lathori OAZ, Vellenga E, et al. Platelet kinetic studies in patients with idiopathic thrombocytopenic purpura. Am J Med 1999;106:430–4.

[7] Takahashi R, Sekine N, Nakatake T. Influence of monoclonal antiplatelet glycoprotein antibodies on in vitro human megakaryocyte colony formation and proplatelet formation. Blood 1999;93:1951–8.

[8] Cremer M, Schulze H, Linthorst G, et al. Serum levels of thrombopoietin, IL-11, and IL-6 in pediatric thrombocytopenias. Ann Hematol 1999;78:401–7.

[9] Payne BA, Pierre RV. Pseudothrombocytopenia: a laboratory artifact with potentially serious consequences. Mayo Clin Proc 1984;59:123–5.

[10] Lowe EJ, Buchanan GR. Idiopathic thrombocytopenic purpura diagnosed during the second decade of life. J Pediatr 2002;141:253–8.

[11] Drachman JG. Inherited thrombocytopenia: when a low platelet count does not mean ITP. Blood 2004;103:390–8.

[12] Kühne T, Imbach P, Bolton-Maggs PHB, et al. Newly diagnosed idiopathic thrombocytopenic purpura in childhood: an observational study. Lancet 2001;358:2122–5.

[13] Kühne T, Buchanan GR, Zimmerman S, et al. A prospective comparative study of 2540 infants and children with newly diagnosed idiopathic thrombocytopenic purpura (ITP) from the Intercontinental Childhood ITP Study Group. J Pediatr 2003;143:605–8.

[14] Bolton-Maggs PHB, Moon I. Assessment of UK practice for management of acute childhood idiopathic thrombocytopenia purpura against published guidelines. Lancet 1997;350: 620–3.

[15] Sutor AH, Harms A, Kaufmehl K. Acute immune thrombocytopenia (ITP) in childhood: retrospective and prospective survey in Germany. Semin Thromb Hemost 2001;27:253–67.

[16] Rosthoj S, Hedlund-Treutiger I, Rajantie J, et al. Duration and morbidity of newly diagnosed idiopathic thrombocytopenic purpura in children. A prospective Nordic study of an unselected cohort. J Pediatr 2003;143:302–7.

[17] Oski FA, Naiman JL. Effect of live measles vaccine on the platelet count. N Engl J Med 1966;275:352–6.

[18] Miller E, Waight P, Farrington CP, et al. Idiopathic thrombocytopaenic purpura and MMR vaccine. Arch Dis Child 2001;84:227–9.

[19] Black C, Kaye JA, Jick H. MMR vaccine and idiopathic thrombocytopenic purpura. Br J Clin Pharmacol 2003;55:107–11.

[20] Choi SI, McClure PD. Idiopathic thrombocytopenic purpura in childhood. Can Med Assoc J 1967;97:562–8.

[21] Lusher JM, Zuelzer WW. Idiopathic thrombocytopenic purpura in childhood. J Pediatr 1966;68:971–9.

[22] Blanchette VS, Carcao M. Childhood acute immune thrombocytopenic purpura: 20 years later. Semin Thromb Hemost 2003;29:605–17.

[23] Edslev PW, Rosthøj S, Treutiger I, et al. A clinical score predicting a brief and uneventful course of newly diagnosed idiopathic thrombocytopenic purpura in children. Br J Haematol 2007;138:513–6.

[24] Imbach P, Kühne T, Müller D, et al. Childhood ITP: 12 months follow-up data from the prospective Registry I of the Intercontinental Childhood ITP Study Group (ICIS). Pediatr Blood Cancer 2006;46:351–6.

[25] Reid MM. Chronic idiopathic thrombocytopenic purpura: incidence, treatment and outcome. Arch Dis Child 1995;72:125–8.

[26] Imbach P, Akatsuka J, Blanchette V, et al. Immunthrombocytopenic purpura as a model for pathogenesis and treatment of autoimmunity. Eur J Pediatr 1995;154(Suppl 3): S60–4.

[27] Lilleyman JS, on behalf of the Paediatric Haematology Forum of the British Society of Haematology. Intracranial haemorrhage in idiopathic thrombocytopenic purpura. Arch Dis Child 1994;71:251–3.

[28] Lee MS, Kim WC. Intracranial hemorrhage associated with idiopathic thrombocytopenic purpura: report of seven patients and a meta-analysis. Neurology 1998;50:1160–3.

[29] Butros LJ, Bussel JB. Intracranial hemorrhage in immune thrombocytopenic purpura: a retrospective analysis. J Pediatr Hematol Oncol 2003;25:660–4.

[30] Woerner SJ, Abildgaard CF, French BN. Intracranial hemorrhage in children with idiopathic thrombocytopenic purpura. Pediatrics 1981;67:453–60.

[31] Medeiros D, Buchanan GR. Major hemorrhage in children with idiopathic thrombocytopenic purpura: immediate response to therapy and long-term outcome. J Pediatr 1998;133: 334–9.

[32] Bolton-Maggs PHB, Dickerhoff R, Vora AJ. The non-treatment of childhood ITP (or "The art of medicine consists of amusing the patient until nature cures the disease"). Semin Thromb Hemost 2001;27:269–75.

[33] Eden OB, Lilleyman JS, on behalf of the British Paediatric Haematology Group. Guidelines for management of idiopathic thrombocytopenic purpura. Arch Dis Child 1992;67:1056–8.

[34] Lilleyman JS. Management of childhood idiopathic thrombocytopenic purpura. Br J Haematol 1999;105:871–5.

[35] De Mattia D, Del Principe D, Del Vecchio GC, et al. Acute childhood idiopathic thrombocytopenic purpura: AIEOP concensus guidelines for diagnosis and treatment. Haematologica 2000;85:420–4.

[36] Provan D, Newland A, Norfolk D, et al. Working Party of the British Committee for Standards in Haematology General Haematology Task Force. Guidelines for the investigation and management of idiopathic thrombocytopenic purpura in adults, children and in pregnancy. Br J Haematol 2003;120:574–96.

[37] Dickerhoff R, von Ruecker A. The clinical course of immune thrombocytopenic purpura in children who did not receive intravenous immunoglobulins or sustained prednisone treatment. J Pediatr 2000;137:629–32.

[38] Sartorius JA. Steroid treatment of idiopathic thrombocytopenic purpura in children. Preliminary results of a randomized cooperative study. Am J Pediatr Hematol Oncol 1984;6:165–9.

[39] Buchanan GR, Holtkamp CA. Prednisone therapy for children with newly diagnosed idiopathic thrombocytopenic purpura. A randomized clinical trial. Am J Pediatr Hematol Oncol 1984;6:355–61.

[40] Özsoylu S, Sayli TR, Öztürk G. Oral megadose methylprednisolone versus intravenous immunoglobulin for acute childhood idiopathic thrombocytopenic purpura. Pediatr Hematol Oncol 1993;10:317–21.

[41] Suarez CR, Rademaker D, Hasson A, et al. High-dose steroids in childhood acute idiopathic thrombocytopenia purpura. Am J Pediatr Hematol Oncol 1986;8:111–5.

[42] van Hoff J, Ritchey AK. Pulse methylprednisolone therapy for acute childhood idiopathic thrombocytopenic purpura. J Pediatr 1988;113:563–6.

[43] Jayabose S, Patel P, Inamdar S, et al. Use of intravenous methylprednisolone in acute idiopathic thrombocytopenic purpura. Am J Pediatr Hematol Oncol 1987;9:133–5.

[44] Carcao MD, Zipursky A, Butchart S, et al. Short-course oral prednisone therapy in children presenting with acute immune thrombocytopenic purpura (ITP). Acta Paediatr Suppl 1998;424:71–4.

[45] Beck CE, Nathan PC, Parkin PC, et al. Corticosteroids versus intravenous immune globulin for the treatment of acute immune thrombocytopenic purpura in children: a systematic review and meta-analysis of randomized controlled trials. J Pediatr 2005;147:521–7.

[46] Imbach P, Barandun S, d'Apuzzo V, et al. High-dose intravenous gammaglobulin for idiopathic thrombocytopenic purpura in childhood. Lancet 1981;1228–31.

[47] Blanchette VS, Luke B, Andrew M, et al. A prospective, randomized trial of high-dose intravenous immune globulin G therapy, oral prednisone therapy, and no therapy in childhood acute immune thrombocytopenic purpura. J Pediatr 1993;123:989–95.

[48] Blanchette V, Imbach P, Andrew M, et al. Randomised trial of intravenous immunoglobulin G, intravenous anti-D and oral prednisone in childhood acute immune thrombocytopenic purpura. Lancet 1994;344:703–7.

[49] Imbach P, Wagner HP, Berchtold W, et al. Intravenous immunoglobulin versus oral corticosteroids in acute immune thrombocytopenic purpura in childhood. Lancet 1985;464–8.

[50] Salama A, Mueller-Eckhardt C, Kiefel V. Effect of intravenous immunoglobulin in immune thrombocytopenia. Competitive inhibition of reticuloendothelial system function by sequestration of autologous red blood cells? Lancet 1983;193–5.

[51] Scaradavou A, Woo B, Woloski BMR, et al. Intravenous anti-D treatment of immune thrombocytopenic purpura: experience in 272 patients. Blood 1997;89:2689–700.

[52] Tarantino MD, Young G, Bertolone SJ, et al. Single dose of anti-D immune globulin at 75 μg/kg is as effective as intravenous immune globulin at rapidly raising the platelet count in newly diagnosed immune thrombocytopenic purpura in children. J Pediatr 2006;148:489–94.

[53] Newman GC, Novoa MV, Fodero EM, et al. A dose of 75 μg/kg/d of i.v. anti-D increases the platelet count more rapidly and for a longer period of time than 50 μg/kg/d in adults with immune thrombocytopenic purpura. Br J Haematol 2001;112:1076–8.

[54] Gaines AR. Disseminated intravascular coagulation associated with acute hemoglobinemia or hemoglobinuria following $Rh_o(D)$ immune globulin intravenous administration for immune thrombocytopenic purpura. Blood 2005;106:1532–7.

[55] Calpin C, Dick P, Poon A, et al. Is bone marrow aspiration needed in acute childhood idiopathic thrombocytopenic purpura to rule out leukemia? Arch Pediatr Adolesc Med 1998;152:345–7.

[56] Blanchette VS, Price V. Childhood chronic immune thrombocytopenic purpura: unresolved issues. J Pediatr Hematol Oncol 2003;25:S28–33.

[57] Mantadakis E, Buchanan GR. Elective splenectomy in children with idiopathic thrombocytopenic purpura. J Pediatr Hematol Oncol 2000;22:148–53.

[58] Ben-Yehuda D, Gillis S, Eldor A, et al. Clinical and therapeutic experience in 712 Israeli patients with idiopathic thrombocytopenic purpura. Acta Haematol 1994;91:1–6.

[59] Blanchette VS, Kirby MA, Turner C. Role of intravenous immunoglobulin G in autoimmune hematologic disorders. Semin Hematol 1992;29:72–82.

[60] Aronis S, Platokouki H, Avgeri M, et al. Retrospective evaluation of long-term efficacy and safety of splenectomy in chronic idiopathic thrombocytopenic purpura in children. Acta Paediatr 2004;93:638–42.

[61] Kühne T, Blanchette V, Buchanan GR, et al. Splenectomy in children with idiopathic thrombocytopenic purpura: a prospective study of 134 children from the Intercontinental Childhood ITP Study Group. Pediatr Blood Cancer 2007;49:829–34.

[62] Wang T, Xu M, Ji L, et al. Splenectomy for chronic idiopathic thrombocytopenic purpura in children: a single centre study in China. Acta Haematol 2006;115:39–45.

[63] Najean Y, Rain J-D, Billotey C. The site of destruction of autologous [111] In-labelled platelets and the efficiency of splenectomy in children and adults with idiopathic thrombocytopenic purpura: a study of 578 patients with 268 splenectomies. Br J Haematol 1997;97: 547–50.

[64] Holt D, Brown J, Terrill K, et al. Response to intravenous immunoglobulin predicts splenectomy response in children with immune thrombocytopenic purpura. Pediatrics 2003; 111:87–90.

[65] Bussel JB, Kaufmann CP, Ware RE, et al. Do the acute platelet responses of patients with immune thrombocytopenic purpura (ITP) to IV anti-D and to IV gammaglobulin predict response to subsequent splenectomy? Am J Hematol 2001;67:27–33.

[66] Price VE, Dutta S, Blanchette VS, et al. The prevention and treatment of bacterial infections in children with asplenia or hyposplenia: practice considerations at the Hospital for Sick Children, Toronto. Pediatr Blood Cancer 2006;46:597–603.

[67] Baumann MA, Menitove JE, Aster RH, et al. Urgent treatment of idiopathic thrombocytopenic purpura with single-dose gammaglobulin infusion followed by platelet transfusion. Ann Intern Med 1986;104:808–9.

[68] Barnes C, Blanchette V, Canning P, et al. Recombinant FVIIa in the management of intracerebral haemorrhage in severe thrombocytopenia unresponsive to platelet-enhancing treatment. Transfus Med 2005;15:145–50.

[69] Wang WC. Evans syndrome in childhood: pathophysiology, clinical course, and treatment. Am J Pediatr Hematol Oncol 1988;10:330–8.

[70] Savaşan S, Warrier I, Ravindranath Y. The spectrum of Evans' syndrome. Arch Dis Child 1997;77:245–8.

[71] Mathew P, Chen G, Wang W. Evans syndrome: results of a national survey. J Pediatr Hematol Oncol 1997;19:433–7.

[72] Blouin P, Auvrignon A, Pagnier A, et al. [Evans' syndrome: a retrospective study from the ship (french society of pediatric hematology and immunology) (36 cases)]. Arch Pediatr 2005;12:1600–7 [in French].

[73] Calderwood S, Blanchette V, Doyle J, et al. Idiopathic thrombocytopenia and neutropenia in childhood. Am J Pediatr Hematol Oncol 1994;16:95–101.

[74] Norton A, Roberts I. Management of Evans syndrome. Br J Haematol 2005;132:125–37.

[75] Scaradavou A, Bussel J. Evans syndrome: results of a pilot study utilizing a multiagent treatment protocol. J Pediatr Hematol Oncol 1995;17:290–5.

[76] Uçar B, Akgün N, Aydoğdu SD, et al. Treatment of refractory Evans' syndrome with cyclosporine and prednisone. Pediatr Int 1999;41:104–7.

[77] Williams JA, Boxer LA. Combination therapy for refractory idiopathic thrombocytopenic purpura in adolescents. J Pediatr Hematol Oncol 2003;25:232–5.

[78] Cunningham-Rundles C. Hematologic complications of primary immune deficiencies. Blood Rev 2002;16:61–4.

[79] Michel M, Chanet V, Galicier L, et al. Autoimmune thrombocytopenic purpura and common variable immunodeficiency. Analysis of 21 cases and review of the literature. Medicine 2004;83:254–63.

[80] Knight AK, Cunningham-Rundles C. Inflammatory and autoimmune complications of common variable immune deficiency. Autoimmun Rev 2006;5:156–9.

[81] Brandt D, Gershwin ME. Common variable immune deficiency and autoimmunity. Autoimmun Rev 2006;5:465–70.

[82] Wang J, Cunningham-Rundles C. Treatment and outcome of autoimmune hematologic disease in common variable immunodeficiency (CVID). J Autoimmun 2005;25:57–62.

[83] Sneller MC, Dale JK, Straus SE. Autoimmune lymphoproliferative syndrome. Curr Opin Rheumatol 2003;15:417–21.

[84] Oliveira JB, Fleischer T. Autoimmune lymphoproliferative syndrome. Curr Opin Allergy Clin Immunol 2004;4:497–503.

[85] Rao VK, Straus SE. Causes and consequences of the autoimmune lymphoproliferative syndrome. Hematology 2006;11:15–23.

[86] Worth A, Thrasher AJ, Gaspar HB. Autoimmune lymphoproliferative syndrome: molecular basis of disease and clinical phenotype. Br J Haematol 2006;133:124–40.

[87] Savaşan S, Warrier I, Buck S, et al. Increased lymphocyte Fas expression and high incidence of common variable immunodeficiency disorder in childhood Evans' syndrome. Clin Immunol 2007;125:224–9.

[88] Teachey DT, Manno CS, Axsom KM, et al. Unmasking Evans syndrome: T-cell phenotype and apoptotic response reveal autoimmune lymphoproliferative syndrome (ALPS). Blood 2005;105:2443–8.

[89] Rao VK, Dugan F, Dale JK, et al. Use of mycophenolate mofetil for chronic, refractory immune cytopenias in children with autoimmune lymphoproliferative syndrome. Br J Haematol 2005;129:534–8.

[90] Vesely SK, Perdue JJ, Rizvi MA, et al. Management of adult patients with persistent idiopathic thrombocytopenic purpura following splenectomy. A systematic review. Ann Intern Med 2004;140:112–20.

[91] Arnold DM, Dentali F, Crowther MA, et al. Systematic review: efficacy and safety of rituximab for adults with idiopathic thrombocytopenic purpura. Ann Intern Med 2007;146:25–33.

[92] Bennett CM, Rogers ZR, Kinnamon DD, et al. Prospective phase 1/2 study of rituximab in childhood and adolescent chronic immune thrombocytopenic purpura. Blood 2006;107: 2639–42.

[93] Cooper N, Stasi R, Cunningham-Rundles S, et al. The efficacy and safety of B-cell depletion with anti-CD20 monoclonal antibody in adults with chronic immune thrombocytopenic purpura. Br J Haematol 2004;125:232–9.

[94] Perrotta AL. Re-treatment of chronic idiopathic thrombocytopenic purpura with Rituximab: literature review. Clin Appl Thromb Hemost 2006;12:97–100.

[95] Larrar S, Guitton C, Willems M, et al. Severe hematological side effects following Rituximab therapy in children. Haematologica 2006;91:101–2.

[96] Anonymous. Rituxan warning. FDA Consum 2007;41:2.

[97] Kaushansky K. Thrombopoietin. N Engl J Med 1998;339:746–54.

[98] Li J, Yang C, Xia Y, et al. Thrombocytopenia caused by the development of antibodies to thrombopoietin. Blood 2001;98:3241–8.

[99] Erickson-Miller CL, DeLorme E, Tian SS, et al. Discovery and characterization of a selective, nonpeptidyl thrombopoietin receptor agonist. Exp Hematol 2005;33:85–93.

[100] Kuter DJ. New thrombopoietic growth factors. Blood 2007;109:4607–16.

[101] Newland A, Caulier MT, Kappers-Klunne M, et al. An open-label, unit dose-finding study of AMG 531, a novel thrombopoiesis-stimulating peptibody, in patients with immune thrombocytopenic purpura. Br J Haematol 2006;135:547–53.

[102] Bussel JB, Kuter DJ, George JN, et al. AMG 531, a thrombopoiesis-stimulating protein, for chronic ITP. N Engl J Med 2006;355:1672–81.

[103] Bussel JB, Cheng G, Saleh MN, et al. Eltrombopag for the treatment of chronic idiopathic thrombocytopenic purpura. N Engl J Med 2007;357:2237–47.

[104] Bolton-Maggs PHB. Management of immune thrombocytopenic purpura. Paediatr Child Health 2007;17:305–10.

[105] Buchanan GR, Adix L. Outcome measures and treatment endpoints other than platelet count in childhood idiopathic thrombocytopenic purpura. Semin Thromb Hemost 2001; 27:277–85.

[106] Barnard D, Woloski M, Feeny D, et al. Development of disease-specific health-related quality of life instruments for children with immune thrombocytopenic purpura and their parents. J Pediatr Hematol Oncol 2003;25:56–62.

[107] von Mackensen S, Nilsson C, Jankovic M, et al. Development of a disease-specific quality of life questionnaire for children and adolescents with idiopathic thrombocytopenic purpura (ITP-QoL). Pediatr Blood Cancer 2006;47:688–91.

[108] Klaassen RJ, Blanchette VS, Barnard D, et al. Validity, reliability and responsiveness of a new measure of health-related quality of life in children with immune thrombocytopenic purpura: the Kids' ITP Tools. J Pediatr 2007;150:510–5.

[109] Buchanan GR, Adix L. Grading of hemorrhage in children with idiopathic thrombocytopenic purpura. J Pediatr 2002;141:683–8.

[110] Page KL, Psaila B, Provan D, et al. The immune thrombocytopenic purpura (ITP) bleeding score: assessment of bleeding in patients with ITP. Br J Haematol 2007;138:245–8.

[111] O'Brien SH, Ritchey AK, Smith KJ. A cost-utility analysis of treatment for acute childhood idiopathic thrombocytopenic purpura (ITP). Pediatr Blood Cancer 2007;48:173–80.

[112] Cines DB, Bussel JB. How I treat idiopathic thrombocytopenic purpura (ITP). Blood 2005; 106:2244–51.

PEDIATRIC CLINICS

OF NORTH AMERICA

ELSEVIER
SAUNDERS

Pediatr Clin N Am 55 (2008) 421–445

Blood Component Therapy

Ross Fasano, MD[a,c], Naomi L.C. Luban, MD[b,c],*

[a]Children's National Medical Center, Department of Hematology/Oncology,
111 Michigan Avenue NW, Washington, DC 20010, USA
[b]Children's National Medical Center, Department of Laboratory Medicine,
111 Michigan Avenue, NW, Washington, DC 20010, USA
[c]The George Washington University Medical Center, Washington, DC, USA

Blood component transfusion is an integral part of the treatment of many infants and children cared for by general pediatricians, surgeons, intensivists, and hematologists/oncologists. Technologic advances in blood collection, separation, anticoagulation, and preservation have resulted in component preparation of red blood cells (RBCs), platelets, white blood cells (WBCs), and plasma, which are superior to whole blood (WB) used in the past. Recent advances in donor selection, infectious disease testing, use of leukoreduction filters, and gamma irradiation also deem today's products safer than the past. Physicians prescribing blood components not only should have a basic understanding of the indications (and contraindications) for their use but also should be cognizant of the methods of preparation, the proper storage conditions, and the requirements for further modification of blood products to prevent potential adverse effects.

Blood component preparation and modification

Blood components are prepared from blood collected by WB or apheresis donations. Transfusion of WB is uncommon in modern medicine. Uses for WB or reconstituted WB units include blood priming for extracorporeal circuits (ie, therapeutic apheresis in small patients, cardiovascular bypass, extracorporeal membrane oxygenation, and continuous hemoperfusion), neonatal exchange transfusions, and patients who have active bleeding and massive volume loss. Given that platelet function is poor after 24 hours

* Corresponding author. Children's National Medical Center, Department of Laboratory Medicine, 111 Michigan Avenue, NW, Washington, DC 20010.
E-mail address: nluban@cnmc.org (N.L.C. Luban).

of storage and that coagulation factors (especially V and VIII) decrease throughout storage, most blood centers rarely collect WB for allogeneic use. In situations when RBC and coagulation factor replacement are needed, components can be given in the form of "reconstituted" WB (RBC unit and a plasma unit in one bag).

Component preparation from whole blood donation

One unit of WB contains approximately 450 mL of blood collected from a healthy adult donor into a sterile plastic bag containing 63 mL of anticoagulant/preservative (AP) solution. Because RBCs, platelets, and plasma have different specific gravities, they can be separated from each other via centrifugation. In North America, this is done most commonly initially by performing a soft spin, which separates the heavier RBCs from platelet-rich plasma. The RBCs then are collected into a sterile satellite bag containing an anticoagulant solution. For separation of platelets from plasma, a hard spin then is performed. One unit of platelet concentrate (PC), which contains a minimum of 5.5×10^{10} platelets in approximately 50 mL of remaining plasma, is the result. The resulting PC can be stored as multiples of single units or pooled with other donor PCs. The typical volume of a unit of plasma collected from WB is approximately 250 mL. In order for the plasma to be labeled as fresh frozen plasma (FFP), the unit must be separated from the other blood components and stored at $-18°C$ within 8 hours of collection.

Component preparation by apheresis

An alternative to WB collection and separation of blood components is to collect a specific component via apheresis. This entails a process where an automated apheresis instrument draws blood into an external circuit, separates the components by centrifugation or filtration, collects the desired component, and returns the remaining blood components to the donor. Although traditionally this has been used for platelet, plasma, and granulocyte collection, newer methods support RBC collection. These methods provide larger quantities of the desired component than WB collection methods. For example, a single apheresis platelet unit contains approximately the same number of platelets as a pool of six to eight random donor platelet units collected from WB (3×10^{11} platelets/U for single donor apheresis platelets versus 5.5×10^{10} platelets/U for single donor WB collected platelets). "Double" collections also are possible for platelets and RBCs. Because platelet and red cell apheresis products expose recipients to fewer donors, there also is a theoretic advantage of decreasing the risk for alloimmunization and transfusion-transmitted diseases in chronically transfused patients. Regarding donors, because RBC loss is minimal during platelet apheresis, donation can be performed more often than with WB collection.

Anticoagulant/preservative solutions

When RBCs are stored for transfusion, several prerequisites must be met: the product must be sterile, the cellular components must remain viable during storage, their in vivo survival after storage must be greater than 75% 24 hours after transfusion, and hemolysis should be less than 1%. RBC viability and functional activity require that RBCs be preserved in solutions that support their metabolic demands. All anticoagulant solutions contain citrate, phosphate, and dextrose (CPD). These constituents function as an anticoagulant, a buffer, and a source of metabolic energy for the RBCs, respectively. Recent advances in the development of AP solutions largely are the result of the addition of nutrients that stabilize the RBC membrane and maintain 2,3-diphosphoglycenate and ATP within the erythrocyte. Mannitol is used in some AP solutions because it stabilizes RBC membranes, and adenine enters RBCs and is incorporated within the nucleotide pools resulting in higher levels of ATP within the RBC products. The use of AP solutions has increased the shelf life of RBCs from 21 days for CPD to 35 days for citrate-phosphate-dextrose-adenine (CPDA)-1 and to 42 days for the newer AP solutions (Adsol, Optisol, and Nutricell).

The concentrations of the additives of products licensed for use in the United States are safe for most children and neonates receiving simple transfusions; however, extremely ill premature neonates requiring massive transfusion (ie, exchange transfusion, extracorporeal membrane oxygenation, or cardiopulmonary bypass), or those who have significant renal or hepatic insufficiency may be at risk for metabolic abnormalities [1–3]. The amounts of adenine and mannitol in small volume transfusions (15 mL/kg RBCs) to neonates using anticoagulant/preservative solution #1 (AS-1) equates to less than one tenth the toxic dose [4]. There are no clinical data, however, on metabolic abnormalities in massive transfusion for neonates. Therefore, some experts recommend avoiding use of RBCs stored in extended-storage media (Adsol, Optisol, or Nutricell) until such data are published. Several options for reducing the AP exist, including inverted storage, centrifugation, or even washing of the RBC product.

Leukocyte reduction of blood components

The American Association of Blood Banks (AABB) states that in order for a blood product to be labeled "leukoreduced," it must contain fewer than 5×10^6 total WBCs per unit [5]. Current third-generation leukocyte reduction filters consistently provide a 3 to 4 log or 99.9% reduction of WBC content to fewer than 5×10^6 WBCs and, with some filters, fewer than 1×10^6 per product. This leukocyte reduction step is performed best prestorage per manufacturer's requirements with good quality control techniques.

Febrile nonhemolytic transfusion reactions (FNHTRs) typically are caused by reactions to donor WBCs or to cytokines present in the product.

Leukocyte reduction reduces the incidence of FNHTRs, especially when prestorage leukoreduction is used, because lower levels of cytokines are present in prestorage leukocyte-reduced products [6–8]. Alloimmunization to foreign HLA class I antigens is a significant concern for patients who may require repeated platelet transfusions. Because platelets also express HLA class I antigens, patients sensitized to such antigens can become refractory to platelet transfusions. Leukocyte reduction also is proved to reduce the incidence of HLA alloimmunization [9].

Leukocyte reduction also is used to reduce transmission of cytomegalovirus (CMV) in high-risk patient populations. Recipient groups at increased risk for post-transfusion CMV-related morbidity and mortality include [10]

Premature, seronegative neonates less than 1250 g who require blood component support
Recipients of hematopoietic stem cell and solid-organ transplants
Fetuses who receive intrauterine transfusions
Other individuals who are severely immunocompromised

Although the use of CMV-seronegative blood is considered the gold standard, such products often are difficult to obtain depending on donor demographics in a specific area. Because CMV is harbored within WBCs, manipulation of leukocyte number and viability should reduce transmission of CMV. Irradiation of blood products (discussed later) is not shown to prevent post-transfusion CMV infection; however, leukocyte reduction ($<5 \times 10^6$ WBCs/U) is effective in preventing CMV infection in adults who have hematopoietic malignancies, neonates, and patients post stem cell transplant. Whether or not leukocyte reduction is as efficacious as CMV-seronegative blood is debated widely. In a landmark study, Bowden and colleagues [11] found equivalent rates of post-transfusion CMV infection in an allogeneic hematopoietic stem cell population (1.4% for seronegative versus 2.4% for leukocyte reduction). Although this study's conclusions are debated widely, no formal consensus on the debate of equivalency has been formulated. A subsequent study by Nichols and colleagues [12] demonstrated that although leukocyte-reduced platelet products were deemed similar to CMV-seronegative products regarding transfusion transmission of CMV, leukocyte-depleted RBCs were not. The investigators warned against the practice of abandoning "dual inventory" blood products for CMV-seronegative and -seropositive units. Nonetheless, variable practices exist depending on donor demographics and the number of high-risk patients treated at a given center [10,13]. Many institutions use algorithms based on (pretransplant) serostatus of recipients, serostatus of hematopoietic stem cell donors, and donor demographics within the area. It is unlikely that further randomized controlled trials will be performed to assess comparability of CMV-seronegative versus leukoreduced products.

Gamma irradiation of blood components

Transfusion-associated graft-versus-host disease (TA-GVHD) occurs when an immunosuppressed or immunodeficient patient receives cellular blood products that possess immunologically competent lymphocytes. The transfused donor lymphocytes are able to proliferate and engraft in the immunologically incompetent recipient because they are unable to detect and reject foreign cells. The degree of similarity between HLA antigens also increases the ability of donor lymphocytes to engraft with the recipient. This explains why TA-GVHD can occur in situations of directed donation from family members. In the event where a donor is homozygous and a recipient is heterozygous for a particular HLA antigen, the donor lymphocytes may escape immune surveillance and thus are able to engraft in the immunocompetent host, resulting in TA-GVHD. This situation also may occur in populations with limited HLA variability, such as in Japan, necessitating universal gamma irradiation of all cellular components in specific situations.

Clinical symptoms of TA-GVHD include fever, an erythematous rash that may progress to bullae and desquamation, anorexia, and diarrhea, which develop within 3 to 30 days of receiving cellular blood components. Because the hematopoietic progenitor cells (HPCs) in particular are affected, severe cytopenia usually is present. Mild hepatitis to fulminant liver failure may occur. Mortality for TA-GVHD is 90% in the pediatric population. Patients at high risk for TA-GVHD include [14]

Patients who have congenital immunodeficiencies of cellular immunity
Those receiving intrauterine transfusion followed by neonatal exchange transfusion
Bone marrow transplant recipients
Recipients of HLA-matched cellular components or blood components from blood-related donors
Patients who have hematologic malignancies and cancer patients undergoing intense chemotherapy or immunomodulatory therapy (ie, fludarabine and other purine analogs)

Neonates, especially those who are extremely premature, are considered by many to be at high risk for TA-GVHD. Whereas some neonatal centers irradiate all cellular blood products for infants less than 4 months of age, others irradiate only blood products given to preterm infants born weighing less than or equal to 1.2 kg [15]. Given the lack of clinical studies on the incidence of TA-GVHD in the neonatal population, however, and the concern for failing to recognize infants who have an undiagnosed congenital immunodeficiency, there exists no standard of care regarding irradiation of blood products for otherwise non–high-risk infants born with a weight greater than 1200 g.

TA-GVHD can be prevented by gamma irradiation of cellular blood components at 2500 cGy [16]. Because in vivo recovery of irradiated

RBCs is decreased compared with nonirradiated RBCs, at 42 days of storage, the Food and Drug Administration recommends a 28-day expiration for irradiated RBCs [17]. Potassium and free hemoglobin (Hb) are increased after irradiation and storage of RBCs. Therefore, it is preferable to irradiate in a time frame close to administration rather than prolonged refrigerator storage products, especially for neonates, who may not be able to tolerate a large potassium load. Irradiation of platelets does not affect function, and although superoxide production and phagocytic function is shown to be decreased in granulocytes irradiated at 2500 cGy, most authorities recommend irradiating granulocytes before administering.

Red blood cell products

RBCs are prepared by removal of 200 to 250 mL of plasma from 1 unit of WB. RBCs collected in CPDA-1 have a volume of approximately 250 mL and a hematocrit of 70% to 80%. When RBCs are supplemented with additional preservative solutions (ie, Adsol, Nutricell, or Optisol) the volume is increased to approximately 350 mL and the hematocrit is reduced to 50% to 60%. These RBC components have approximately 50 mL of plasma and the advantage of longer storage shelf life (42 days versus 35 days) and lower viscosity; therefore, they flow more rapidly than the traditional CPD and CPDA components. Notice must be taken by today's practitioners of the lower hematocrit of the current AP-based RBC products when calculating Hb increments post transfusion. For example, using the formula: Volume of RBCs to be transfused = TBV × ([desired Hb]−[actual Hb])/[Hb] of RBC unit, where *TBV* (total blood volume) is 70 to 75 mL/kg by 3 months of age.

Although approximately 10 mL/kg increases the Hb concentration by 3 g/dL for individuals receiving RBCs in CPDA (hematocrit 69%), approximately 12.5 to 15 mL/kg is necessary to attain the same Hb concentration increment for individuals receiving RBCs in AS-1 (hematocrit 54%).

In addition to leukocyte reduction and gamma irradiation, RBC products can be washed using sterile saline to rinse away the remaining plasma proteins within an RBC unit or frozen using high glycerol concentrations for long-term storage of RBC units with unique phenotypes. RBC washing removes plasma proteins, microaggregates, and cytokines and is indicated for severe, recurrent allergic reactions to blood components despite premedication with antihistamines, because these reactions usually are the result of reactions from foreign plasma proteins. Patients who have IgA deficiency and anti-IgA are at risk for anaphylaxis from donor IgA within the plasma and may benefit from washed RBCs [18]. RBC washing should not be considered a substitute for leukoreduction because the washing process removes by only 1 log versus the 3 to 4 log depletion attained by third-generation leukoreduction filters. Given that the average total WBC content in a standard RBC unit is 2 to 5×10^9, washed RBCs contain an average of 5×10^8 WBC/U versus 5×10^6 WBCs/U via leukoreduction. Washed RBC units also are used for some neonates receiving large volume transfusions (>20 mL/kg) with RBCs that are older than 14 days or that have been irradiated before storage. The washing process removes approximately 20% of the RBCs for a final volume of 180 to 200 mL and hematocrit of 70% to 80%. The washing process itself causes electrolyte leakage from RBCs, especially when washing an already irradiated RBC unit, so the unit should be transfused as soon as possible after being washed [19]. Regardless of irradiation, the RBC product needs to be transfused within 24 hours of being washed, because the washing process itself creates an open system.

In cases when a RBC unit is found to have a unique phenotype, it may be frozen and cryopreserved by the use of glycerol. Once frozen, these units have a shelf life of 10 years at less than or equal to $-65°C$. When needed, the unit is deglycerolized, which entails defrosting and washing. This entire process reduces the WBC/U by 100-fold (2 log). As with washed RBC units, defrosted-deglycerolized RBCs must be transfused within 24 hours of preparation. These RBC units are suspended in approximately 250 mL of saline with a hematocrit of 55% to 70% (Table 1).

Special considerations and indications for red blood cell transfusion

Although published clinical guidelines for RBC transfusions exist in the pediatric literature, they often are based on expert panel consensus rather than scientific data because of a relative void of randomized controlled trials on RBC transfusion thresholds for children and neonates. In cases of acute hemorrhage, RBC transfusion should be administered if the amount of bleeding exceeds 15% of TBV [20]. In acutely bleeding patients, the measured Hb concentration does not reflect an accurate assessment of the RBC mass. Therefore, careful assessment of the amount of blood loss and signs of circulatory decompensation are imperative. In contrast to acute hemorrhage, patients who have hemolysis usually are normovolemic, and the measured Hb concentration is a more accurate gauge of the level of anemia. The indication for RBC transfusion in this setting depends on Hb concentration, the rate of decrease of the Hb, the underlying etiology for hemolysis, and whether or not alternative management options (eg, steroids or intravenous immunoglobulin G for autoimmune hemolytic anemia) are exhausted. The use of crossmatch compatible RBCs always is preferred, but on rare occasions, crossmatch "least incompatible" blood must be considered because of the presence of warm-reactive autoantibodies or multiple alloantibodies [21]. Consultation with a transfusion medicine physician in these cases is paramount. In life-threatening autoimmune hemolytic anemia, transfusion of crossmatch incompatible blood often is necessary. If children

Table 1
Blood component characteristics

Component	Storage	Volume	Expiration	Dose
RBC (CPDA-1)	1°C–6°C	250 mL	35 days	10–20 mL/kg
RBC (AP)	1°C–6°C	300–350 mL	42 days	10–20 mL/kg
RBC (washed)	1°C–6°C	180–200 mL	24 hours	10–20 mL/kg
RBC (deglycerolized)	Frozen: <−65°C Deglycerolized: 1°C–6°C	250 mL	Frozen: 10 years Deglycerolized: 24 hours	10–20 mL/kg
PC	20°C–24°C with agitation	50–75 mL	5 days	1–2 U/10 kg[a]
Apheresis platelets	20°C–24°C with agitation	200–400 mL	5 days	1–2 U/10 kg[a]
FFP	Frozen: <−18°C Thawed: 1°C–6°C	200–500 mL	Frozen: 1 year Thawed: 24 hours	10–20 mL/kg
Fresh plasma	Frozen: <−18°C Thawed: 1°C–6°C	200–500 mL	Frozen: 1 year Thawed: 24 hours	10–20 mL/kg
Cryoprecipitate	Frozen: <−18°C Thawed: 20°C–24°C	10–15 mL	Frozen: 1 year Thawed: 6 hours[b]	1 U/5 kg
Granulocyte concentrate	20°C–24°C (no agitation)	200–300 mL	24 hours	$1–2 \times 10^9$ PMNs/kg/d[c]

[a] Neonates: 10–15 mL/kg.
[b] 4 hours if pooled.
[c] 4 to 8×10^{10} PMNs per day for older children/adults.

Data from Luban NL. Basics of transfusion medicine. In: Furman B, Zimmerman JJ, editors. Pediatric critical care. 3rd edition. Philadelphia: Mosby; 2006. p. 1185–98.

have signs of cardiac failure, partial exchange transfusion should be considered to avoid circulatory overload.

Congenital hemoglobinopathies

Individuals who have sickle hemoglobinopathies (HbSS, HbSC, and HbS/β-thalassemia) are unique in that the reason for RBC transfusion not always is to increase the oxygen-carrying capacity and delivery; it also decreases the percentage of Hb S relative to Hb A. Raising the total Hb concentration while lowering the Hb S percentage to 30% is effective in the management of acute cerebrovascular accident (CVA), acute chest syndrome, splenic sequestration, and recurrent priapism. In a large multicenter trial, Vichinsky and colleagues [22] showed that preoperative transfusion to a total Hb concentration of 10 g/dL was equivalent to more aggressive preoperative exchange transfusion with a goal of reducing the Hb S to 30% of total Hb. Because transfusion-related complications were twice as common in the preoperative exchange group, simple transfusion to a total Hb of 10 g/dL is considered by some to be appropriate management to prevent significant morbidity and mortality in patients who have preoperative sickle-cell disease (SCD). A retrospective cohort study of children who had SCD showed that in the absence of concurrent medical events associated with first CVA, recurrent CVA within 5 years was 22% for those not on a chronic transfusion versus 1.9% for those who received regularly scheduled blood transfusions after first CVA [23]. The Stroke Prevention Trial in Sickle Cell Anemia (STOP) showed that children who had SCD and abnormal transcranial Doppler (blood flow greater than 200 cm per second in internal carotid or middle cerebral artery) are at increased risk for initial CVA and that initiation of chronic transfusions in these high-risk patients significantly decreases the risk (14.9% versus 1.6%) [24]. In the STOP II follow-up study, discontinuation of transfusion for the prevention of stroke in children who had SCD resulted in a high rate of reversion to abnormal blood flow velocities on Doppler studies and CVA [25]. Although there is a paucity of clinical studies, chronic transfusions may be indicated in patients who have SCD who have experienced recurrent episodes of severe acute chest syndrome or severe splenic sequestration.

Children who have thalassemia major require chronic transfusions to alleviate anemia and to suppress extramedullary erythropoeisis, which leads to poor growth and bony abnormalities. The common practice involves RBC transfusions every 3 to 4 weeks with the goal to keep the pretransfusion Hb concentration at 9 to 10 g/dL [18,21]. Although all children receiving chronic transfusions are at significant risk for developing iron overload, patients who have thalassemia are at even greater risk because of increased intestinal iron absorption.

Alloimmunization

RBC alloimmunization is estimated to occur in 18% to 47% of pediatric patients who have SCD versus 5% to 11% of chronically transfused thalassemia patients and 0.2% to 2.6% of the general population [26]. It is believed that alloimmunization rates are higher in patients who have SCD because of the disparity between RBC antigens and possibly also an altered immunologic response to foreign antigens. Almost two thirds of clinically significant antibodies are directed toward the rhesus (Rh) and Kell blood group antigens. Methods to reduce the risk for alloimmunization in high-risk populations vary; however, phenotypically matching for Rh (D, C, E, c, and e) and Kell (K and k) decreases the incidence of alloantibodies per unit transfused and the incidence of hemolytic reactions in chronically transfused SCD patients [27]. Extended RBC antigen phenotyping (ABO, Rh, Kell, Kidd, Duffy, Lewis, and MNS blood group systems) for all patients who have SCD should be performed before initiating transfusion therapy, and more extensive red cell antigen matching may be used for those patients who develop multiple alloantibodies. Other strategies include methods to increase African American donor recruitment so as to racially match blood for patients who have SCD. This strategy capitalizes on the different RBC antigen frequencies that exist in those of European and those of African origin [28]. Recent technologic advances in blood group antigen genotyping using molecular methods may enhance the ability to match red cell antigens in this high-risk patient population.

Neonates

Transfusion indications for neonates, especially premature neonates, are controversial because there are few randomized controlled studies. Current guidelines take into account the level of anemia in lieu of the overall cardio-respiratory support, which is required by neonates (Table 2) [20,29]. Recently, two studies addressed liberal versus restrictive guidelines for RBC transfusions in preterm infants [30,31]. Although they are different in design and outcome, neither study establishes unequivocally an appropriate Hb target. Although the multi-institutional Canadian Premature Infants in Need of Transfusion study [30] demonstrated no advantage for liberal transfusion, Bell and coworkers' study [31] suggested that restrictive transfusion is more likely to result in neurologic events and apneic episodes.

Transfusion of neonates is complicated by neonatal blood containing variable amounts of maternal immunoglobulins in the serum, which may be directed against A, B, or both antigens, depending on the maternal blood group and type and the amount of maternal antibody transferred via the placenta. For this reason, some blood banks choose to transfuse group O RBCs to all neonates whereas others use group-specific blood if a neonate's serum is free of maternal antibodies directed toward the neonate's RBC ABO antigens. In cases when reconstituted WB is needed for exchange transfusion or cardiopulmonary bypass, a neonate may be given plasma

Table 2
Red blood cell transfusion guidelines for patients less than 4 months of age

United States guidelines [20]	
Clinical status	Hemoglobin concentration
Severe pulmonary or cyanotic heart disease/congestive heart failure	<15 g/dL
CPAP/MV with mean airway pressure > 6–8 cm H_2O[a] FIO_2 > 35% via oxygen hood	<12 g/dL
CPAP/MV with mean airway pressure < 6 cm H_2O FIO_2 < 35% via oxygen hood On nasal canula Significant apnea/bradycardia, tachypnea, tachycardia[b] Low weight gain (<10 g/d over 4 days)	<10 g/dL
Low reticulocyte count and symptoms of anemia[c]	<7 g/dL
British guidelines [29]	
Clinical status	Hemoglobin concentration
Anemia in first 24 hours of life	<12 g/dL
Neonate receiving intensive care	<12 g/dL
Chronic oxygen dependency	<11 g/dL
Late anemia, stable patient	<7 g/dL
Acute blood loss	10% TBV
Cumulative blood loss in 1 week, neonate requiring intensive care	10% TBV

Abbreviations: FIO_2, fraction of inspired oxygen; TBV, total blood volume.

[a] Continuous positive airway pressure/mechanical ventilation.

[b] Heart rate greater than 180 beats per minute and respiratory rate greater than 80 breaths per minute over 24 hours.

[c] Poor feeding, tachycardia, tachypnea.

Data from Robitaille N, Hume HA. Blood components and fractional plasma products: preparations, indications, and administration. In: Arceci RJ, Hann IM, Smith OP, editors. Pediatric hematology. 3rd edition. New York: Wiley Blackwell; 2006. p. 693–708.

that is ABO compatible with the neonate's RBCs but receive RBCs that are compatible with maternal serum. To limit donor exposure in these situations, some blood centers advocate using low-titer group O WB. Because of the immaturity of neonates' immune system, antibody screens and serologic crossmatch do not need to be repeated until 4 months of age [18,20,21].

Because premature neonates have small blood volumes and often require multiple RBC transfusions throughout their hospitalizations, many pediatric transfusion services have adopted a system in which aliquots from one RBC unit are reserved for and dispensed to one or more neonates for each RBC transfusion. This practice theoretically reduces donor exposure to neonates and reduces the amount of wastage. This is accomplished by use of sterile connecting devices to assure that the original RBC unit remains in a closed system.

Platelets

Platelets may be prepared by one of two methods: WB collection and separation via centrifugation or apheresis. Platelets prepared by centrifugation of individual units of WB often are referred to as random-donor platelets. Each PC usually contains approximately 7.5×10^{10} platelets but must contain at least 5.5×10^{10} platelets in 50 to 70 mL of plasma. Apheresis platelets (often called single-donor platelets) are collected from a donor by selectively removing platelets in a volume of approximately 200 to 400 mL of plasma whereas the rest of the blood components are returned to the donor during the cytapheresis procedure. This technique allows collection of platelets with a minimum of 3×10^{11} platelets per 250-mL bag (see Table 1). This limits the amount of donor exposure per platelet transfusion because this technique collects the equivalent of a pool of six to eight random donor platelets. Regardless of the method of collection, all platelet units must be stored at 20°C to 24°C under constant agitation because storage at cold temperatures is detrimental to platelet function. As a result of these warmer storage temperatures, the shelf life of platelet products is only 5 days because of the risk for bacterial contamination. In compliance with AABB standards, all blood banks and transfusion services must have methods in place to limit and detect bacterial contamination [5].

Platelets express intrinsic ABO antigens but not Rh antigens. Whenever possible, ABO-compatible platelets should be administered, especially for small children and neonates, because of reports of intravascular hemolysis after transfusion of ABO-incompatible platelets. If ABO-incompatible platelets are to be transfused, selection of low isoagglutinin (anti-A, anti-B) titer units or volume reduction should be considered. With volume reduction, however, approximately 20% of platelets are lost in the final product. Patients who are RhD negative (especially women) should be transfused "Rh-negative" platelets because RBCs are present in small amounts (apheresis platelets 0.001 mL per unit versus 0.3 mL in WB-derived platelets) [32]. The minimal volume reported to cause Rh alloimmunization in D-volunteer subjects is 0.03 mL as a result of the manufacturing process [33]. In cases when Rh-negative platelets are unavailable, Rh immune globulin may be administered within 72 hours of transfusion at a dose of 120 IU/mL of RBCs intramuscularly (90 IU/mL of RBCs intravenously). Although the exact immunizing dose in pediatric patients is unknown, certain patient groups, such as pediatric oncology patients, require further study to confirm their limited ability to mount an anti-D response [34].

Platelet transfusion is indicated for the treatment of qualitative and quantitative platelet abnormalities. Clinical factors considered when assessing the need for a platelet transfusion include the primary diagnosis; the bone marrow function and its ability to compensate or recover; the presence of fever, sepsis, or splenomegaly, which increases platelet consumption; and the presence of uremia or medications that may alter platelet function. Until recently, physicians transfused patients platelets for platelet counts under 20,000/µL. Several large prospective studies, however, mainly of acute leukemia, showed no difference in bleeding risk between transfusion thresholds of 10,000/µL and 20,000/µL. Most recommend, therefore, that for prophylaxis, platelets should be maintained greater than 10,000/μL for adults and children who do not have additional bleeding risk factors [35–37]. Platelet counts greater than 20,000/μL are indicated for invasive procedures and greater than 50,000/μL for major surgeries or invasive procedures with significant bleeding risk. For central nervous system bleeding or planned central nervous system surgery, the platelet count should be maintained greater than 100,000/μL [20]. Because of the risk for intraventricular hemorrhage in sick neonates, many physicians traditionally have adopted a fairly aggressive platelet threshold for transfusion. Although there is little data on the appropriate threshold for platelet transfusion in (preterm) neonates, Murray and colleagues [38], in their retrospective study of 53 neonates (44 preterm) who had severe thrombocytopenia, concluded that a threshold of 30,000/μL without other risk factors or previous intraventricular hemorrhagic is safe for the majority of patients in neonatal ICUs.

Platelet refractoriness

A calculated platelet dose of 5 to 10 mL/kg for neonates and 0.1 to 0.2 U/kg for children over 10 kg should result in a platelet increment of 50,000/μL to 100,000/μL if no predisposing risk factors for refractoriness exist. Few data exist as to the difference in platelet increment that result from the use of apheresis versus PCs. An attenuated result can be the result, however, of a host of causes, which can be immune related or nonimmune related. Nonimmune causes include splenomegaly, fever, sepsis, disseminated intravascular coagulation (DIC), bleeding, antibiotic therapy (eg, vancomycin), and use of immunosuppressive agents. Immune causes include autoantibodies, such as immune thrombocytopenic purpura, or alloantibodies to HLA class I antigens or uncommonly to platelet-specific antigens (eg, HPA-1a). Evaluation of platelet refractoriness entails evaluation of the platelet increment (PI) at 1 hour and 24 hours post transfusion and calculation of the calculated count increment (CCI). The CCI can be calculated as follows: CCI = (PI × BSA)/number of platelets transfused (in units of 10^{11}), where BSA is body surface area.

Two consecutive transfusions with a CCI less than 7500/uL are evidence of the refractory state. Although immune-mediated refractoriness has minimal increment at 1 hour and 24 hours post transfusion, nonimmune-mediated refractoriness traditionally has an adequate initial increment at 1 hour but with poor platelet increment at 24 hours post transfusion. No special platelet product can improve platelet increments in cases of nonimmune refractoriness. Patients who have immune refractoriness after ABO-identical platelets should be screened for the presence of HLA antibodies and, if positive, their specificity determined.

Support of patients who have platelet refractoriness from HLA antibodies generally involves the use of HLA-matched platelets, crossmatched platelets, or platelets selected that lack the specific antigen to which the patients have antibodies. HLA-matched apheresis platelets are graded on a scale of A (most identical) to D (least identical). This must be considered when judging responses to HLA-matched pheresis platelets, because "HLA-matched" platelets rarely are identical [39]. Crossmatching apheresis platelet samples with an immunized patient's serum can detect compatible platelet products without requiring an HLA phenotype or antibody identification; however, a compatible crossmatch is predictive of successful platelet incre-ments in only 50% to 60% of transfusions [40]. Because the shelf life of platelets is only 5 days, crossmatching must be performed frequently for al-loimmunized patients requiring chronic support. HLA-matched and cross-matched platelets are hindered by the fact that finding exact matches using these methods is challenging, even in large blood centers with a wealth of donors. Selection of antigen-negative platelets, as first described by Petz and colleagues [41], is analogous to selection of red cell products for those who are alloimmunized to red cell antigens. Patients' sera are combined with panels of lymphocytes of known HLA phenotype and observed for cy-totoxicity. Phenotyped apheresis platelets that lack the antigens to which antibody is present are considered compatible for transfusion to alloimmu-nized patients. This approach expands the number of compatible platelet products and seems as efficacious as crossmatching [39,42]. Regardless of the method used, excellent communication between clinicians and transfu-sion medicine specialists is critical for success in managing alloimmunized patients.

Plasma products

Fresh frozen plasma

Plasma is prepared by WB separation by centrifugation or by apheresis. When prepared by the former method, one unit contains a volume of 200 to 250 mL, whereas when prepared by the latter method, a volume up to 500 mL can be collected from one donor. To be labeled as FFP, the plasma product needs to be stored at $-18°C$ or colder within 8 hours of collection. FFP can be stored at this temperature for up to 1 year. Another plasma product, frozen plasma (FP), is plasma frozen within 24 hours of collection. Although FP has less factor V (FV) and factor VIII (heat labile factors) ac-tivity, it is considered clinically similar to FFP and used interchangeably [18]. Because FFP undergoes a freezing process in the absence of a cryopro-tectant, the majority of WBCs are killed or nonfunctional. Therefore, leu-koreduction and irradiation are unnecessary for prevention of CMV reactivation and TA-GVHD, respectively, in high-risk patients. FFP should be ABO compatible with recipient RBCs; however, Rh type does not need to be considered nor does a crossmatch need to be done before administering [43]. FFP is the blood product used most commonly. Indications include [18,21]

Multiple coagulation factor deficiencies (eg, liver failure, vitamin K deficiency from malabsorbtion or biliary disease, or DIC)

Reversal of warfarin emergently when vitamin K is deemed untimely

Dilutional coagulopathy from massive transfusion

Replacement of rare single congenital factor deficiencies when specific concentrates are not available (eg, protein C or factor II, V, X, XI, or XIII deficiency)

Replacement of C1 esterase inhibitor in patients who have hereditary angioedema

As a component of WB priming for small children for apheresis

Thrombotic thrombocypenic purpura as simple transfusion, as part of therapeutic plasma exchange, or as "cryopoor plasma" (prepared by removing cryoprecipitate that is rich in high molecular weight von Willebrand multimers from FFP)

FFP should not be used before invasive procedures for patients who have less than 1.5 times the midpoint of normal range for prothrombin time (PT) or activated partial thromboplastin time (aPTT) because clinical experience suggests that FFP does not prevent bleeding in this setting. FFP also is contraindicated for intravascular volume expansion, correction/prevention of protein malnutrition, and when specific factor concentrates are available; alternative products that have undergone viral inactivation through complex manufacturing processes are preferable.

When single factor replacement is needed, the amount of FFP needed can be calculated based on the following, where HCT is hematocrit and TPV is total plasma volume:

1 mL of factor activity = 1 mL FFP
TBV = weight $\times$ 70 mL/kg
TPV = TBV $\times$ (1 $-$ HCT)
Unit of factor needed = TPV (desired factor [%] $-$ initial factor [%])

For example, if a 10-kg child who has an initial FV of 10 U/mL and hematocrit 40% is going to surgery and the goal is a FV of greater than 50 U/mL for hemostasis, then

TBV = 700 mL and TPV = 420 mL
Units of factor needed = 420 $\times$ (0.50 $-$ 0.10) = 168 mL
Amount of FFP needed = 170 mL (or 17mL/kg)

Using these calculations, it is evident that 20 mL/kg of FFP replaces approximately 50% of most factors immediately after transfusion. It is important for clinicians to know the half-lives of the factors for which replacement is sought to plan a dosing schedule because not all factors have equivalent half-lives (eg, FVII half-life: 2 to 6 hours versus FV: 20 hours) [21]. It also is important to know that normal values of certain factors (eg, vitamin K–dependent factors) in neonates may be lower than in older children and adults; therefore, the PT and aPTT are prolonged similarly, rendering correlation of laboratory values to clinical status of patients more complicated.

Cryoprecipitate

Cryoprecipitated antihemophilic factor, or cryoprecipitate, is prepared by thawing FFP at 1°C to 6°C, removing the supernatant, and refreezing at −18°C for up to 1 year. The resulting small volume of precipitate contains concentrated levels of factor VIII, factor XIII, factor VIII: von willebrand's factor (VWF), fibrinogen, and fibronectin. Each cryoprecipitate unit (sometimes referred to as a "bag" of cryoprecipitate, 10 to 15 mL) contains a minimum of 80 units of factor VIII activity and 150 mg of fibrinogen. Because there are no standards for the quantity of the other factors, and because the Food and Drug Administration has licensed viral-inactivated, pooled, plasma-derived and recombinant factor concentrates, cryoprecipitate should not be considered first-line treatment for hemophilia A and B or von Willebrand disease (VWD). In emergent cases of bleeding, however, when these commercially available products are unavailable, cryoprecipitate may be used for replacement. Cryoprecipitate is indicated for treatment for active bleeding in patients who have dysfibrinogenemia, hypofibrinogenemia (<150 mg/dL), or afibrinogenemia with active bleeding. For complex coagulation factor deficiency states (ie, DIC and dilutional coagulopathy), cryoprecipitate may be needed along with FFP to normalize fibrinogen levels. For correcting states of hypofibrinogenemia, the same replacement formula can be applied, but in general, 1 U/5 kg should increase a small child's fibrinogen by approximately 100 mg/dL (see Table 1).

Plasma derivatives

Plasma derivatives are concentrates of plasma proteins prepared from large donor pools (10,000 to 60,000) of plasma or cryoprecipitate. The specific protein of interest is purified and concentrated and cell fragments, cytokines, and viruses are inactivated or removed. Methods of viral inactivation include solvent-detergent treatment, pasteurization, immunoaffinity chromatography, and nanofiltration. Factor concentrates can be human plasma derived or produced in vitro using genetically engineered cell lines (recombinant). Human-derived and recombinant factor VIII and IX preparations are available for short-term and prophylactic treatment of bleeding in patients who have hemophilia A or B. Because the newer recombinant products (Recombinate, Kogenate, Advate, Benefix, and Novoseven) have limited or no albumin as a human protein, they are considered extremely safe for transmitting human infectious organisms and, therefore, are the preferred products when available for specific single factor replacement. Certain selected human-derived factor VIII preparations (Humate-P and Koate-HP) contain significant amounts of VWF and are used for treatment of significant bleeding in VWD rather than cryoprecipitate when available. The VWF activity and dosing are expressed as ristocetin cofactor units. Recombinant factor VIIa (Novoseven) is indicated for the use of acute bleeding and prophylaxis for patients with hemophilia A or B, who have inhibitors to FVIII and FIX, respectively, and congenital factor VII deficiency. Reports also have documented off-label use for treatment of acute bleeding in patients who have qualitative platelet disorders, such as Glanzmann's thrombasthenia, severe liver disease, and massive bleeding in the trauma setting [44,45]. Activated prothrombin complex (FEIBA) is a human plasma–derived factor IX complex that in addition to factor IX contains various amounts of activated factors II, VII, and X and trace amounts of factor VIII. Although traditionally used for patients who have hemophilia A and who have inhibitors, FEIBA has been replaced by recombinant factor VIIa because of a higher thrombotic risk at higher doses and because the small amounts of factor VIII present within the product can stimulate anamnesis, thereby increasing inhibitor titers in patients who have hemophilia and who are considered for immune tolerance therapy [46].

Granulocytes

Granulocytes are the least used blood component for many reasons, including the logistics of collection, limited storage viability (24 hours), and lack of conclusive evidence of efficacy in various clinical settings. Granulocytes are collected by apheresis from "stimulated" donors to collect higher numbers and more activated granulocytes. Donors can be stimulated with steroids, granulocyte colony-stimulating factor (GCSF), or both. Although studies show that costimulation with GCSF and steroids is superior in terms of granulocyte yield (increase collections to 6 to 8 $\times$ 10^{10} granulocytes per procedure), stimulation of donors is not performed by all blood banks and transfusion centers. All granulocyte components are stored at 20°C to 24°C without agitation, and contain at least 1 $\times$ 10^{10} granulocytes per product, with variable numbers of lymphocytes, platelets, and RBCs in 200 to 400 mL plasma. Because of this, units must be ABO compatible and preferably RhD negative for RhD-negative recipients. Granulocyte function deteriorates rapidly during storage and, therefore, should be transfused as soon as possible after collection and no later than 24 hours after collection. This may require that physicians waive, in writing, viral serologic testing of the product and obtain separate consent from recipients.

Granulocyte transfusion should be used as an adjunct to other medical therapies, including the use of granulocyte-stimulating factors, antibiotics, and antifungals. Because of the lack of randomized controlled trials addressing efficacy and the recent developments of better antimicrobial agents, the Infectious Disease Society of America does not recommend the routine use of granulocyte transfusions for prolonged refractory neutropenic infections

[21]. Meta-analysis of the efficacy and safety of granulocyte infusion as adjuncts to antibiotic therapy in treatment of neutropenic neonates who have sepsis was inconclusive that granulocyte infusions reduce morbidity and mortality in septic neutropenic newborns [47]. It generally is accepted, however, to strongly consider granulocyte transfusion in severe (or progressive) bacterial or fungal infection in patients who are severely neutropenic and who have no response to appropriate aggressive antimicrobial treatment and no expected recovery of neutrophil count for more than 7 days [48,49]. For neonates and small children, daily infusion of 1 to 2×10^9 polymorphonuclear cells (PMNs)/kg, and for larger children, an absolute daily dosage of at least 4 to 8×10^{10} PMNs, are recommended until recovery (see Table 1) [18,21,48].

Granulocyte transfusions frequently are accompanied by fevers, chills, and allergic reactions. More severe reactions, such as hypotension, respiratory distress, and lung injury, occur in 1% to 5% of transfusions; previously HLA-alloimmunized patients are at the greatest risk [48]. Patients should be tested for the presence of HLA and antineutrophil antibodies before the first granulocyte transfusion and periodically during prolonged courses of transfusions or when there is concern for alloimmunization (eg, poor post-transfusion increments in WBC or platelets, pulmonary infiltrates, or frequent febrile transfusion reactions). An additional concern regarding alloimmunization entails the likelihood of future patients who have bone marrow transplantation of finding a suitable HLA match. This is important especially when family members are considered as donors; these individuals should not be considered as granulocyte donors for patients before bone marrow transplantation. If alloimmunization does occur, HLA-matched granulocytes may be sought. Because granulocyte concentrates contain lymphocytes, all components should be gamma irradiated and CMV negative if appropriate to recipients, because leukoreduction is contraindicated.

Acute transfusion reactions

There are many benefits to transfusion therapy; however, there are risks that may be incurred acutely or in the long term. It is important for physicians to be aware of their incidence and to be able to recognize these adverse reactions swiftly so as to take proper action to prevent significant morbidity and mortality as a result of them. Some adverse reactions are discussed previously (eg, TA-GVHD, alloimmunization, and CMV reactivation) and are not discussed further. Discussed later are adverse reactions that take place at the time of, or within 24 hours after, transfusion. Although most acute reactions in pediatric patients are immune related, nonimmune-related complications, such as bacterial contamination, transfusion-associated circulatory overload (TACO), and thermal/mechanical hemolysis, always should be considered. When an acute transfusion reaction occurs, it is imperative to stop the transfusion immediately, maintain intravenous access, verify that the correct unit was transfused to the patient, treat the patient's symptoms, and notify the transfusion service for further investigation.

Febrile reactions

Fever is a common symptom of transfusion reactions. When a fever develops, serious transfusion reactions, such as bacterial contamination, acute hemolysis of ABO incompatible red cells, or transfusion-related acute lung injury (TRALI), should be considered; the transfusion should be stopped and the transfusion service notified so as to initiate the appropriate evaluation and quarantine any further products from the suspected donor unit. A common less severe etiology includes FNHTRs, which can result from the transfusion of RBCs, platelets, or plasma [16]. In the past, FNHTRs occurred in up to 30% of transfusions; however, since the advent of leukoreduction, the incidence is only 0.1% to 3% for all products [6–8,16]. Although FNHTRs are relatively harmless, they may be uncomfortable for recipients. A fever ($>1°C$ increase in temperature) often is accompanied by chills, rigors, and overall discomfort making it difficult to discern this entity from other more serious etiologies. FNHTRs are believed to result from the release of pyrogenic cytokines, interleukin (IL)-1β, IL-6, and IL-8 and tumor necrosis factor α, by leukoctyes within the plasma during storage. Prestorage leukoreduction is shown to decrease the incidence of FNHTRs in patients receiving RBCs and platelet products [6–8]. In severe or recalcitrant cases, washing the blood product may be considered. The usefulness of premedication with antipyretics to prevent FNHTRs is controversial. Retrospective analysis showed no difference in the incidence of FNHTRs between those who received premedication versus those who received placebo [50].

Allergic reactions

Allergic transfusion reactions (ATRs) are the most common of all acute transfusion reactions. The severity of the allergic reaction can range from mild localized urticaria, pruritis, and flushing to bronchospasm and anaphylaxis. Unlike other acute transfusion reactions, fever usually is absent, and if the symptoms are mild and resolve with stopping the transfusion and administering antihistamines, the transfusion may be restarted. Most patients who have ATRs respond to antihistamines and pretreatment may help to prevent recurrence. These reactions are caused by an antibody response in recipients to soluble plasma proteins within the blood product. Leukoreduction is not shown to decrease the incidence of ATRs as it has for FNHTRs [8,51]. Severe ATRs leading to anaphylaxis often are the result of the development of anti-IgA antibodies in recipients who are IgA deficient. Long-term management of individuals who have had severe ATRs is difficult.

Pretransfusion medication with antihistamines and steroids is recommended and washed RBCs and platelets should be used because they remove most of the plasma responsible for the ATR. Epinephrine should be readily available during subsequent transfusions. In patients who are IgA deficient and have documented anti-IgA antibodies, IgA-deficient plasma products may be obtained through rare donor registries if time permits [51].

Acute hemolytic transfusion reactions

An acute hemolytic transfusion reaction (AHTR) occurs when RBCs are transfused to a recipient who has preformed antibodies to antigens on the transfused RBCs. Most reactions are the result of antibodies to the RBC major blood group antigens A or B resulting from clerical errors. Infants under 4 months are not considered at risk for AHTRs because of the absence of A and B isoagglutinins and other RBC antigens (alloantibodies); however, maternal IgG antibodies can cross the placenta causing hemolysis of transfused RBCs and, therefore, should be considered when transfusing infants. Less commonly, nonimmune causes of acute hemolysis may occur. These include hemolysis from mechanical devices, such as blood warmers, infusion devices, filters, and catheters; improper storage; or bacterial contamination [10].

Signs and symptoms of AHTRs include fever, chills, nausea, vomiting, shortness of breath, chest pain, hypotension, vasoconstriction, and hemoglobinuria, with potential progression to DIC and acute renal failure. When AHTR is suspected, the transfusion should be stopped immediately and a full transfusion evaluation initiated, which includes obtaining blood cultures from the units, comparing the direct antibody test from the patient's pretransfusion crossmatch to the post-transfusion direct antibody test, and a clerical check to verify the correct unit was given to the correct patient. Aggressive intravenous fluid therapy is required to maintain intravascular volume and to prevent acute renal failure. The severity of the reaction and mortality rate are correlated directly to the rate and amount of incompatible blood transfused. Mortality reaches 44% in individuals receiving larger volumes of incompatible blood [51].

Transfusion-related acute lung injury

TRALI is an uncommon yet potentially fatal acute immune-related transfusion reaction that recently has become the leading cause of death from transfusion in the United States. It typically occurs during or within 4 hours of transfusion and presents with respiratory distress resulting from noncardiogenic pulmonary edema (normal central venous pressure and pulmonary capillary wedge pressure), hypotension, fever, and severe hypoxemia (O_2 saturation < 90% in room air) [10,52]. Transient leukopenia can be observed within a few hours of the reaction and can distinguish

TRALI from TACO, an acute, nonimmune transfusion reaction that presents with respiratory distress, cardiogenic pulmonary edema, and hypertension resulting from volume overload. TRALI usually improves after 48 to 96 hours from onset of symptoms, but aggressive respiratory support is required in 75% of patients and 10% to 15% of patients who have TRALI have a fatal outcome. Although patients who have TACO often respond to diuresis, patients who have TRALI may require fluid or vasopressor support in the face of hypotension, and diuretics should be avoided [52].

Although the exact mechanism of TRALI remains uncertain, two not mutually exclusive hypotheses are proposed: the antibody-mediated hypothesis and the neutrophil priming hypothesis. According to the antibody-mediated hypothesis, antineutrophil or anti–HLA I or II antibodies (from donor or recipient) attach to the corresponding antigen on neutrophils, causing sequestration and activation of neutrophils within the lungs, resulting in endothelial damage and vascular leakage. Many reports clearly document the presence of these antibodies in TRALI reactions [53]. In 85% to 90% of the cases, the antibodies were present within the donor blood unit, whereas in approximately 10% of the cases, the antibodies were found present in the recipient. Leukoreduction of cellular blood products decreases the incidence of TRALI caused by recipient leukocyte antibodies to incompatible donor leukocyte antigens [6,52]. The neutrophil priming hypothesis is proposed to account for the cases of TRALI in which no antibody is identified. In this two-hit mechanism, the first event is the clinical situation within the recipient surrounding the transfusion, which primes neutrophils (eg, surgery, infection, or trauma). The second event consists of the transfusion of "bioactive factors," such as cytokines, IL-6, IL-8, bioactive lipids (ie, lysophosphatidylcholines), or anti-HLA/antineutrophil antibodies, which produces neutrophil sequestration with the endothelium of the lungs. Some reports show that cases of TRALI in adults, in which antibodies were not identified in the donor or recipient, had less severe courses than those associated with antibodies [52,53].

TRALI is reported as a consequence of all blood product transfusions; however, plasma products (FFP and FP) account for the majority (50%–63%) of TRALI fatalities [52,53]. TRALI is reported in pediatric patients, albeit in a limited number of case reports. High-risk pediatric populations consist of those with hematologic malignancy, post–bone marrow transplant, and autoimmune disorders. In the largest epidemiologic study on TRALI, which included 15 pediatric patients, the most common setting surrounding the reaction in children was induction chemotherapy for acute lymphoblastic leukemia [54]. There are no definitive cases of TRALI documented in the neonatal population.

Recent data from the United Kingdom's serious hazards of transfusion initiative and the American Red Cross have shown that the majority of TRALI cases resulting from high-volume plasma products (FFP and apheresis platelets) involved an antileukocyte antibody-positive female donor

[55,56]. This is attributed to an increase in antileukocyte and anti-HLA antibodies present in multiparous women. Although the United Kingdom has adopted a policy of minimizing transfusion of high-volume plasma products from female donors and subsequently has seen a dramatic decrease in the incidence of TRALI, somewhat different procedures have been adopted in the United States [55]. These include use of male-only, high-volume plasma products or the use of male and female donor products after selecting for donors who have a low likelihood of having been alloimmunized by pregnancy or transfusions. Performing leukocyte antibody testing on female-donor, high-volume plasma products is a suggested alternative measure [57].

Future directions

Since the advent of transfusion medicine, many technologic advances have made the collection of blood products safer and more efficient. Ongoing research, however, is underway to improve several aspects of blood component collection and administration. Advances in DNA technology are changing the understanding of blood group antigens and HLA serotypes and allowing blood centers to solve compatibility problems among alloimmunized/refractory patients. The implications of DNA-based RBC and HLA genotyping are only beginning to become apparent in clinical practice. Nucleic acid amplification testing is beginning to replace serologic testing for several blood-borne infectious agents in blood products, and ongoing research involving multipathogen microarray technology for donor screening may reform the current infectious disease donor screening interventions. Pathogen inactivation is successful in eliminating enveloped virus transmission in plasma derivatives. Considerable effort continues to be invested in the development of universal pathogen inactivation techniques using nucleic acid inactivating agents, given that no single technique has proved effective for all blood components, and their effect on the final blood product is not fully known.

As a result of dramatic developments in apheresis technology, separation of every blood component, including HPCs, can be accomplished from a single donor. HPC transplantation increasingly is used in place of bone marrow transplantation in childhood malignancies and other diseases because of the increased safety and availability of this technique of stem cell collection. In addition, the use of umbilical cord blood as a source of HPCs, whose collection and processing parallels that of peripheral blood stem cell techniques, rapidly is expanding the inventory of viable graft options for children and adults who have these disorders. Refinements in bioengineering and apheresis technology are expanding the ability to grow, proliferate, and collect many bone marrow–derived cells, which may show promise in cellular immunotherapy.

Lastly, a call for a national hemovigilance system, similar to those established in European countries, has been proposed for the United States. Once established, transfusion safety can be monitored at several levels to prevent adverse transfusion events with ongoing monitoring and early recognition of undesirable trends within the community.

References

[1] Luban NL. Basics of transfusion medicine. In: Furman B, Zimmerman JJ, editors. Pediatric critical care. 3rd edition. Philadelphia: Mosby; 2006. p. 1185–98.

[2] Luban NL, Strauss RG, Hume HA. Commentary on the safety of red cells preserved in extended storage media for neonatal transfusions. Transfusion 1991;31:229–35.

[3] Strauss RG, Burneister LF, Johnson K, et al. Feasibility and safety of AS-3 red blood cells for neonatal transfusions. J Pediatr 2000;136:215–9.

[4] Jain R, Jarosz C. Safety and efficacy of AS-1 red blood cell use in neonates. Transfus Apher Sci 2001;24(2):111–5.

[5] Price TH, editor. Standards for blood banks and transfusion services. 25th edition. Bethesda (MD): American Association of Blood Banks; 2008.

[6] Yazer MH, Podlosky L, Clarke G, et al. The effect of prestorage leukoreduction on the rates of febrile nonhemolytic transfusion reactions to PC and RBC. Transfusion 2004;44:10–5.

[7] Paglino JC, Pomper GJ, Fisch G, et al. Reduction of febrile but not allergic reactions to red cells and platelets following conversion to universal prestorage leukoreduction. Transfusion 2004;44:16–24.

[8] King TE, Tanz W, Shirey S, et al. Universal leukoreduction decreases the incidence of febrile nonhemolytic transfusion reactions to red cells. Transfusion 2004;44:25–9.

[9] Technical manual of the American Association of Blood Banks. 14th edition. Bethesda (MD): American Association of Blood Banks; 2003.

[10] Luban NL, Wong EC. Hazards of transfusion. In: Arceci RJ, Hann IM, Smith OP, editors. Pediatric hematology. 3rd edition. New York: Wiley Blackwell; 2006. p. 724–44.

[11] Bowden RA, Slichter SJ, Sayers M, et al. A comparison of filtered leukocyte-reduced and cytomegalovirus (CMV) seronegative blood products for the prevention of transfusion-associated CMV infection after marrow transplant. Blood 1995;86:3598–603.

[12] Nichols WG, Price TH, Gooley T, et al. Transfusion-transmitted cytomegalovirus infection after receipt of leukoreduced blood products. Blood 2003;101:4195–220.

[13] Narvios AB, de Lima M, Shah H, et al. Transfusion of leukoreduced cellular blood components from cytomegalovirus-unscreened donors in allogeneic hematopoietic transplant recipients: analysis of 72 recipients. Bone Marrow Transpl 2005;35:499–501.

[14] Special products. In: Roseff SD, editor. Pediatric transfusion: a physician's handbook. 2nd edition. Bethesda (MD): American Association of Blood Banks; 2006. p. 179–94.

[15] Strauss RG. Data-driven blood banking practices for neonatal RBC transfusions. Transfusion 2000;40(12):1528–40.

[16] Pelsynski MM, Moroff G, Luban NL, et al. Effect of gamma irradiation of red blood cell units on T-cell inactivation as assessed by limiting dilution analysis: implications for preventing transfusion-associated graft-versus-host disease. Blood 1994;83(6):1683–9.

[17] Davey RJ, McCoy NC, Yu M, et al. The effect of prestorage irradiation on posttransfusion red cell survival. Transfusion 1992;32(6):525–8.

[18] Blood components. In: Roseff SD, editor. Pediatric transfusion: a physician's handbook. 2nd edition. Bethesda (MD): American Association of Blood Banks; 2006. p. 1–52.

[19] Weiskopf RB, Schnapp S, Rouine-Rapp K, et al. Extracellular potassium concentration in red blood cell suspensions after irradiation and washing. Transfusion 2005;45:1295–301.

[20] Roseff SD, Luban NL, Manno CS. Guidelines for assessing appropriateness of pediatric transfusion. Transfusion 2002;42:1398–413.

[21] Robitaille N, Hume HA. Blood components and fractionated plasma products: preparations, indications, and administration. In: Arceci RJ, Hann IM, Smith OP, editors. Pediatric hematology. 3rd edition. New York: Wiley Blackwell; 2006. p. 693–706.

[22] Vichinsky EP, Haberkern CM, Neumayer L, et al. A comparison of conservative and aggressive transfusion regimens in the perioperative management of sickle cell disease. N Engl J Med 1995;333:206–13.

[23] Scotborn DJ, Price C, Schwartz D, et al. Risk of recurrent stroke in children with sickle cell disease receiving blood transfusion therapy for at least five years after initial stroke. J Pediatr 2002;140:348–54.

[24] Adams RJ, McKie VC, Hsu L, et al. Prevention of first stroke by transfusions in children with sickle cell anemia and abnormal results on transcranial Doppler ultrasonagraphy. N Engl J Med 1998;339:5–11.

[25] Adams RJ, Brambilla D. Discontinuing prophylactic transfusions used to prevent stroke in sickle cell disease. N Engl J Med 2005;353:2769–78.

[26] Smith-Whitley K. Alloimmunization in patients with sickle cell disease. In: Manno CS, editor. Pediatric transfusion therapy. Bethesda (MD): AABB Press; 2002. p. 249–82.

[27] Vichinsky EP, Luban NC, Wright E, et al. Prospective RBC phenotype matching in a stroke-prevention trial in sickle cell anemia: a multicenter transfusion trial. Transfusion 2001;41:1086–92.

[28] Alloimmune cytopenias. In: Roseff SD, editor. Pediatric transfusion: a physician's handbook. 2nd edition. Bethesda (MD): American Association of Blood Banks; 2006. p. 53–97.

[29] British Committee for Standards in Hematology, Blood Transfusion Task Force. Transfusion guidelines for neonates and older children. Br J Haematol 2004;124:433–53.

[30] Kirpalani H, Whyte RK, Anderson C, et al. The Premature Infants in Need of Transfusion (PINT) study: a randomized, controlled trial of a restrictive (low) versus liberal (high) transfusion threshold for extremely low birth weight infants. J Pediatr 2006;149:301–7.

[31] Bell EF, Strauss RG, Widness JA, et al. Randomized trial of liberal versus restrictive guidelines for red blood cell transfusion in preterm infants. J Pediatr 2005;115:1685–91.

[32] Cid J, Lozano M. Risk of Rh(D) alloimmunization after transfusion of platelets from D+ donors to D- recipients. Transfusion 2005;45:453.

[33] Klein HG, Anstee DJ, editors. Mollison's blood transfusion in clinical medicine. 11th edition. Blackwell; 2005. p. 187–91.

[34] Molnar R, Johnson R, Sweat LT, et al. Absence of D alloimmunization in D- pediatric oncology patients receiving D-incompatible single-donor platelets. Transfusion 2002;42:177–82.

[35] Gil-Fernandez JJ, Alegre A, FernandezVillalta MJ, et al. Clinical results of a stringent policy on prophylactic platelet transfusion: Non-randomized comparative analysis of 190 bone marrow transplant patients from a single institution. Bone Marrow Transplant 1996;18:931–5.

[36] Heckman KD, Weiner GJ, Davis CS. Randomized study of prophylactic platelet transfusion threshold during induction therapy for adult acute leukemia: 10,000 microL versus 20,000 microL. J Clin Oncol 1997;15:1143–9.

[37] Wandt H, Frank M, Ehninger G, et al. Safety and cost effectiveness of 10 x 109/L trigger for prophylactic platelet transfusion compared with the traditional 20 x 109/L trigger: a prospective comparative trial in 105 patients with acute myeloid leukemia. Blood 1998;91:3601–6.

[38] Murray NA, Horwarth LJ, McCloy MP, et al. Platelet transfusion in the management of severe thrombocytopenia in neonatal intensive care unit patients. Transfus Med 2002;12:35–41.

[39] Vassallo RR. New paradigms in the management of alloimmune refractoriness to platelet transfusions. Curr Opin Hematol 2007;14:655–63.

[40] Perotta PL, Pisciotto PT, Snyder EL. Platelets and related products. In: Hillyer CD, Silberstein LE, Ness PM, et al, editors. Blood banking and transfusion medicine basic principles and practice. 1st edition. Philadelphia: Churchill Livingstone; 2003. p. 181–206.

[41] Petz LD, Garatty G, Calhoun L, et al. Selecting donors of platelets for refractory patients on the basis of HLA antibody specificity. Transfusion 2000;40:1446–56.

[42] Delaflor-Weiss E, Mintz PD. The evaluation and management of platelet refractoriness and alloimmunization. Transfus Med Rev 2000;14:180–96.

[43] British Committee for Standards in Hematology, Blood Transfusion Task Force. Amendments and corrections to the 'transfusion guidelines for neonates and older children' (BCSH, 2004a); and to the 'Guidelines for the use of fresh frozen plasma, cryoprecipitate and cryosupernatent' (BCSH, 2004b). Br J Haematol 2006;136:514–6.

[44] Mathew P. The use of rVIIa in non-hemophilia bleeding conditions in paediatrics. A systematic review. Thromb Haemost 2004;92:738–46.

[45] Mathew P, Young G. Recombinant factor VIIa in paediatric bleeding disorders—a 2006 review. Haemophilia 2006;12:457–72.

[46] Green D. Complications associated with the treatment of haemophiliacs with inhibitors. Haemophilia 1999;5(Suppl 3):11–7.

[47] Mohan P, Brocklehurst P. Granulocyte transfusions for neonates with confirmed or suspected sepsis and neutropenia. Cochrane Database Syst Rev 2003;4:CD003956.

[48] Bishton M, Chopra R. The role of granulocyte transfusions in neutropenic patients. Br J Haematol 2004;127:501–8.

[49] Vamvakas EC, Pineda AA. Determinants of the efficacy of prophylactic granulocyte transfusions: a meta-analysis. J Clin Apheresis 1997;12:74–81.

[50] Sanders RP, Maddirala SD, Geiger TL, et al. Premedication with acetaminophen or diphenhydramine for transfusion with leucoreduced blood products in children. Br J Haematol 2005;130:781–7.

[51] Davenport RD. Hemolytic transfusion reactions. In: Popovsky MA, editor. Transfusion reactions. 3rd edition. 2007. p. 1–56.

[52] Kopko PM, Popovsky MA. Transfusion related acute lung injury. In: Popovsky MA, editor. Transfusion reactions. 3rd edition. 2007. p. 207–28.

[53] Sanchez R, Toy P. Transfusion related acute lung injury: a pediatric perspective. Pediatr Blood Cancer 2005;45:248–55.

[54] Silliman CC, Boshkov LK, Meddizadehkashi Z, et al. Transfusion-related acute lung injury: epidemiology and a prospective analysis of etiologic factors. Blood 2003;101:454–62.

[55] Serious Hazards of Transfusion (SHOT). Annual report. 2006. Manchester, UK: SHOT Scheme, 2006. Available at: http://www.shotuk.org/SHOTREPORT2006.PDF. Accessed March 12, 2008.

[56] Eder AF, Herron R, Strupp A, et al. Transfusion related acute lung injury surveillance (2003–2005) and the potential impact of the selective use of plasma from male donors in the American Red Cross. Transfusion 2007;47:599–607.

[57] Transfusion-related acute lung injury Association bulletin #06-07. Bethesda (MD): AABB; 2006. Available at: http://www.aabb.org/content/Members_Area/Association_Bulleins/ab06-07.htm. Accessed March 12, 2008.

ELSEVIER
SAUNDERS

PEDIATRIC CLINICS
OF NORTH AMERICA

Pediatr Clin N Am 55 (2008) 447–460

Update on Thalassemia: Clinical Care and Complications

Melody J. Cunningham, MD

*Thalassemia Research Program, Division of Hematology/Oncology, Children's Hospital
Boston, 300 Longwood Avenue, Fegan 7, Boston, MA 02115, USA*

β-Thalassemia, originally named Cooley anemia, initially was described by Dr. Cooley in 1925 in Detroit as an inherited blood disease [1]. It is speculated that thalassemia was first recognized in the United States and not in its area of highest prevalence (the Mediterranean) because its presentation as a distinct clinical entity was masked by the fact that malaria, with its similar clinical picture of hemolysis, anemia, and splenomegaly, was ubiquitous in that region [1]. Thus, patients who had this clinical triad were assumed to have malaria, not thalassemia [1]. Now it is recognized that various types of thalassemia are inherited anemias caused by mutations at the globin gene loci on chromosomes 16 and 11, affecting the production of α- or β-globin protein, respectively [2,3].

The thalassemia syndromes are named according to the globin chain affected or the abnormal hemoglobin produced. Thus, β-globin gene mutations give rise to β-thalassemia and α-globin mutations cause α-thalassemia. In addition, the thalassemias are characterized by their clinical severity (phenotype). Thalassemia major (TM) refers to disease requiring more than eight red blood cell (RBC) transfusions per year and thalassemia intermedia (TI) to disease that requires no or infrequent transfusions [4]. Thalassemia trait refers to carriers of mutations; such individuals have microcytosis and hypochromia but no or only mild anemia [5,6]. Untreated TM uniformly is fatal in the first few years of life [1]. In addition, TM and severe TI can lead to considerable morbidity affecting nearly all organ systems [7–9]. The combination of early diagnosis, improvements in monitoring for organ complications, and advances in supportive care, however, have enabled many patients who have severe thalassemia syndromes to live productive, active lives well into adulthood [9–11].

E-mail address: melody.cunningham@childrens.harvard.edu

doi:10.1016/j.pcl.2008.02.002   *pediatric.theclinics.com*

Epidemiology

Similar to sickle cell disease and G6PD deficiency, the high prevalence of α- and β-thalassemia genotypes is believed a consequence of an evolutionary protection of heterozygotes against death from *Plasmodium falciparum* malaria [11,12]. Before the twentieth century, thalassemia tracked with areas of malarial prevalence. β-Thalassemia arose in the Mediterranean, Middle East, South and Southeast Asia, and southern China. α-Thalassemia originated in Africa, the Middle East, China, India, and Southeast Asia [13–15]. Immigration and emigration, however, have led to changing demographics, and patients who have thalassemia syndromes and heterozygote carriers now reside in all parts of the world [16,17]. Thus, it is important for pediatricians, obstetrician, and hematologists to be aware of a possible diagnosis of thalassemia wherever they practice and for any patients they evaluate who have anemia. Consideration of the diagnosis allows proper diagnosis and management of individual patients and identification of carriers and ensures necessary testing and counseling to the population at risk for having children who have thalassemia.

Diagnosis

Understanding how thalassemia can be diagnosed requires a review of the structure of hemoglobin and the genetics of the thalassemia syndromes. Normal human hemoglobin is comprised of two α-like and two β-like globin chains. Adult hemoglobin consists of hemoglobin A ($\alpha_2\beta_2$) plus small amounts of hemoglobin A_2 ($\alpha_2\delta_2$) and hemoglobin F ($\alpha_2\gamma_2$). Genetic mutations in one of the globin genes (α or β) result in decreased or absent production of that globin chain and a relative excess of the other. These mutations can result in no globin production (β° or α°) or decreased globin production (β^+ or α^+).

The α-globin gene is duplicated on chromosome 16; thus, each diploid cell carries four copies. The clinical syndromes of α-thalassemia reflect the number of inherited genes that are mutated. The α-thalassemia syndromes are silent carrier, α-thalassemia trait, hemoglobin H disease, and hydrops fetalis and reflect inheritance of 1, 2, 3, or 4 α-globin gene mutations, respectively. In contrast, a single β-globin gene resides on each chromosome 11. The four clinical syndromes of β-thalassemia, namely silent carrier, thalassemia trait, TI, and TM, correspond to the degree of expression of the two β-globin genes that encode β-globin and not the number of mutated genes.

α-Thalassemia has a wide spectrum of syndromes due to the possibility of one, two, three, or four allelic mutations. Mutation in one of the four alleles results in the silent carrier, with no clinical symptoms, normal complete blood cell count, and hemoglobin electrophoresis results past infancy. If two of the four α-globin alleles are mutated, affected individuals have α-thalassemia trait, with no clinical symptoms, but microcytosis and hypochromia and only mild anemia. The newborn screen often reports hemoglobin Bart, a fast-migrating hemoglobin that appears only in cord and neonatal blood when there is a deletion of one or more of the four α-globin alleles. Hemoglobin Bart is a γ_4 homotetramer that disappears rapidly in the neonatal period; its amount at birth corresponds to the number of affected alleles [18]. Three α-gene mutations cause hemoglobin H disease with anemia characterized by microcytosis and hypochromia. Complete absence of α-globin chain production (all four alleles affected) leads to hydrops fetalis, which usually results in death in utero if intrauterine transfusions are not available [6,18].

β-Thalassemia has a similar spectrum of clinical phenotypes that reflect the underlying allelic mutations in the β-globin genes. If only a single β-globin gene is affected, then the resulting β-thalassemia silent carrier or trait results from partial (β^+) or absent (β°) gene expression, respectively. Similar to α-thalassemia trait, patients who have β-thalassemia trait typically have mild anemia, microcytosis, and hypochromia. When both β-globin genes are affected, then the resulting phenotype is more severe, depending on the degree of gene expression and relative imbalance of globin chains. For example, β^+/β^+ genotypes typically are associated with an intermediate phenotype (TI), whereas the β°/β° genotype leads to the more severe TM.

Specific mutations in the α or β genes may lead to production of unique hemoglobins on electrophoresis, two of which have unusual features worth discussing in the context of thalassemia. Hemoglobin Constant Spring (Hb CS) is an α-globin gene variant caused by a mutation in the normal stop codon. The resulting elongated α-globin chain forms an unstable hemoglobin tetramer. Hb CS often occurs in conjunction with α-thalassemia so is associated with the more severe α-thalassemia phenotypes. Hemoglobin E (HbE) is caused by a nucleotide change in the β-globin gene, which leads to a single amino acid substitution (Glu26Lys) and diminished expression with a β^+ phenotype. HbE thus is an unusual "thalassemic hemoglobinopathy" that can lead to clinically severe phenotypes when paired with other forms of β-thalassemia.

Pathophysiology

The thalassemia syndromes were among the first genetic diseases to be understood at the molecular level. More than 200 β-globin and 30 α-globin mutations deletions have been identified; these mutations result in decreased or absent production of one globin chain (α or β) and a relative excess of the other. The resulting imbalance leads to unpaired globin chains, which precipitate and cause premature death (apoptosis) of the red cell precursors within the marrow, termed ineffective erythropoiesis. Of the damaged but viable RBCs that are released from the bone marrow, many are removed by the spleen or hemolyzed directly in the circulation due to the hemoglobin precipitants. Combined RBC destruction in the bone marrow, spleen, and periphery causes anemia and, ultimately, an escalating cycle of pathology resulting in the clinical syndrome of severe thalassemia.

Damaged erythrocytes enter the spleen and are trapped in this low pH and low oxygen environment; subsequent splenomegaly exacerbates the trapping of cells and worsens the anemia. Anemia and poor tissue oxygenation stimulate increased kidney erythropoietin production that further drives marrow erythropoiesis, resulting in increased ineffective marrow activity and the classic bony deformities associated with poorly managed TM and severe TI [19]. Anemia in the severe thalassemia phenotypes necessitates multiple RBC transfusions and, over time, without proper chelation, results in transfusion-associated iron overload. In addition, ineffective erythropoiesis enhances gastrointestinal iron absorption and can result in iron overload, even in untransfused patients who have TI [20–22]. It has long been recognized that the severity of ineffective erythropoiesis affects the degree of iron loading, but until the recent discovery of hepcidin and understanding, its role in iron metabolism the link was not understood.

Hepcidin, an antimicrobial hormone, is recognized as playing a major role in iron deficiency and overload [23]. Hepcidin initially was discovered due to its role in the etiology of anemia of chronic inflammation or chronic disease [24]. Elevated levels, associated with increased inflammatory markers, maintain low levels of circulating bioavailable iron in two important ways: (1) by preventing iron absorption and transport from the gut and (2) by preventing release and recycling of iron from macrophages and the reticuloendothelial system [23]. Conversely, inadequate hepcidin allows increased gastrointestinal absorption of iron and ultimately may lead to excess iron sufficient to result in organ toxicity [22,25,26].

Iron not bound to transferrin, also referred to as nontransferrin-bound iron, damages the endocrine organs, liver, and heart [27]. Nontransferrin-bound iron can result in myocyte damage leading to arrhythmias and congestive heart failure, the primary causes of death in patients who have thalassemia [9,10,28]. Appropriate chelation therapy and close monitoring of cardiac siderosis can avoid this devastating complication (see the article by Kwiatkowski elsewhere in this issue for discussion of iron chelators).

Changing demographics and carrier screening

The clinical spectrum of thalassemia in the developed world has changed dramatically in the 3 decades since the introduction of deferoxamine chelation [9,10]. In addition, new treatment options and prevention strategies to avoid complications of the disease and its compulsory treatments, coupled with immigration changes, have altered the demography of thalassemia in North America [16,17]. Younger patients are now predominantly of Asian descent, whereas the aging population of patients who have thalassemia are of Mediterranean descent (Fig. 1). According to the United States Census Bureau, the number of Asians increased significantly from 1980 to a total

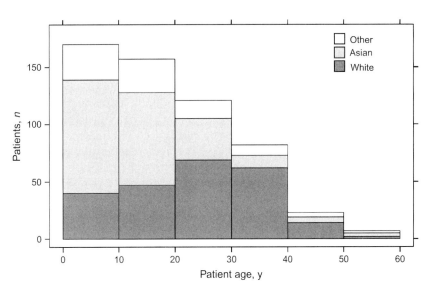

Fig. 1. Changing demographics of patients who have thalassemia in the North American Thalassemia Clinical Research Network. Patients of Asian descent predominate in the younger population. (*From* Vichinsky EP, Macklin EA, Waye JS, et al. Changes in the epidemiology of thalassemia in North America: a new minority disease. Pediatrics 2005;116(6):e818–25; with permission.)

of 6.9 million in the census count in 1990. Coupled with other changes that have occurred over the past few decades, it is estimated that up to 100 million people of African, Hispanic, Southern and Eastern European, Middle Eastern, and Asian ethnic backgrounds reside in the United States. Similarly, it is estimated that approximately one sixth of the Canadian population is foreign born. This includes a considerable influx of Asians: in the 1990s more than 2 million people immigrated to Canada, approximately half from Asia. Many of the ethnic immigrants who relocated to North America are carriers of globin gene mutations, which have important implications for carrier screening. Recent reports reveal births of children who have severe α- or β-thalassemia in which appropriate screening and counseling was not offered to the parents [18].

Screening is inexpensive and simple but requires clinicians to be astutely attentive and aware of potential carriers. A complete blood cell count identifies microcytosis and hypochromia, which are present in nearly all thalassemia carriers at risk for having babies who have a severe thalassemia syndrome. In an adult, a mean corpuscular volume of less than 80 fL and mean corpuscular hemoglobin of less than 27 pg should alert a clinician to perform further screening, specifically hemoglobin electrophoresis and, in some cases, globin genotype testing. In addition, β-thalassemia carriers have elevated hemoglobin A_2 on adult electrophoresis unless there is concomitant iron deficiency, which may falsely normalize the hemoglobin

A2 (HbA$_2$) level [29]. Once confirmed, genetic counseling should be offered to parents or potential parents [18].

A newborn hemoglobinopathy screen can be helpful in the recognition and diagnosis of potential thalassemia syndromes. Severe β-thalassemia with absent β production due to two β° mutations has only fetal hemoglobin (HbF) as there is no hemoglobin A ($\alpha_2\beta_2$) produced. This abnormal "HbF only" result should prompt a clinician to follow the baby's hemoglobin and growth to determine at what age the baby will need to initiate transfusions to prevent the complications of severe anemia. The anticipated severity of the α-thalassemia syndromes not always is determined easily by the results of a newborn screen. These babies all have an elevated percentage of hemoglobin Bart (γ_4) at birth but the level does not always correspond directly to the number of affected genes. This should alert pediatricians, however, to counsel parents to receive personal testing to determine the number of abnormal α-globin genes in each parent. If each parent has only one mutated α-globin gene, the most clinically significant outcome results in the birth of a baby who has a two-gene α-thalassemia (α-thalassemia trait), which has no clinical consequences. Conversely, if each parent has a two-gene mutation on the same chromosome, termed a *cis* mutation, there exists a risk for the most severe form of α-thalassemia, four-gene deletion, leading to hydrops fetalis, which often results in fetal demise without in utero transfusion [30,31].

Clinical complications

Transfusion-associated issues

Iron overload

The primary long-term complication of chronic RBC transfusions for thalassemia is iron loading and the resultant parenchymal organ toxicity. Cardiac iron-overload leading to cardiac failure or arrhythmias is the most common fatal complication seen in chronically transfused patients who have thalassemia [9]. Adherence to chelation can prevent cardiac damage and death from cardiac injury. Patients who present with cardiac arrythmias or failure due to iron injury often can be rescued by continuous infusion deferoxamine although adherence to the regimen of subcutaneous deferoxamine delivered 24 hours per day, 7 days per week, is difficult [32].

In addition, the endocrine organs are exquisitely sensitive to the toxic effects of iron and this may result in hypogonadotropic hypogonadism, pituitary damage, diabetes [4,8,33], osteopenia, and osteoporosis. Hypogonadotrophic hypogonadism is common in young adults who have TM and is believed to contribute to low fertility in this population [34,35]. Additionally, cardiac complications of iron overload may exacerbate pregnancy and delivery complications in women who have thalassemia. Case reports and small published series reveal, however, that successful pregnancy and delivery of healthy babies is possible in women who have TM [33,35,36]. Spontaneous pregnancy without hormonal assistance is reported [33,35]. Recent literature on hypogonadotrophic hypogonadism suggests that early intervention with hormonal therapy and aggressive iron chelation therapy to prevent permanent damage may help preserve innate fertility. The effect of chelation on preservation of gonadal function currently is being investigated. For example, deferasirox, which provides extended blood chelator levels, may have a protective effect against toxicity to the endocrinologic organs, but further research remains necessary.

Alloimmunization

Chronic transfusions may result in the development of anti-RBC antibodies, alloantibodies and autoantibodies, in a variety of diseases [37]. Although several studies have investigated the rates of alloimmunization in patients who had sickle cell disease [37,38], the thalassemia population is less well studied. Small retrospective analyses have suggested alloimmunization rates of 2.7% to 37% in patients who had thalassemia [39,40]. Rates of alloimmunization are suggested as higher for transfusions with donor/recipient ethnic disparity [41] and in splenectomized patients [42]. Because of the risk for alloimmunization and autoimmunization, it is recommended that extended RBC antigen phenotyping be performed before initiation of RBC transfusions, so that patients can be transfused safely in the event of anti-RBC autoantibody or alloantibody formation. If a patient then develops autoantibodies directed against ubiquitous RBC antigens or multiple alloantibodies, blood that is matched more fully can be transfused more safely. For sickle cell patients requiring chronic transfusions, Rh and Kell antigen matching is considered standard of care and performed by many, but not all, care centers. For patients who have thalassemia, this matching strategy is not performed routinely. One recent study suggests, however, that matching for Rh and Kell in this population can decrease the alloantibody rate by 53% [42]. Unlike most patients who have sickle cell disease, patients who have thalassemia usually initiate chronic transfusions at 6 months to 2 years of age. Many clinicians believe that chronic transfusions early in life may allow development of tolerance to foreign RBC antigens and prevent development of alloimmunization. Further prospective studies in this area are required to determine the appropriate transfusion strategy in patients who have thalassemia.

Viral infection

The transmission of infections, in particular HIV, hepatitis B, and hepatitis C, remains a serious complication and a significant problem in some developing countries [43]. For now the sole use of volunteer donors who have no financial incentive to donate and thus are likely to answer a detailed donor questionnaire honestly provides the greatest protection against transfusion transmission of infections. Additionally, serologic and nucleic acid testing, used in the developed world, augment the safety of blood products [44]. When these safety measures are in place, the risk for transfusion-transmission of known infections is extraordinarily low [45].

The development of the hepatitis B vaccine, identification of the hepatitis C virus (HCV), and a serologic test to screen donors has greatly minimized the risk for transfusion-transmitted hepatitis B virus and HCV. The prevalence of HCV in patients who have thalassemia is disparate and depends on the screening procedures and donor pool. In the developing world, the prevalence is 20% to 64% [46], with recent data demonstrating continued exposure and infection to patients who have thalassemia receiving transfusions, including many pediatric patients [46]. In the North American population studied in the National Heart, Lung, and Blood Institute–sponsored Thalassemia Clinical Research Network, the prevalence of exposure was 70% in patients over 25 years of age but only 5% in patients under 15 years of age [4].

Chronic active hepatitis can lead to fibrosis, cirrhosis, and hepatocellular carcinoma (HCC) if untreated [9]. Treatment with interferon-α and ribavirin is the standard of care for patients who have chronic hepatitis C. Because ribavirin causes hemolysis and thus increases transfusion requirements and concomitant iron exposure, the package guidelines for ribavirin still recommend that it not be used to treat chronic hepatitis in patients who are chronically transfused. Small studies have demonstrated, however, that ribavirin can be given safely and effectively to patients who have thalassemia [47–50]. Because hepatic cirrhosis, liver failure, and HCC all are potential consequences of chronic active hepatitis, the majority of clinicians who care for these patients recommend treatment with interferon and ribavirin.

HCV-infected patients who have thalassemia are living long enough to develop prolonged chronic active hepatitis and be at risk for developing HCC. A multicenter retrospective review by Borgna-Pignatti and colleagues reported 22 patients who had HCC from a cohort of approximately 5000 patients who had thalassemia followed in 52 Italian centers [51]. These numbers likely underestimate, however, the true risk for cirrhosis and HCC to patients who have thalassemia and are infected with hepatitis C, because many succumbed to cardiac complications before living long enough to develop frank cirrhosis or HCC [9]. Patients who do not have evidence of hepatitis C exposure should have annual screening for HCV. Patients who have chronic hepatitis and are at risk for HCC should undergo routine screening with serum α-fetoprotein and liver ultrasound because survival in patients who have HCC is inversely proportional to the size of the tumor [52].

Thrombosis and hypercoagulable state

Data compiled from many series present compelling clinical evidence for increased risk for thrombosis in patients who have β-TI, β-TM, α-thalassemia syndromes, or hemoglobin E/β-thalassemia [53–55]. The risk for thromboses is increased in patients who are nontransfused or infrequently transfused and in patients who are splenectomized. This is believed to result in part from increased proportion of defective, innate RBCs [56]. Defective RBCs have disrupted membranes resulting in exposure of negatively charged lipids, including phosphatidylserine, on the external cell surface, which are believed thrombogenic. In the absence of the splenic removal of senescent cells, more of these defective cells are circulating, which increases the risk for thrombosis. In addition, markers studied show increased platelet activation, which also is believed to increase thrombotic risk [57]. The difficulty in ascertaining absolute clinical risk and determining appropriate preventive strategies is that many patients reported in the literature do not have exact transfusion regimens known [55]. More frequent transfusions result in an increased ratio of normal transfused RBCs to disrupted innate RBCs, thus decreasing the clinical risk for thrombosis based on current knowledge of risk factors.

Data in hemolytic states, including sickle cell disease and thalassemia, suggest depletion of nitric oxide resulting from chronic hemolysis and increased plasma levels of free hemoglobin [58]. Nitric oxide is a smooth muscle relaxant and decreased levels are believed to cause increased peripheral vascular resistance and ultimately pulmonary hypertension. Nitric oxide scavenging by free hemoglobin is implicated in the pulmonary arterial disease of sickle cell anemia and data suggest that this is a possible factor in thalassemia. Studies aimed at increasing the levels of nitric oxide and decreasing pulmonary hypertension [59] are ongoing and will be critical in determining clinical approaches to this problem in the aging thalassemia population.

Improvements in prognosis and survival

Survival

Historically, patients who had thalassemia had a poor prognosis. In a United States cohort born between 1960 and 1976, the median survival was 17 years [32]. In an Italian cohort born in the mid-1960s, the median survival was 12 years [9]. Remarkable and promising improvement in survival of patients who have thalassemia has been made, however, as demonstrated in two reports by Pearson and collagues [60,61]. In the first 1973 manuscript, before the era of deferoxamine chelation, they reported the ages of 243 patients who had thalassemia in 12 North American centers. In this cohort, 22% were younger than 5 years of age and 2.1% older than 25. The precipitous decrease in number of living patients who had thalassemia began at 15 years of age. Just over a decade later, in 1985, the same centers were surveyed and of the 303 patients, 11% were younger than 5 years and the population of patients older than 25 years had increased to 11% ($P < .01\%$).

More recently, Borgna-Pignatti and colleagues [28] published cohort survival data for nearly 1100 patients who had TM from seven centers in Italy. Kaplan-Meier survival curves were evaluated for 5-year birth cohorts (Fig. 2). The curves demonstrated a statistically significant difference in survival in patients in the later birth cohorts. Patients born between 1960 and 1964 had a greater than 60% mortality rate at 30 years of age as compared with the rate of 10% at 25 years of age in the cohort born from 1975 to 1979. The majority of the deaths resulted from cardiac hemosiderosis.

Curative therapies

Bone marrow transplantation

Successful cure of β-thalassemia by bone marrow transplantation first was reported by Thomas and associates in 1982 [62]. Subsequently, several centers have explored the use of this modality as definitive therapy [63–65]. The most extensive published experience with bone marrow transplantation in β-thalassemia is that of Lucarelli and coworkers in Italy [65]. Early on they reported thalassemia-free survival of only 53% in the older patients who had thalassemia with hepatomegaly, liver fibrosis, and inadequate pre-transplant chelation [65]. More recent data, however, even in patients considered at high-risk for transplant, demonstrate significant improvements [66]. Survival for the most recently transplanted 33 pediatric patients was 93% and the rate of graft rejection decreased from 30% to 8% [66]. Adults treated with this protocol demonstrated improved thalassemia-free survival, from 62% to 67%, and transplant-related mortality decreased from 37% but still was significant at 27%.

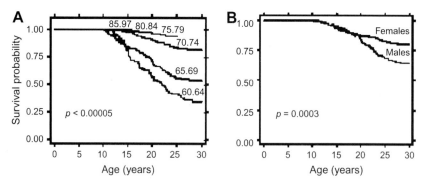

Fig. 2. Kaplan-Meier survival curves after the first decade of life by birth cohort (*A*) and gender (*B*) of 977 patients who had thalassemia in Italy. This demonstrates the dramatic improvement in the younger cohort born between 1985 and 1997. Because they have not had sufficient time to age into the fourth and fifth decades, it makes it difficult to determine the life expectancy of patients treated in developed countries who have access to appropriate chelation therapy and adequate medical care. (*From* Borgna-Pignatti C, Rugolotto S, De SP, et al. Survival and complications in patients with thalassemia major treated with transfusion and deferoxamine. Haematologica 2004;89(10):1187–93; with permission.)

On the basis of available data, bone marrow transplantation may be recommended to patients receiving adequate chelation without evidence of liver disease who have an HLA-matched sibling donor. Many of these patients can be cured [67–69]. Chronic graft-versus-host disease still is a potential long-term complication of successful allogeneic transplantation. A current limitation to the general applicability of this therapy is the availability of a related HLA-matched donor. Only one in four siblings on average is HLA identical. Improved management of graft-versus-host disease and the development of technologies for bone marrow transplantation from unrelated donors may expand the pool of potential donors in the near future. The use of cord blood stem cells and unrelated donors is extending the donor pool and number of patients who may receive bone marrow transplantation [70–72].

Gene therapy

Treatment of hematologic and other diseases through gene therapy is actively studied in murine and primate models [73,74]. The obstacles to success of this therapeutic modality and the availability of this therapy for humans include the need for improved efficiency of gene delivery, regulated and sustained expression of introduced genes, and insertion of the gene into non-oncogenic sites. Although gene therapy is an area of active clinical investigation, the aforementioned obstacles currently preclude its use in the management of thalassemia or sickle cell anemia. Nonetheless, the successful transfer of globin genes into hematopoietic cells of primates and humans has been demonstrated and is encouraging [75]. A phase I human gene therapy trial for thalassemia and sickle cell disease has been initiated in France but clinical data are not yet available.

References

[1] Weatherall DJ, Clegg JB. Historical perspectives: the many and diverse routes to our current understanding of the thalassaemias. In: Weatherall DJ, Clegg JB, editors. The thalassaemia syndromes. 4th edition. Oxford (England): Blackwell Science; 2001. p. 3–62.

[2] Deisseroth A, Nienhuis A, Turner P, et al. Localization of the human alpha-globin structural gene to chromosome 16 in somatic cell hybrids by molecular hybridization assay. Cell 1977; 12(1):205–18.

[3] Deisseroth A, Nienhuis A, Lawrence J, et al. Chromosomal localization of human beta globin gene on human chromosome 11 in somatic cell hybrids. Proc Natl Acad Sci U S A 1978; 75(3):1456–60.

[4] Cunningham MJ, Macklin EA, Neufeld EJ, et al. Complications of beta-thalassemia major in North America. Blood 2004;104(1):34–9.

[5] Cao A. Carrier screening and genetic counselling in beta-thalassemia. Int J Hematol 2002; 76(Suppl 2):105–13.

[6] Galanello R, Sanna MA, Maccioni L, et al. Fetal hydrops in Sardinia: implications for genetic counselling. Clin Genet 1990;38(5):327–31.

[7] Calleja EM, Shen JY, Lesser M, et al. Survival and morbidity in transfusion-dependent thalassemic patients on subcutaneous desferrioxamine chelation. Nearly two decades of experience. Ann N Y Acad Sci 1998;850:469–70.

[8] Mohammadian S, Bazrafshan HR, Sadeghi-Nejad A. Endocrine gland abnormalities in thalassemia major: a brief review. J Pediatr Endocrinol Metab 2003;16(7):957–64.

[9] Borgna-Pignatti C, Cappellini MD, De SP, et al. Survival and complications in thalassemia. Ann N Y Acad Sci 2005;1054:40–7.

[10] Olivieri NF, Nathan DG, MacMillan JH, et al. Survival in medically treated patients with homozygous beta-thalassemia. N Engl J Med 1994;331(9):574–8.

[11] Clegg JB, Weatherall DJ. Thalassemia and malaria: new insights into an old problem. Proc Assoc Am Physicians 1999;111(4):278–82.

[12] Weatherall DJ. Thalassaemia and malaria, revisited. Ann Trop Med Parasitol 1997;91(7): 885–90.

[13] Flint J, Hill AV, Bowden DK, et al. High frequencies of alpha-thalassaemia are the result of natural selection by malaria. Nature 1986;321(6072):744–50.

[14] Kanavakis E, Tzotzos S, Liapaki K, et al. Molecular basis and prevalence of alpha-thalassemia in Greece. Birth Defects Orig Artic Ser 1988;23(5B):377–80.

[15] Falusi AG, Esan GJ, Ayyub H, et al. Alpha-thalassaemia in Nigeria: its interaction with sickle-cell disease. Eur J Haematol 1987;38(4):370–5.

[16] Vichinsky EP. Changing patterns of thalassemia worldwide. Ann N Y Acad Sci 2005;1054: 18–24.

[17] Vichinsky EP, Macklin EA, Waye JS, et al. Changes in the epidemiology of thalassemia in North America: a new minority disease. Pediatrics 2005;116(6):e818–25.

[18] Lorey F, Cunningham G, Vichinsky EP, et al. Universal newborn screening for Hb H disease in California. Genet Test 2001;5(2):93–100.

[19] Logothetis J, Economidou J, Constantoulakis M, et al. Cephalofacial deformities in thalassemia major (Cooley's anemia). A correlative study among 138 cases. Am J Dis Child 1971; 121(4):300–6.

[20] Kearney SL, Nemeth E, Neufeld EJ, et al. Urinary hepcidin in congenital chronic anemias. Pediatr Blood Cancer 2007;48(1):57–63.

[21] Detivaud L, Nemeth E, Boudjema K, et al. Hepcidin levels in humans are correlated with hepatic iron stores, hemoglobin levels, and hepatic function. Blood 2005;106(2):746–8.

[22] Gardenghi S, Marongiu MF, Ramos P, et al. Ineffective erythropoiesis in beta-thalassemia is characterized by increased iron absorption mediated by down-regulation of hepcidin and up-regulation of ferroportin. Blood 2007;109(11):5027–35.

[23] Ganz T. Hepcidin, a key regulator of iron metabolism and mediator of anemia of inflammation. Blood 2003;102(3):783–8.

[24] Weinstein DA, Roy CN, Fleming MD, et al. Inappropriate expression of hepcidin is associated with iron refractory anemia: implications for the anemia of chronic disease. Blood 2002; 100(10):3776–81.

[25] Breda L, Gardenghi S, Guy E, et al. Exploring the role of hepcidin, an antimicrobial and iron regulatory peptide, in increased iron absorption in beta-thalassemia. Ann N Y Acad Sci 2005;1054:417–22.

[26] De FL, Daraio F, Filippini A, et al. Liver expression of hepcidin and other iron genes in two mouse models of beta-thalassemia. Haematologica 2006;91(10):1336–42.

[27] Porter JB, Abeysinghe RD, Marshall L, et al. Kinetics of removal and reappearance of non-transferrin-bound plasma iron with deferoxamine therapy. Blood 1996;88(2):705–13.

[28] Borgna-Pignatti C, Rugolotto S, De SP, et al. Survival and complications in patients with thalassemia major treated with transfusion and deferoxamine. Haematologica 2004; 89(10):1187–93.

[29] Aghai E, Shabbad E, Quitt M, et al. Discrimination between iron deficiency and heterozygous beta-thalassemia in children. Am J Clin Pathol 1986;85(6):710–2.

[30] Lie-Injo LE, Jo BH. A fast-moving haemoglobin in hydrops foetalis. Nature 1960;185:698.

[31] Kan YW, Allen A, Lowenstein L. Hydrops fetalis with alpha thalassemia. N Engl J Med 1967;276(1):18–23.

[32] Ehlers KH, Giardina PJ, Lesser ML, et al. Prolonged survival in patients with beta-thalassemia major treated with deferoxamine. J Pediatr 1991;118(4 Pt 1):540–5.

[33] Karagiorga-Lagana M. Fertility in thalassemia: the Greek experience. J Pediatr Endocrinol Metab 1998;11(Suppl 3):945–51.

[34] Skordis N, Petrikkos L, Toumba M, et al. Update on fertility in thalassaemia major. Pediatr Endocrinol Rev 2004;2(Suppl 2):296–302.

[35] Skordis N, Christou S, Koliou M, et al. Fertility in female patients with thalassemia. J Pediatr Endocrinol Metab 1998;11(Suppl 3):935–43.

[36] Pafumi C, Farina M, Pernicone G, et al. At term pregnancies in transfusion-dependent beta-thalassemic women. Clin Exp Obstet Gynecol 2000;27(3–4):185–7.

[37] Hmida S, Mojaat N, Maamar M, et al. Red cell alloantibodies in patients with haemoglobinopathies. Nouv Rev Fr Hematol 1994;36(5):363–6.

[38] Olujohungbe A, Hambleton I, Stephens L, et al. Red cell antibodies in patients with homozygous sickle cell disease: a comparison of patients in Jamaica and the United Kingdom. Br J Haematol 2001;113(3):661–5.

[39] Economidou J, Constantoulakis M, Augoustaki O, et al. Frequency of antibodies to various antigenic determinants in polytransfused patients with homozygous thalassaemia in Greece. Vox Sang 1971;20(3):252–8.

[40] Wang LY, Liang DC, Liu HC, et al. Alloimmunization among patients with transfusion-dependent thalassemia in Taiwan. Transfus Med 2006;16(3):200–3.

[41] Vichinsky EP, Earles A, Johnson RA, et al. Alloimmunization in sickle cell anemia and transfusion of racially unmatched blood. N Engl J Med 1990;322(23):1617–21.

[42] Singer ST, Wu V, Mignacca R, et al. Alloimmunization and erythrocyte autoimmunization in transfusion-dependent thalassemia patients of predominantly asian descent. Blood 2000; 96(10):3369–73.

[43] Moroni GA, Piacentini G, Terzoli S, et al. Hepatitis B or non-A, non-B virus infection in multitransfused thalassaemic patients. Arch Dis Child 1984;59(12):1127–30.

[44] Allain JP, Thomas I, Sauleda S. Nucleic acid testing for emerging viral infections. Transfus Med 2002;12(4):275–83.

[45] O'Brien SF, Yi QL, Fan W, et al. Current incidence and estimated residual risk of transfusion-transmitted infections in donations made to Canadian Blood Services. Transfusion 2007;47(2):316–25.

[46] Ansar MM, Kooloobandi A. Prevalence of hepatitis C virus infection in thalassemia and haemodialysis patients in north Iran-Rasht. J Viral Hepat 2002;9(5):390–2.

[47] Butensky E, Pakbaz Z, Foote D, et al. Treatment of hepatitis C virus infection in thalassemia. Ann N Y Acad Sci 2005;1054:290–9.

[48] Inati A, Taher A, Ghorra S, et al. Efficacy and tolerability of peginterferon alpha-2a with or without ribavirin in thalassaemia major patients with chronic hepatitis C virus infection. Br J Haematol 2005;130(4):644–6.

[49] Telfer PT, Garson JA, Whitby K, et al. Combination therapy with interferon alpha and ribavirin for chronic hepatitis C virus infection in thalassaemic patients. Br J Haematol 1997; 98(4):850–5.

[50] Wonke B, Hoffbrand AV, Bouloux P, et al. New approaches to the management of hepatitis and endocrine disorders in Cooley's anemia. Ann N Y Acad Sci 1998;850: 232–41.

[51] Borgna-Pignatti C, Vergine G, Lombardo T, et al. Hepatocellular carcinoma in the thalassaemia syndromes. Br J Haematol 2004;124(1):114–7.

[52] Ren FY, Piao XX, Jin AL. Efficacy of ultrasonography and alpha-fetoprotein on early detection of hepatocellular carcinoma. World J Gastroenterol 2006;12(29):4656–9.

[53] Borgna PC, Carnelli V, Caruso V, et al. Thromboembolic events in beta thalassemia major: an Italian multicenter study. Acta Haematol 1998;99(2):76–9.

[54] Cappellini MD. Coagulation in the pathophysiology of hemolytic anemias. Hematology Am Soc Hematol Educ Program 2007;2007:74–8.

[55] Eldor A, Rachmilewitz EA. The hypercoagulable state in thalassemia. Blood 2002;99(1): 36–43.

[56] Borenstain-Ben YV, Barenholz Y, Hy-Am E, et al. Phosphatidylserine in the outer leaflet of red blood cells from beta-thalassemia patients may explain the chronic hypercoagulable state and thrombotic episodes. Am J Hematol 1993;44(1):63–5.

[57] Eldor A, Krausz Y, Atlan H, et al. Platelet survival in patients with beta-thalassemia. Am J Hematol 1989;32(2):94–9.

[58] Reiter CD, Gladwin MT. An emerging role for nitric oxide in sickle cell disease vascular homeostasis and therapy. Curr Opin Hematol 2003;10(2):99–107.

[59] Machado RF, Martyr S, Kato GJ, et al. Sildenafil therapy in patients with sickle cell disease and pulmonary hypertension. Br J Haematol 2005;130(3):445–53.

[60] Pearson HA, Rink L, Guiliotis DK. Thalassemia major in Connecticut: a 20-year study of changing age distribution and survival. Conn Med 1994;85(5):259–60.

[61] Pearson HA, Guiliotis DK, Rink L, et al. Patient age distribution in thalassemia major: changes from 1973 to 1985. Pediatrics 1987;80(1):53–7.

[62] Thomas ED, Buckner CD, Sanders JE, et al. Marrow transplantation for thalassaemia. Lancet 1982;2(8292):227–9.

[63] Hongeng S, Pakakasama S, Chuansumrit A, et al. Reduced intensity stem cell transplantation for treatment of class 3 Lucarelli severe thalassemia patients. Am J Hematol 2007; 82(12):1095–8.

[64] La NG, Argiolu F, Giardini C, et al. Unrelated bone marrow transplantation for beta-thalassemia patients: the experience of the Italian Bone Marrow Transplant Group. Ann N Y Acad Sci 2005;1054:186–95.

[65] Lucarelli G, Galimberti M, Polchi P, et al. Bone marrow transplantation in patients with thalassemia. N Engl J Med 1990;322(7):417–21.

[66] Sodani P, Gaziev D, Polchi P, et al. New approach for bone marrow transplantation in patients with class 3 thalassemia aged younger than 17 years. Blood 2004;104(4):1201–3.

[67] Lucarelli G, Andreani M, Angelucci E. The cure of the thalassemia with bone marrow transplantation. Bone Marrow Transplant 2001;28(Suppl 1):S11–3.

[68] Walters MC, Quirolo L, Trachtenberg ET, et al. Sibling donor cord blood transplantation for thalassemia major: experience of the Sibling Donor Cord Blood Program. Ann N Y Acad Sci 2005;1054:206–13.

[69] Bhatia M, Walters MC. Hematopoietic cell transplantation for thalassemia and sickle cell disease: past, present and future. Bone Marrow Transplant 2008;41(2):109–17.

[70] Adamkiewicz TV, Szabolcs P, Haight A, et al. Unrelated cord blood transplantation in children with sickle cell disease: review of four-center experience. Pediatr Transplant 2007;11(6): 641–4.

[71] Adamkiewicz TV, Boyer MW, Bray R, et al. Identification of unrelated cord blood units for hematopoietic stem cell transplantation in children with sickle cell disease. J Pediatr Hematol Oncol 2006;28(1):29–32.

[72] Walters MC. Cord blood transplantation for sickle cell anemia: bust or boom? Pediatr Transplant 2007;11(6):582–3.

[73] Nishino T, Tubb J, Emery DW. Partial correction of murine beta-thalassemia with a gammaretrovirus vector for human gamma-globin. Blood Cells Mol Dis 2006;37(1):1–7.

[74] Rivella S, May C, Chadburn A, et al. A novel murine model of Cooley anemia and its rescue by lentiviral-mediated human beta-globin gene transfer. Blood 2003;101(8):2932–9.

[75] Sadelain M, Lisowski L, Samakoglu S, et al. Progress toward the genetic treatment of the beta-thalassemias. Ann N Y Acad Sci 2005;1054:78–91.

PEDIATRIC CLINICS
OF NORTH AMERICA

Pediatr Clin N Am 55 (2008) 461–482

Oral Iron Chelators

Janet L. Kwiatkowski, MD, MSCE[a,b,*]

[a]University of Pennsylvania School of Medicine, 34th Street and Civic Center Boulevard,
Philadelphia, PA 19104, USA
[b]Division of Hematology, The Children's Hospital of Philadelphia, 34th Street and Civic
Center Boulevard, Children's Seashore House, 4th Floor, Hematology,
Philadelphia, PA 19104, USA

Transfusion-related iron overload

Regular red cell transfusions are used in the management of many hematologic disorders in children. In β-thalassemia major, transfusions relieve severe anemia, suppress compensatory bone marrow hyperplasia, and prolong survival. Regular red cell transfusions also are used frequently in children who have sickle cell disease, primarily to prevent and treat devastating complications, such as stroke [1]. Other conditions that may be treated with transfusion therapy include Diamond-Blackfan anemia that is poorly responsive to steroids; Fanconi anemia; hemolytic anemias, such as pyruvate kinase deficiency; sideroblastic anemias; congenital dyserythropoietic anemias; and myelodysplastic syndromes.

In humans, iron is required for many essential functions, including oxygen transport, oxidative energy production, mitochondrial respiration, and DNA synthesis [2]. Iron loss is limited to small amounts in the stool, urine, desquamated nail and skin cells, and menstrual losses in women, and humans lack physiologic mechanisms to excrete excess iron. Chronic red cell transfusion therapy leads to progressive iron accumulation in the absence of chelation therapy because the iron contained in the transfused red cells is not excreted efficiently.

Each milliliter of packed red cells contains approximately 1.1 mg of iron. A regular transfusion regimen usually consists of 10 to 15 mL/kg of packed red cells administered every 3 to 4 weeks to maintain a trough hemoglobin level of 9 to 10 g/dL in patients who have thalassemia and other congenital

---

* Division of Hematology, The Children's Hospital of Philadelphia, 34th Street and Civic Center Boulevard, Children's Seashore House, 4th Floor, Hematology, Philadelphia, PA 19104.
E-mail address: kwiatkowski@email.chop.edu

0031-3955/08/$ - see front matter © 2008 Elsevier Inc. All rights reserved.
doi:10.1016/j.pcl.2008.01.005 *pediatric.theclinics.com*

anemias and to maintain the hemoglobin S percentage at less than 30% in children who have sickle cell disease. This leads to an average iron accumulation of approximately 0.3 to 0.5 mg/kg per day, although there is considerable interpatient variability in iron loading. In addition, gastrointestinal iron absorption is increased greatly in patients who have ineffective erythropoiesis, such as thalassemia, and in some red cell enzyme deficiencies, in particular pyruvate kinase deficiency. The increased absorption of dietary iron can cause iron overload even in the absence of transfusions, although at a slower rate than that associated with chronic transfusions. Serial phlebotomy may be used to treat iron overload in some patients who have congenital anemia, but chelation therapy is needed to remove iron for those who have more severe anemia or transfusion dependence.

Hereditary hemochromatosis

Iron overload can result from hereditary causes that lead to increased intestinal absorption of dietary iron. Hepcidin, a small peptide produced by the liver in response to high iron levels and inflammation, inhibits iron absorption [3]. Dysregulation of hepcidin now seems central in many of the hereditary forms of hemochromatosis. The most common form of hereditary hemochromatosis is caused by mutations in the HFE gene, which prevent the appropriate up-regulation of hepcidin expression in response to increased iron levels [4]. A mutation causing a cysteine-to-tyrosine substitution (C282Y) in the HFE protein is common in those of Northern European ancestry and a second mutation causing a histidine-to-aspartic acid substitution (H63D) is distributed worldwide. Homozygosity for the C282Y mutation or compound heterozygosity for C282Y/H63D is associated with the development of iron overload, although clinical penetrance is variable. Clinical manifestations, including bronzing of the skin, cirrhosis, arthropathies, diabetes mellitus, and endocrinopathies, usually do not develop until middle age. Cardiac disease also can occur, although less commonly than with transfusional iron overload (discussed later). Mutations in the hepcidin gene or in another protein involved in hepcidin regulation, hemojuvelin, lead to a juvenile form of hemochromatosis with symptoms presenting by the third decade of life [5]. The standard treatment for hereditary hemochromatosis is phlebotomy to reduce iron stores, although iron chelation therapy may be used in patients who are unable to tolerate the procedure.

Organ toxicity related to iron overload

Free iron is toxic to cells and, therefore, iron normally is shielded by forming tight complexes with proteins. In plasma, iron is bound to transferrin, which transports iron to the cells. The main storage form of iron is ferritin, whereas hemosiderin is another iron storage protein, consisting of large iron-salt aggregates. Both are found principally in the liver, reticuloendothelial cells, and red cell precursors, but ferritin also is found in the blood, where it can be measured readily. In iron overload states, high levels of iron exceed the iron-carrying capacity of transferrin within the plasma, leading to accumulation of nontransferrin-bound iron [6]. The nontransferrin-bound iron is taken up into cells, including liver, heart, and endocrine cells. Within the cells, the iron storage proteins become saturated, and instead, iron is bound only weakly to various low molecular weight proteins, known as labile iron [7]. Iron that is not tightly bound can participate in the generation of free radicals that damage the cells leading to organ toxicity.

Most knowledge of the complications of iron overload comes from patients who have thalassemia who require lifelong red blood cell transfusions. Whether or not patients who have different diseases requiring chronic transfusions, in particular sickle cell disease, develop the same complications remains to be determined [8,9]. Given the lack of substantial information about disease-specific responses to iron overload, data from the thalassemia population continue to guide monitoring and treatment for other transfused patient populations.

Iron overload leads to many clinical complications. Cardiac toxicity, including congestive heart failure and arrhythmias, is the leading cause of death related to iron overload in patients who have thalassemia major [10]. Excess iron deposition in the liver leads to inflammation, fibrosis, and cirrhosis [11], which may be exacerbated by concomitant transfusion-acquired viral hepatitis. Iron is toxic to the endocrine organs, leading to growth failure, delayed puberty [12], diabetes mellitus, hypothyroidism, and hypoparathyroidism [13]. In a report of 342 North American patients who had thalassemia major, 38% of subjects had at least one endocrinopathy, most commonly hypogonadism, and 13% had more than one endocrinopathy [13]. Moreover, in that study, the prevalence of endocrine abnormalities increased with age, likely reflecting an accumulating iron burden. The goal of chelation therapy is to maintain the body iron at levels low enough to prevent the development of these organ toxicities. Once organ toxicity has developed, chelation therapy can reverse some of the complications, such as the cardiac complications (discussed later), although the endocrinopathies usually are not reversible.

Measurement of iron levels

There are several methods of assessing the degree of iron overload and each method has benefits and limitations (Table 1). Thus, combinations of measurements, including serial measurements, are used in clinical practice to determine individual iron burden and response to iron chelation therapy over time.

The serum ferritin level is the test that is available most widely and easiest to perform. Because it is a simple blood test, many measurements can be

Table 1
Comparison of techniques to measure iron burden

Method	Advantages	Disadvantages
Serum ferritin	Inexpensive Widely available Repeated measurements possible	Imprecise correlation with total body iron Value altered by inflammation, infection, ascorbate deficiency Less reliable in sickle cell disease and nontransfusional secondary iron overload disease states
Liver iron concentration by biopsy	Correlates well with total body iron burden Allows for assessment of liver histology High levels predict risk for cardiac disease, endocrine complications, and death	Invasive Accuracy affected by sample size (>1 mg dry weight is best) Sampling errors due to fibrosis and uneven distribution of iron Cardiac disease may be present when liver iron is low
Liver iron concentration by SQUID	Noninvasive Well tolerated Correlates well with liver iron concentration	Expensive Complex equipment Very limited availability Cardiac disease may be present when liver iron is low
Liver iron concentration by MRI	Noninvasive More widely available Correlates well with liver iron concentration by biopsy	Expensive Variety of techniques and analytic programs may limit comparability among sites Cardiac disease may be present when liver iron is low
Cardiac iron loading by MRI	Noninvasive Correlates with risk for cardiac disease	Expensive Difficult to validate with biopsy specimen

performed without difficulty to establish trends in iron burden over time. In transfusional iron overload, the ferritin level correlates with total body iron burden, although the correlation is not precise, especially at higher values [14]. Changes in the serum ferritin level in response to chelation have been shown to parallel changes in liver iron concentration measured by liver biopsy and noninvasive means [15,16]. Thus, trends in serum ferritin levels may be useful for monitoring adequacy of chelation therapy. In addition, the ferritin level has prognostic significance for patients who have thalassemia major receiving chelation therapy with deferoxamine. Sustained levels of over 2500 μg/L are associated with an increased risk for organ toxicity and death [17,18]. Thus, optimal chelation regimens should maintain the ferritin level at least lower than this value.

A limitation of the ferritin level is that a variety of disease states, including infection, inflammation, and ascorbate deficiency, can raise or lower serum ferritin levels. The limitation of ferritin in predicting iron stores is relevant particularly for patients who have sickle cell disease. In an analysis of 50 children who had sickle cell disease and were receiving regular red cell transfusions for primary stroke prevention in the Stroke Prevention Trial in Sickle Cell Anemia (STOP), great variability in the rate of rise of serum ferritin despite similar transfusion regimens was found among patients [19]. Serum ferritin levels also underestimate liver iron concentration in patients who have thalassemia-intermedia and nontransfusion-associated iron overload [20].

Given that the liver is the major target organ for iron accumulation after multiple transfusions, the liver iron concentration is a good indicator of total iron burden [21]. Various methods are available to estimate liver iron concentration, but liver biopsy generally is considered the gold standard for accurate iron measurement. In addition, this procedure allows direct assessment of liver inflammation and fibrosis. Liver iron concentration is a useful predictor of prognosis in patients who have thalassemia: levels in excess of 15 mg/g dry weight are associated with an increased risk for cardiac complications and death [22]. Maintenance of the liver iron concentration between 3 and 7 mg/g dry weight in those receiving chelation therapy is considered ideal [23]. Several limitations to liver biopsy exist, however. First, it is an invasive procedure, which restricts the acceptability to patients and its frequent use to monitor trends over time. In addition, liver fibrosis and cirrhosis cause an uneven distribution of iron, which may lead to an underestimation of liver iron in patients who have advanced liver disease [24]. Finally, although high levels of liver iron predict an increased risk for cardiac disease, the converse not always is true: low levels do not always predict a low risk for cardiac disease [25]. This may reflect the different organ-specific rates of iron accumulation and iron removal in response to chelation therapy. In patients who have a history of poor chelation and high iron levels in the past who subsequently use chelation, hepatic iron may be removed more rapidly then cardiac iron, so liver iron levels can fall before cardiac iron levels improve [26].

The superconducting quantum interference device (SQUID) technique uses magnetometers to measure very small magnetic fields and can be used as a noninvasive technique to measure ferritin and hemosiderin in the liver [27]. Estimation of liver iron concentration by SQUID correlates linearly with concentrations measured by liver biopsy [27]. Because this is a noninvasive technique, repetitive iron concentration measurements by SQUID have been used to monitor the efficacy of chelation in several studies [16,28–30]. A major limitation to using SQUID is that it is a highly specialized and expensive approach. In addition, in recent clinical trials of the oral chelator, deferasirox, SQUID measurements underestimated liver iron concentrations obtained by biopsy by approximately 50% [15]. Currently, only four sites worldwide offer the technology, limiting accessibility to patients.

MRI increasingly is used to monitor iron overload. This technique takes advantage of local inhomogeneities of the magnetic field caused by iron deposition in tissues [31]. Magnetic resonance scanners are more widely available than SQUID, which should allow greater accessibility to patients. Differences in the type of machine, the strength of the magnetic field, and the analytic measurements, however, can limit accuracy and comparability among different sites. Although MRI may be used to estimate iron levels in a variety of organs, including the pituitary, pancreas, and bone marrow, it is used most commonly to measure hepatic [32] and cardiac iron [25,33]. MRI images darken at a rate proportional to the iron concentration. The darkening can be measured by two different techniques, spin-echo imaging and gradient-echo imaging. T2 refers to the time constant (half-life) of darkening for spin echo and T2* for gradient echo, with values inversely proportional to the amount of iron accumulation. The reciprocals of T2 and T2*, known as R2 and R2*, respectively, refer to rates of signal decay and are directly proportional to iron concentration [34]. Studies using R2 to estimate liver iron show good correlation with iron levels determined by liver biopsy and reproducibility across different scanners [32,35]. Other approaches using T2* or R2* also are promising for determining liver iron content [25,36]. Cardiac iron levels also can be assessed using MRI, most commonly with T2* measurements. Determination of cardiac iron may be of greater clinical relevance than liver iron measurements because cardiac disease is the leading cause of death in patients who have thalassemia and transfusional iron overload [10]. Cardiac T2* values below 20 ms indicate cardiac iron overload, whereas levels below 10 ms are associated with an increased risk for cardiac disease, including ventricular dysfunction and arrhythmias [25,33]. Thus, patients who have very low cardiac T2* values may benefit from intensification of chelation therapy.

History of iron chelation

Deferoxamine, a naturally occurring iron chelator produced by *Streptomyces pilosus*, was the first iron chelator approved for human use [37]. It is a hexadentate iron chelator that binds iron stably in a 1:1 ratio (Table 2). Deferoxamine is absorbed poorly from the gastrointestinal tract and has an extremely short half-life [38]. Thus, it must be administered parenterally, usually as a continuous subcutaneous infusion (25 to 50 mg/kg given over 8 to 12 hours, 5 to 7 days per week). Iron bound to deferoxamine is excreted in urine and feces.

The efficacy of deferoxamine is well established. In the 1960s, the ability of deferoxamine to induce substantial iron excretion and a net negative iron balance was demonstrated [39]. Subsequently, in the 1970s, deferoxamine therapy was shown to reduce hepatic iron content and prevent progression of fibrosis [40]. Most importantly, the use of deferoxamine is associated with a reduced incidence of cardiac complications and death [17,37,41]. In addition, cardiac disease secondary to iron overload can be reversed with the use of deferoxamine, typically administered as a 24-hour infusion

Table 2
Comparison of iron chelators

Property	Deferoxamine	Deferiprone	Deferasirox
Chelator:iron binding	1:1	3:1	2:1
Route of administration	Subcutaneous or intravenous	Oral	Oral
Usual dosage	25–50 mg/kg per day	75 mg/kg per day	20–30 mg/kg per day
Schedule	Administered over 8–24 hours, 5–7 days per week	Three times a day	Daily
Primary route(s) of excretion	Urine/feces	Urine	Feces
Adverse effects	Local reactions Ophthalmologic Auditory Bone abnormalities Pulmonary Neurologic Allergic reactions	Agranuloctyosis/ neutropenia Gastrointestinal disturbances Transminase elevations Arthralgia	Gastrointestinal disturbances Transaminase elevations Rise in serum creatinine Proteinuria Rash
Advantages	Long-term data available	May be superior in removal of cardiac iron	The only oral chelator licensed for use in United States
Disadvantages	Compliance problems may be greater	Not licensed for use in United States Variable efficacy in removal of hepatic iron	Long-term data lacking Efficacy at cardiac iron removal not known
Special monitoring considerations	Long bone films in growing children Annual ophthalmology exam Annual audiology exam	Weekly complete blood count with differential	Monthly blood urea nitrogen, creatinine, hepatic transaminases, and urinalysis

Adapted from Kwiatkowski JL, Cohen AR. Iron chelation therapy in sickle cell disease and other transfusion-dependent anemias. Hematol Oncol Clin N Am 2004;18(6):1355–77; with permission.

[42]. Chelation therapy with deferoxamine prevents other organ toxicities, such as diabetes [37].

Local infusion site reactions, including induration and erythema, commonly are seen with administration of deferoxamine. Low zinc levels also can develop with deferoxamine use. Other adverse effects, including high frequency hearing loss, ophthalmologic toxicity [43], growth retardation, and skeletal changes, including rickets-like lesions and genu valgum [44], are more common when patients receive high doses of deferoxamine relative to their total body iron burden and can be minimized by maintaining an optimal chelator dose [45]. Acute pulmonary toxicity with respiratory distress and hypoxemia and a diffuse interstitial pattern on chest roentgenogram is reported with the administration of high doses of deferoxamine (10 to 20 mg/kg per hour) [46].

The major limitation to deferoxamine is the need to administer the drug parenterally, which is painful and time consuming. As a result, poor compliance remains a significant problem with administration of this drug, and preventable, premature deaths related to iron overload continue to occur [47,48].

Characteristics of an ideal chelator

The limitations of treatment with deferoxamine have led investigators to search for more acceptable iron chelators to be used in the management of iron overload. An optimal chelator should have adequate gastrointestinal absorption to allow oral administration, a long half-life permitting once or twice daily dosing, and a high affinity for iron with lesser affinities for other metals. The chelator should be able to induce iron excretion at a rate of at least 0.5 mg/kg per day to offset the amount of transfusional iron loading, and should be able to remove excess cardiac iron. Finally, toxicities associated with the drug should be minimal and manageable.

Deferiprone

Pharmacology

Deferiprone, or 1,2 dimethyl-3-hydroxypyrid-4-1 (Ferriprox), was the first orally active chelator studied extensively for the treatment of transfusional iron overload, introduced into clinical trials 20 years ago (see Table 2). Most studies have been open-label, noncomparative studies, often including patients who had a history of inadequate iron chelation, but a few randomized trials comparing deferiprone to deferoxamine are reported. A substantial amount of data on the safety and efficacy of the drug has been acquired, but considerable controversy surrounding the drug exists. In the European Union, deferiprone is approved for use for patients in whom deferoxamine therapy is contraindicated or inadequate, but the drug is not approved for use in North America and currently is available only to a limited number of patients through expanded access programs or research trials.

Deferiprone is a bidentate chelator, which forms a 3:1 chelator:iron complex. Given its short plasma half-life of 1.5 to 2.5 hours [49,50], the drug usually is dosed 3 times daily, although regimens of 2 or 4 times daily have been explored [51]. The usual daily dose is 75 mg/kg per day, but higher doses have been studied [51]. Deferiprone induces iron excretion almost exclusively in the urine, with minimal contribution from fecal elimination [52,53].

Efficacy

Urinary iron excretion with deferiprone at 75 mg/kg is comparable to that induced by deferoxamine at a dose of 50 mg/kg [52,53]. Given that deferoxamine induces fecal iron excretion, total iron excretion with deferiprone is approximately 60% of that with deferoxamine at these doses [52]. The mean urinary iron excretion with deferiprone at 75 mg/kg was 0.48 mg/kg per day in one study, a level predicted to maintain or decrease iron stores in most patients [52]. Significant interpatient variability exists, however, so not all patients can achieve a negative iron balance at this dose. For example, in one study, urinary iron excretion ranged from 11.2 to 74.9 mg per day at a 75 mg/kg dosing level [54]. Higher doses of deferiprone, 90 to 119 mg/kg, induced greater urinary iron excretion and may be beneficial for patients who have inadequate responses at lower doses [51,54,55].

Short-term studies of deferiprone generally show a reduction [51,56–58] or stabilization [59] in serum ferritin levels over a treatment period of 1 year or less. Similarly, studies that assessed the response to deferiprone over longer treatment periods, of 3 to 4 years, show reduced [30,54,60,61] or stable [62,63] mean serum ferritin levels. Similar responses are shown across different disease states, including sickle cell disease and thalassemia.

A small proportion of patients demonstrated a significant increase in serum ferritin levels while receiving long-term deferiprone [30,61–63]. In a group of 151 Italian patients who received deferiprone for 3 years or more, 20% of subjects had clinically significant rises in ferritin levels during the first year of treatment [61]. In general, patients who had higher baseline ferritin levels showed a greater reduction in serum ferritin than those who had lower pretreatment ferritin levels. In a long-term, multicenter study, 84 patients received deferiprone for 4 years at a mean daily dosage of 73 mg/kg. Mean serum ferritin levels declined significantly from 3661 to 2630 μg/L in the group whose baseline serum ferritin was above 2500 μg/L, whereas ferritin levels remained stable in those with baseline values less than 2500 μg/L [63].

Studies on the effect of chelation with deferiprone on liver iron content have mixed results [30,57,62,64,65]. In a report of 21 patients who received deferiprone (75 mg/kg per day), mean liver iron concentration assessed by biopsy or SQUID decreased from 15 to 8.7 mg/g dry weight after an average of 3.1 years of treatment [30]. Eight of 10 patients who had initial liver iron concentrations associated with a high risk for cardiotoxicity (> 15 mg/g dry weight) had levels that fell to below that threshold with deferiprone treatment, and no patient who had lower initial hepatic iron concentrations rose above this threshold. With longer follow-up of a mean of 4.6 years in 18 patients, although there was an overall reduction in liver iron concentration from baseline (16.5 to 12.1 mg/g dry weight, $P = .07$), in seven patients, the liver iron concentration remained above 15 mg/g liver dry weight [65]. In another report of 20 patients who received deferiprone (70 mg/kg daily) for 1 year or more, the mean liver iron content increased from 16 to 21 mg/g dry weight, although this change did not reach statistical significance [64]. Liver iron content decreased in seven patients, rose in 12 patients, and remained the same in one patient. Thus, the data suggest that chelation with deferiprone (at a dose of 75 mg/kg per day) does not reduce liver iron concentration effectively in some patients.

Few randomized clinical trials have compared the efficacy of deferiprone directly to deferoxamine for the treatment of iron overload. In one study of 144 patients randomized to receive deferiprone (75 mg/kg per day) or deferoxamine (50 mg/kg per day), the reduction in serum ferritin levels after 1 year was similar between the two treatment groups [57]. In a subset of 36 patients who underwent liver biopsy at the beginning and end of treatment, the mean reduction in liver iron content also was not significantly different between the two groups. In a more recent study, 61 Italian and Greek patients were randomized to receive deferoxamine (50 mg/kg daily for 5 days a week) or deferiprone (75 mg/kg per day initially, increasing to 100 mg/kg per day) [66]. The changes over a 1-year period in serum ferritin level and liver iron content assessed by SQUID did not differ significantly between the two treatment groups. In contrast, in a third study, in which 30 children were randomized into three groups to receive deferoxamine (40 mg/kg per day, 5 days per week), deferiprone (75 mg/kg daily), or combination treatment with deferiprone (75 mg/kg daily) and deferoxamine (40 mg/kg per day, twice weekly), after 6 months of treatment, those receiving deferoxamine alone had a significant reduction in serum ferritin, whereas the other two groups had a slight rise in ferritin levels [67].

The lack of reduction in serum ferritin or liver iron concentration in some patients receiving deferiprone may be explained by a variety of reasons, including poor compliance, variability in drug metabolism rate, or higher transfusional iron burden. The latter two problems potentially might be overcome by treating with a higher dosage of deferiprone. In one study, increasing the daily dose of deferiprone (from 75 mg/kg to 83 to 100 mg/kg) resulted in a fall in serum ferritin level in nine patients who had had inadequate chelation at the lower dose [55]. Although no significant increased toxicity has been found in small studies using higher doses of deferiprone (up to 100 mg/kg daily) [66,68], larger studies are needed to determine the long-term safety and efficacy of doses greater than 75 mg/kg per day.

Cardiac iron removal

A growing body of evidence supports the theory that deferiprone may be more effective than deferoxamine at removing iron from the heart and reducing iron-related cardiotoxicity [66,69–71]. In one retrospective study, cardiac T2* and cardiac function were compared between 15 patients who had thalassemia and were receiving long-term deferiprone and 30 matched controls receiving long-term deferoxamine [69]. Patients receiving deferiprone had significantly less cardiac iron (median T2* 34 ms versus 11.4 ms, $P = .02$). Furthermore, T2* values less than 20 ms, a level associated with excess cardiac iron, were found in only 27% of patients receiving deferiprone compared with 67% of those receiving deferoxamine ($P = .025$), despite a significantly greater liver iron concentration in those receiving deferiprone. Left ventricular ejection fraction also was significantly higher in the deferiprone-treated group. Moreover, in a multicenter, retrospective study of patients who had thalassemia major, the risk for cardiac complications (cardiac failure or arrhythmia requiring drug treatment) was compared between 359 subjects who received only deferoxamine and 157 patients who received deferiprone [70]. Fifty-two patients (14.5%) developed cardiac events, including 10 deaths from cardiac causes, during therapy with deferoxamine whereas no patients developed cardiac events during treatment with deferiprone or within 18 months of discontinuing therapy.

A few prospective trials have compared the effect of deferiprone to deferoxamine on cardiac iron removal and cardiac function [57,66,72,73]. Two studies comparing deferiprone (75 mg/kg per day) to deferoxamine (50 mg/kg per day, 5–6 days per week) showed no significant difference in the reduction in cardiac iron between treatment groups after 1 year of therapy [57,72]. A third study using similar dosing, however, showed a significantly greater reduction in cardiac iron and improvement in left ventricular ejection fraction with deferiprone than with deferoxamine after 3 years of therapy [73].

More recently, a multicenter, randomized, controlled clinical trial compared deferiprone (average dose 92 mg/kg per day) to deferoxamine (average dose 35 mg/kg per day, 7 days a week) for the treatment of 61 patients who had thalassemia major and abnormal cardiac T2* (<20 ms) [66]. Patients who had severe cardiac iron loading, T2* values less than 8 ms, or left ventricular ejection fraction less than 56% were excluded. A significantly greater improvement in T2* values was seen with deferiprone compared with deferoxamine after 1 year of treatment (27% versus 13%, $P = .023$). Similarly, left ventricular ejection fraction increased more in those treated with deferiprone (3.1% versus 0.3%, $P = .003$).

Adverse effects

The most serious adverse event associated with deferiprone is agranulocytosis. In a multicenter study of 187 patients who had thalassemia major treated with deferiprone in which weekly blood counts were monitored, the incidence of agranulocytosis (absolute neutrophil count $< 500 \times 10^9/L$) was 0.6 per 100 patient-years and the incidence of milder neutropenia (absolute neutrophil count 500 to $1500 \times 10^9/L$) was 5.4 per 100 patient-years [59]. In the largest study reported to date, similar rates for agranulocytosis (0.4 per 100 patient years) and for neutropenia (2.1 per 100 patient years) were reported [61]. Neutropenia usually is reversible with discontinuation of the drug but often recurs with reinstitution of therapy [61,74]. In clinical practice, blood counts should be obtained at least weekly and with all febrile illnesses or significant infections to monitor for this potentially life-threatening side effect. Treatment with deferiprone may not be appropriate for patients who have underlying bone marrow failure syndromes, such as Diamond-Blackfan anemia, who may be more likely to develop agranulocytosis or neutropenia [75,76]. Similarly, caution should be exercised when using this drug in combination with hydroxyurea, interferon, or other drugs that can cause neutropenia.

Gastrointestinal symptoms, including nausea, vomiting, diarrhea, and abdominal pain, are common side effects reported with deferiprone, occurring in 33% of subjects in one large study [63]. These symptoms usually occur in the first few weeks of treatment and rarely require discontinuation of therapy [59,61]. Arthropathy with pain or swelling of the knees and other large joints is another common complication and can occur early or late in treatment [60,61,63]. In a large study of 532 patients, the prevalence of this complication was only 4% [61], but other studies have reported higher rates of up to 38.5% [54,60,63]. The arthropathy usually is reversible with discontinuation of the drug [54,59]. Low plasma zinc levels developed in a minority of patients receiving deferiprone; thus, periodic monitoring of zinc levels is warranted [54,59].

Elevations in serum alanine aminotransferase (ALT) levels are observed in patients receiving deferiprone. This abnormality often is transient and resolves even if the drug continues to be administered at the same or reduced dose [60,61]. Patients who have a higher iron burden [61] and those who have hepatitis C infection [59,61] may be more likely to develop ALT elevations. In addition, concerns have been raised regarding a possible progression of hepatic fibrosis with deferiprone therapy [65]. In a retrospective study, five of 14 patients receiving deferiprone developed progression of liver fibrosis compared with none of 12 patients receiving deferoxamine [65]. Four of the five patients who had worsening liver fibrosis also had antibodies to hepatitis C compared with only two of the nine subjects who did not have progression. In addition, the patients receiving deferiprone had higher baseline hepatic iron concentrations than the group receiving deferoxamine. Given that chronic viral hepatitis and iron overload may result in liver fibrosis, it is difficult to assess the contribution of deferiprone to progression of fibrosis. Other studies fail to show significant hepatic fibrosis attributable to deferiprone [62,77,78]. In the largest study to date, no significant progression of fibrosis was observed in 56 patients (11 seronegative for hepatitis C), with liver biopsy specimens obtained before and after treatment with deferiprone at a mean interval of 3.1 years [78].

Deferiprone and deferoxamine combination therapy

Several studies that explored the use of deferiprone in combination with deferoxamine, using a variety of dose regimens, have been published [55,79,80]. Such an approach could allow deferoxamine to be infused less frequently, which might improve compliance and could overcome the potential inability of deferiprone to induce sufficient hepatic iron clearance in some patients. In addition, combination therapy might remove cardiac iron more rapidly than either drug given alone, thereby improving the treatment of patients who have iron-related cardiac disease. Iron balance studies show an additive or possibly synergistic effect when the two drugs are administered together, possibly because deferiprone, a smaller molecule, can enter cardiac cells, bind iron, and then transfer it to deferoxamine for excretion [81,82]. Significant reduction in serum ferritin levels [79,80] and in cardiac iron stores measured by MRI [80] and significant improvement in left ventricular shortening fraction [79,80] are reported using combination therapy, without unexpected toxicities.

A recently reported randomized, placebo-controlled clinical trial comparing the use of deferoxamine alone or in combination with deferiprone in the treatment of 65 patients who had mild to moderate cardiac iron loading (cardiac T2* 8–20 ms) confirmed the beneficial effect of combination therapy on cardiac iron removal [83]. After a 12-month treatment period, those receiving combination therapy had significantly greater improvement in cardiac T2* and in left ventricular ejection fraction than those receiving deferoxamine alone.

Deferasirox

Pharmacology

Deferasirox (ICL670, Exjade) is the first oral iron chelator approved for use in the United States and it is approved in several other countries (see Table 2). Deferasirox is a triazole compound, designed using computer-aided molecular modeling [84]. Two molecules of deferasirox are needed to bind one molecule of iron fully (tridentate chelator). Deferasirox has a high specificity for iron, with minimal binding to copper and zinc. The drug is supplied as orally dispersible tablets that are dissolved in water or juice and administered best on an empty stomach. Deferasirox is absorbed rapidly, achieving peak plasma levels within 1 to 3 hours after administration. Its plasma half-life with repeated doses ranges from 7 to 16 hours [29] and is longer with higher drug doses [84]. The drug's long half-life supports a once-daily dosing regimen. The deferasirox-iron complex is excreted almost exclusively in the feces, with minimal urinary excretion [84].

Efficacy

An early, short-term treatment study in which 24 adult patients who had thalassemia and transfusional iron overload were treated with deferasirox at doses of 10, 20, or 40 mg/kg daily for a 12-day period showed that mean iron excretion rose linearly related to drug dose [85]. Mean iron excretion was 0.3 mg/kg per day with the 20-mg/kg dose and 0.5 mg/kg per day with the 40-mg/kg dose, suggesting that these doses are sufficient to at least maintain iron balance in many patients receiving chronic transfusions.

The safety and efficacy of deferasirox have been investigated in several phase 2 trials and a pivotal phase 3 study. In an initial phase 2 study, 71 adult patients who had thalassemia were randomized to receive deferasirox (10 mg/kg daily or 20 mg/kg daily) or deferoxamine (40 mg/kg for 5 days per week) [29]. Dose increases or reductions were allowed during the course of the study for rising or very low liver iron concentrations, respectively. Deferasirox (20 mg/kg) had similar efficacy to deferoxamine: the liver iron concentration measured by SQUID was reduced by an average of 2.1 and 2.0 mg/g dry weight, respectively, after 48 weeks of treatment. In contrast, only a minimal reduction of liver iron of 0.4 mg/g dry weight was seen with the 10 mg/kg deferasirox dose group, and more than half of the subjects in this group required dose increases to 20 mg/kg during the course of the study. A phase 2 study of 40 children who had β-thalassemia major, ages 2 to 17 years, treated with deferasirox (10 mg/kg per day), showed that this dose is unlikely to achieve negative iron balance in most patients [28]. In this study, there was an overall rise in liver iron concentration measured by SQUID during the 48 weeks of treatment, and the rise was proportional to the amount of transfusional iron loading.

A single large phase 3 clinical trial compared the efficacy of deferasirox to deferoxamine [15]. In this study, 586 patients who had β-thalassemia major were randomized to receive deferasirox or deferoxamine, and the primary endpoint was change in liver iron concentration by liver biopsy (SQUID was used in 16% of patients). More than half of the patients were under 16 years old, including children as young as 2. The dosing algorithm was based on the baseline liver iron concentration: with deferasirox dosing of 5 to 30 mg/kg daily and deferoxamine dosing of 20 to ≥50 mg/kg, 5 days per week. Patients randomized to receive deferoxamine with lower baseline liver iron concentrations were allowed to remain on their prestudy deferoxamine dose, even if higher than the protocol recommended, resulting in patients receiving proportionately higher deferoxamine than deferasirox doses in the lowest two liver iron concentration groups. The primary objective of noninferiority of deferasirox to deferoxamine across all treatment groups was not attained, likely related to this relative underdosing of deferasirox compared with deferoxamine in the lowest 2 dose groups. Noninferiority of deferasirox, however, was demonstrated at the 20- and 30-mg/kg dose groups. The average reduction in liver iron concentration over the 1-year treatment period with deferasirox at 20 or 30 mg/kg was 5.3 ± 8.0 mg/g dry weight, compared with a reduction of 4.3 ± 5.8 mg/g dry weight, with deferoxamine ($P = .367$). With deferasirox at 20 mg/kg, liver iron concentration remained relatively stable for the 1-year period, whereas with 30 mg/kg, average liver iron concentration fell. Trends in serum ferritin levels over the course of the study paralleled the changes in liver iron concentration, with stable values in those receiving deferasirox at 20 mg/kg and declining values at the 30 mg/kg dose.

Phase 2 studies in patients who had other transfusion-dependent anemias have demonstrated similar results. In a multicenter study, 195 patients who had sickle cell disease were randomized to receive deferasirox (10 to 30 mg/kg daily) or deferoxamine (20 to ≥ 50 mg/kg 5 days per week) with dosing based on the pretreatment liver iron content, measured by SQUID [16]. More than half of the patients studied were younger than 16 years old. With deferasirox, a mean reduction in liver iron concentration of 3 mg/g dry weight was seen after 1 year of treatment, which was similar to the decrease in liver iron concentration seen with deferoxamine (2.8 mg/g dry weight). Similarly, an overall significant reduction in liver iron concentration, measured by SQUID, was seen in a phase 2 study of 184 patients who had myelodysplasia, thalassemia, Diamond-Blackfan anemia, or other rare, transfusion-dependent anemias who received deferasirox at 20 to 30 mg/kg per day for 1 year [86].

Subsequent analyses have shown that the response to deferasirox is dependent on ongoing transfusional requirements. For most patients who had lower transfusional iron intake (averaging < 0.3 mg/kg per day), a dose of 20 mg/kg of deferasirox was effective in reducing liver iron concentration, whereas in over half of patients with the highest iron intake (> 0.5 mg/kg per day), the 20 mg/kg dose did not reduce liver iron content effectively [87]. Some patients who had higher transfusional iron loading did not have adequate reduction in iron stores with deferasirox at doses of 30 mg/kg; thus, higher doses of up to 40 mg/kg are being investigated in the ongoing extension studies. Dosing of deferasirox should be guided by the goal of maintenance or reduction of body iron stores, ongoing transfusional requirements, and trends in ferritin and liver iron content during treatment.

Cardiac iron removal

The ability of deferasirox to chelate cardiac iron and to prevent or reverse cardiac disease is not yet known. Preliminary data suggest, however, that deferasirox may be effective in removing cardiac iron. In cultured heart muscle cells, deferasirox was able to extract intracellular iron and restore iron-impaired contractility [88]. Similarly, in iron-overloaded gerbils, deferasirox was as effective as deferiprone in reducing cardiac iron content [89]. Furthermore, in a preliminary report of 23 patients receiving deferasirox at doses of 10 to 30 mg/kg per day, cardiac iron content measured by T2* MRI improved from an average of 18 ms to 23 ms over a treatment period of 13 months [90]. Further studies are needed to confirm the effect of deferasirox on cardiac iron and cardiac disease.

Adverse effects

The toxicity profile of deferasirox is similar across disease states and seems tolerable. Gastrointestinal disturbances, including nausea, vomiting, and abdominal pain, are common [15]. Although usually transient and dose related, these symptoms have led to discontinuation of the drug in some patients in clinical trials and in actual practice. The gastrointestinal side effects may be related to lactose intolerance as lactose is present in the drug preparation [16]. Diffuse, maculopapular skin rashes are reported in approximately 10% of subjects receiving deferasirox [15,16,28]. The rash often improves, even if the drug is continued. More than one third of patients experience mild elevations in serum creatinine levels, but few patients experience elevations beyond the normal range [15,16]. In some patients, the creatinine returned to baseline without dose modification, whereas in others, elevated or fluctuating levels persisted. Elevations in hepatic transaminases to more than 5 times baseline values also are reported [15,16]. The abnormalities are transient in some, even with continued administration of drug, whereas in others the abnormalities resolved with discontinuation of drug and recurred with drug reinstitution, suggesting causality. Fulminant hepatic failure is reported in rare cases, often in patients who have comorbidities. Cataracts or lenticular opacities and audio-toxicity are reported at low rates, similar to deferoxamine [15,16]. To date, the use of deferasirox is reported for more than 350 pediatric patients and the toxicity profile is similar to that seen in adults [15,16,28,86,91]. In addition, no adverse effects on growth or sexual development have been found, although longer follow-up is needed to assess fully for this potential complication. Agranulocytosis is not seen with deferasirox administration and the rare reports of neutropenia with deferasirox all are believed related to the underlying hematologic disorder and unlikely a drug effect.

Long-term data on treatment with deferasirox are lacking, and less common side effects may become evident only when larger numbers of patients are treated with the drug for a longer duration. Ongoing extension studies and postmarketing surveillance will help better define the long-term efficacy and safety profile of this drug. In addition, the use of deferasirox in combination with other chelators is not yet tested, and studies are needed to evaluate the efficacy and safety of such an approach before combination therapy can be recommended for clinical use.

Other oral chelators in development

Deferitrin (GT56-252) is an orally active tridentate iron chelator. It is a derivative of desferrithiocin, an oral chelator that showed good iron excretion in animal studies but had unacceptable renal toxicity, so the structure of deferitrin was modified to limit this toxicity [92]. In a phase 1 study, 26 adult patients who had thalassemia were treated with at least one dose of deferitrin, ranging from 3 to 15 mg/kg [93]. The drug's half-life was 2 to 4 hours and similar at all dose levels. Thus, once-daily dosing is not adequate with this medication. One serious adverse event occurred: hypoglycemic coma believed unrelated to deferitrin in a patient who had pre-existing diabetes. No significant laboratory abnormalities or electrocardiogram changes occurred. Further early phase clinical trials are ongoing.

Pyridoxal isonicotinoyl hydraxone (PIH) is a tridentate iron chelator introduced in 1979. When orally administered to iron-overloaded rats, PIH analogs were 2.6 to 2.8 times more effective at removing hepatic iron than deferoxamine, but deferoxamine was more effective at removing iron from cultured myocytes [94]. When given in combination with deferoxamine, the PIH analogs had a synergistic effect, suggesting that there may be a future role of this drug in combination chelation therapy [94]. A study in which 30 mg/kg per day of PIH was administered to patients who had thalassemia resulted in mean iron excretion of only 0.12 mg/kg per day, which is lower than the amount required to maintain negative iron balance in most regular transfused patients [95,96]. It is possible, however, that higher doses might increase efficacy. Further studies are needed to evaluate this drug's potential.

Managing chelation therapy

Children who have iron overload who require chelation therapy generally should be managed in conjunction with an experienced hematologist. Special considerations for children include the potential for adverse effects on growth and bone development with excess chelation, and these risks must be balanced against the risk for organ damage with prolonged iron accumulation. A variety of measurements can be used to determine when chelation therapy should be initiated for transfusional iron overload, including a cumulative transfusional iron burden of 120 mL/kg or greater, liver iron concentration of at least 7 mg/g dry weight [97], and serum ferritin levels persistently elevated above 1000 µg/L. Typically, chelation therapy is not administered to children younger than 2 years of age, and often it is deferred until at least 3 or 4 years of age. When administering chelation to children younger than 5 years old, lower doses of chelation usually are used to avoid toxicity [97]. The available chelator options and their toxicities should be discussed with patients and their families. Oral chelation often is used first line in children given that subcutaneous administration is painful, which limits compliance. Serial ferritin and liver and cardiac iron measurements and testing for organ dysfunction are used to monitor efficacy and make dose adjustments. Patient interviews and examinations, serial measurements of growth and pubertal development, appropriate laboratory studies (see Table 2), and annual ophthalmologic examination and audiologic testing are used to monitor for toxicity.

Summary

Effective chelation therapy can prevent or reverse organ toxicity related to iron overload, yet cardiac complications and premature death continue to occur, largely related to difficulties with compliance that may occur in patients who receive parenteral therapy. The use of oral chelators may be able to overcome these difficulties and improve patient outcomes. Two oral agents, deferiprone and deferasirox, have been studied extensively and are in clinical use worldwide, although in North America, deferasirox currently is the only approved oral chelator. Newer oral agents are under study. The chelator's efficacy at cardiac and liver iron removal and side effect profile should be considered in tailoring individual chelation regimens. Broader options for chelation therapy, including possible combination therapy, should improve clinical efficacy and enhance patient care.

References

[1] Adams RJ, McKie VC, Hsu L, et al. Prevention of a first stroke by transfusions in children with sickle cell anemia and abnormal results on transcranial doppler ultrasonography. N Engl J Med 1998;339:5–11.

[2] Lieu PT, Heiskala M, Peterson PA, et al. The roles of iron in health and disease. Mol Aspects Med 2001;22(1–2):1–87.

[3] Hugman A. Hepcidin: an important new regulator of iron homeostasis. Clin Lab Haematol 2006;28(2):75–83.

[4] Bridle KR, Frazer DM, Wilkins SJ, et al. Disrupted hepcidin regulation in HFE-associated haemochromatosis and the liver as a regulator of body iron homoeostasis. Lancet 2003; 361(9358):669–73.

[5] Wallace DF, Subramaniam VN. Non-HFE haemochromatosis. World J Gastroenterol 2007;13(35):4690–8.

[6] Breuer W, Hershko C, Cabantchik ZI. The importance of non-transferrin bound iron in disorders of iron metabolism. Transfus Sci 2000;23:185–92.

[7] Kushner JP, Porter JP, Olivieri NF. Secondary iron overload. Hematology Am Soc Hematol Educ Program 2001;47–61.

[8] Fung EB, Harmatz PR, Lee PD, et al. Increased prevalence of iron-overload associated endocrinopathy in thalassaemia versus sickle-cell disease. Br J Haematol 2006;135(4):574–82.

[9] Wood JC, Tyszka M, Carson S, et al. Myocardial iron loading in transfusion-dependent thalassemia and sickle cell disease. Blood 2004;103(5):1934–6.

[10] Zurlo MG, De Stefano P, Borgna-Pignatti C, et al. Survival and causes of death in thalassaemia major. Lancet 1989;2:27–30.

[11] Jean G, Terzoli S, Mauri R, et al. Cirrhosis associated with multiple transfusions in thalassaemia. Arch Dis Child 1984;59(1):67–70.

[12] Borgna-Pignatti C, De Stefano P, Zonta L, et al. Growth and sexual maturation in thalassemia major. J Pediatr 1985;106:150–5.

[13] Cunningham MJ, Macklin EA, Neufeld EJ, et al. Complications of beta-thalassemia major in North America. Blood 2004;104(1):34–9.

[14] Brittenham GM, Cohen AR, McLaren CE, et al. Hepatic iron stores and plasma ferritin concentration in patients with sickle cell anemia and thalassemia major. Am J Hematol 1993;42:81–5.

[15] Cappellini MD, Cohen A, Piga A, et al. A phase 3 study of deferasirox (ICL670), a once-daily oral iron chelator, in patients with beta-thalassemia. Blood 2006;107(9):3455–62.

[16] Vichinsky E, Onyekwere O, Porter J, et al. A randomised comparison of deferasirox versus deferoxamine for the treatment of transfusional iron overload in sickle cell disease. Br J Haematol 2007;136(3):501–8.

[17] Olivieri NF, Nathan DG, MacMillan JH, et al. Survival in medically treated patients with homozygous beta-thalassemia. N Engl J Med 1994;331(9):574–8.

[18] Telfer PT, Prestcott E, Holden S, et al. Hepatic iron concentration combined with long-term monitoring of serum ferritin to predict complications of iron overload in thalassaemia major. Br J Haematol 2000;110(4):971–7.

[19] Files B, Brambilla D, Kutlar A, et al. Longitudinal changes in ferritin during chronic trans-fusion: a report from the Stroke Prevention Trial in Sickle Cell Anemia (STOP). J Pediatr Hematol Oncol 2002;24(4):284–90.

[20] Pakbaz Z, Fischer R, Fung E, et al. Serum ferritin underestimates liver iron concentration in transfusion independent thalassemia patients as compared to regularly transfused thalasse-mia and sickle cell patients. Pediatr Blood Cancer 2007;49(3):329–32.

[21] Angelucci E, Brittenham GM, McLaren CE, et al. Hepatic iron concentration and total body iron stores in thalassemia major. N Engl J Med 2000;343(5):327–31.

[22] Olivieri NF, Brittenham GM. Iron-chelating therapy and the treatment of thalassemia. Blood 1997;89(3):739–61.

[23] Olivieri NF. The beta-thalassemias. N Engl J Med 1999;341(2):99–109.

[24] Villeneuve JP, Bilodeau M, Lepage R, et al. Variability in hepatic iron concentration measurement from needle-biopsy specimens. J Hepatol 1996;25(2):172–7.

[25] Anderson LJ, Holden S, Davis B, et al. Cardiovascular T2-star (T2*) magnetic resonance for the early diagnosis of myocardial iron overload. Eur Heart J 2001;22(23):2171–9.

[26] Anderson LJ, Westwood MA, Holden S, et al. Myocardial iron clearance during reversal of siderotic cardiomyopathy with intravenous desferrioxamine: a prospective study using T2* cardiovascular magnetic resonance. Br J Haematol 2004;127(3):348–55.

[27] Brittenham GM, Farrell DE, Harris JW, et al. Magnetic-susceptibility measurement of human iron stores. N Engl J Med 1982;307(27):1671–5.

[28] Galanello R, Piga A, Forni GL, et al. Phase II clinical evaluation of deferasirox, a once-daily oral chelating agent, in pediatric patients with beta-thalassemia major. Haematologica 2006; 91(10):1343–51.

[29] Piga A, Galanello R, Forni GL, et al. Randomized phase II trial of deferasirox (Exjade, ICL670), a once-daily, orally-administered iron chelator, in comparison to deferoxamine in thalassemia patients with transfusional iron overload. Haematologica 2006;91(7):873–80.

[30] Olivieri NF, Brittenham GM, Matsui D, et al. Iron-chelation therapy with oral deferiprone in patients with thalassemia major. N Engl J Med 1995;332(14):918–22.

[31] Brittenham GM, Badman DG. Noninvasive measurement of iron: report of an NIDDK workshop. Blood 2003;101(1):15–9.

[32] St. Pierre TG, Clark PR, Chua-Anusorn W, et al. Noninvasive measurement and imaging of liver iron concentrations using proton magnetic resonance. Blood 2005; 105(2):855–61.

[33] Westwood MA, Wonke B, Maceira AM, et al. Left ventricular diastolic function compared with T2* cardiovascular magnetic resonance for early detection of myocardial iron overload in thalassemia major. J Magn Reson Imaging 2005;22(2):229–33.

[34] Wood JC. Magnetic resonance imaging measurement of iron overload. Curr Opin Hematol 2007;14(3):183–90.

[35] Clark PR, Chua-Anusorn W, St. Pierre TG. Proton transverse relaxation rate (R2) images of iron-loaded liver tissue; mapping local tissue iron concentrations with MRI. Magnet Reson Med 2003;49:572–5.

[36] Wood JC, Enriquez C, Ghugre N, et al. MRI R2 and R2* mapping accurately estimates hepatic iron concentration in transfusion-dependent thalassemia and sickle cell disease patients. Blood 2005;106(4):1460–5.

[37] Brittenham GM, Griffith PM, Nienhuis AW, et al. Efficacy of deferoxamine in preventing complications of iron overload in patients with thalassemia major. N Engl J Med 1994; 331(9):567–73.

[38] Lee P, Mohammed N, Marshall L, et al. Intravenous infusion pharmacokinetics of desferrioxamine in thalassaemic patients. Drug Metab Disp 1993;21:640–4.

[39] Pippard MJ, Letsky EA, Callender ST, et al. Prevention of iron loading in transfusion-dependent thalassaemia. Lancet 1978;1(8075):1178–81.

[40] Barry M, Flynn DM, Letsky EA, et al. Long-term chelation therapy in thalassaemia major: effect on liver iron concentration, liver histology, and clinical progress. Br Med J 1974;2: 16–20.

[41] Wolfe L, Oliveri N, Sallan D, et al. Prevention of cardiac disease by sucutaneous deferoxamine in patients with thalassemia major. N Engl J Med 1985;312(25):1600–3.

[42] Davis BA, Porter JB. Long-term outcome of continuous 24-hour deferoxamine infusion via indwelling intravenous catheters in high-risk beta-thalassemia. Blood 2000;95(4): 1229–36.

[43] Olivieri NF, Buncic JR, Chew E, et al. Visual and auditory neurotoxicity in patients receiving subcutaneous deferoxamine infusions. N Engl J Med 1986;314(14):869–73.

[44] De Sanctis V, Pinamonti A, DiPalma A, et al. Growth and development in thalassemia major patients with severe bone lesions due to desferrioxamine. Eur J Pediatr 1996;155: 368–72.

[45] Porter JB, Jaswon MS, Huehns ER, et al. Desferrioxamine ototoxicity: evaluation of risk factors in thalassaemic patients and guidelines for safe dosage. Br J Haematol 1989; 73(73):403–9.

[46] Freedman MH, Grisaru D, Oliveri N, et al. Pulmonary syndrome in patients with thalassemia major receiving intravenous deferoxamine infusions. Am J Dis Child 1990;144:565–9.

[47] Borgna-Pignatti C, Rugolotto S, DeStefano P, et al. Survival and disease complications in thalassemia major. Ann N Y Acad Sci 1998;850:227–31.

[48] Ceci A, Baiardi P, Catapano M, et al. Risk factors for death in patients with beta-thalassemia major: results of a case-control study. Haematologica 2006;91(10):1420–1.

[49] Al-Refaie FN, Sheppard LN, Nortey P, et al. Pharmacokinetics of the oral iron chelator deferiprone (L1) in patients with iron overload. Br J Haematol 1995;89(2):403–8.

[50] Matsui D, Klein J, Hermann C. Relationship between the pharmacokinetics and iron excretion of the new oral iron chelator 1,2-dimethyl-3-hydroxypyrid-4-1 in patients with thalassemia. Clin Pharmacol Ther 1991;50:294–8.

[51] Al-Refaie FN, Wonke B, Hoffbrand AV, et al. Efficacy and possible adverse effects of the oral iron chelator 1,2-dimethyl-3-hydroxypyrid-4-one (L1) in thalassemia major. Blood 1992;80(3):593–9.

[52] Collins AF, Fassos FF, Stobie S, et al. Iron-balance and dose-response studies of the oral iron chelator 1,2-dimethyl-3-hydroxypyrid-4-one (L1) in iron-loaded patients with sickle cell disease. Blood 1994;83(8):2329–33.

[53] Olivieri NF, Koren G, Hermann C, et al. Comparison of oral iron chelator L1 and desferrioxamine in iron-loaded patients. Lancet 1990;336(8726):1275–9.

[54] Agarwal MB, Gupte SS, Viswanathan C, et al. Long-term assessment of efficacy and safety of L1, an oral iron chelator, in transfusion dependent thalassaemia: Indian trial. Br J Haematol 1992;82(2):460–6.

[55] Wonke B, Wright C, Hoffbrand AV. Combined therapy with deferiprone and desferriox-amine. Br J Haematol 1998;103(4):361–4.

[56] Kersten MJ, Lange R, Smeets ME, et al. Long-term treatment of transfusional iron overload with the oral iron chelator deferiprone (L1): a Dutch multicenter trial. Ann Hematol 1996; 73(5):247–52.

[57] Maggio A, D'Amico G, Morabito A, et al. Deferiprone versus deferoxamine in patients with thalassemia major: a randomized clinical trial. Blood Cells Mol Dis 2002;28(2):196–208.

[58] Voskaridou E, Douskou M, Terpos E, et al. Deferiprone as an oral iron chelator in sickle cell disease. Ann Hematol 2005;84(7):434–40.

[59] Cohen AR, Galanello R, Piga A, et al. Safety profile of the oral iron chelator deferiprone: a multicentre study. Br J Haematol 2000;108(2):305–12.

[60] Al-Refaie FN, Hershko C, Hoffbrand AV, et al. Results of long-term deferiprone (L1) therapy: a report by the International Study Group on oral iron chelators. Br Haematol 1995;91(1):224–9.

[61] Ceci A, Baiardi P, Felisi M, et al. The safety and effectiveness of deferiprone in a large-scale, 3-year study in Italian patients. Br J Haematol 2002;118(1):330–6.

[62] Hoffbrand AV, Al-Refaie F, Davis B, et al. Long-term trial of deferiprone in 51 transfusion-dependent iron overloaded patients. Blood 1998;91(1):295–300.

[63] Cohen AR, Galanello R, Piga A, et al. Safety and effectiveness of long-term therapy with the oral iron chelator deferiprone. Blood 2003;102(5):1583–7.

[64] Mazza P, Amurri B, Lazzari G, et al. Oral iron chelating therapy. A single center interim report on deferiprone (L1) in thalassemia. Haematologica 1998;83(6):496–501.

[65] Olivieri NF, Brittenham GM, McLaren CE, et al. Long-term safety and effectiveness of iron-chelation therapy with deferiprone for thalassemia major. N Engl J Med 1998; 339(7):417–23.

[66] Pennell DJ, Berdoukas V, Karagiorga M, et al. Randomized controlled trial of deferiprone or deferoxamine in beta-thalassemia major patients with asymptomatic myocardial sidero-sis. Blood 2006;107(9):3738–44.

[67] Gomber S, Saxena R, Madan N. Comparative efficacy of desferrioxamine, deferiprone and in combination on iron chelation in thalassemic children. Indian Pediatr 2004;41(1):21–7.

[68] Taher A, Sheikh-Taha M, Sharara A, et al. Safety and effectiveness of 100 mg/kg/day deferi-prone in patients with thalassemia major: a two-year study. Acta Haematol 2005;114(3):146–9.

[69] Anderson LJ, Wonke B, Prescott E, et al. Comparison of effects of oral deferiprone and subcutaneous desferrioxamine on myocardial iron concentrations and ventricular function in beta-thalassaemia. Lancet 2002;360(9332):516–20.

[70] Borgna-Pignatti C, Cappellini MD, De Stefano P, et al. Cardiac morbidity and mortality in deferoxamine- or deferiprone-treated patients with thalassemia major. Blood 2006;107(9): 3733–7.

[71] Piga A, Gaglioti C, Fogliacco E, et al. Comparative effects of deferiprone and deferoxamine on survival and cardiac disease in patients with thalassemia major: a retrospective analysis. Haematologica 2003;88(5):489–96.

[72] Galia M, Midiri M, Bartolotta V, et al. Potential myocardial iron content evaluation by magnetic resonance imaging in thalassemia major patients treated with Deferoxamine or Deferiprone during a randomized multicenter prospective clinical study. Hemoglobin 2003;27(2):63–76.

[73] Peng CT, Chow KC, Chen JH, et al. Safety monitoring of cardiac and hepatic systems in beta-thalassemia patients with chelating treatment in Taiwan. Eur J Haematol 2003;70(6):392–7.

[74] Al-Refaie FN, Wonke B, Hoffbrand AV. Deferiprone-associated myelotoxicity. Eur J Haematol 1994;53(5):298–301.

[75] Henter JI, Karlen J. Fatal agranulocytosis after deferiprone therapy in a child with Diamond-Blackfan anemia. Blood 2007;109(12):5157–9.

[76] Hoffbrand AV, Bartlett AN, Veys PA, et al. Agranulocytosis and thrombocytopenia in pa-tient with Blackfan-Diamond anaemia during oral chelator trial. Lancet 1989;2(8660):457.

[77] Tondury P, Zimmerman A, Nielsen P, et al. Liver iron and fibrosis during long-term treatment with deferiprone in Swiss thalassaemic patients. Br J Haematol 1998;101(3):413–5.

[78] Wanless IR, Sweeney G, Dhillon AP, et al. Lack of progressive hepatic fibrosis during long-term therapy with deferiprone in subjects with transfusion-dependent beta-thalassemia. Blood 2002;100(5):1566–9.

[79] Origa R, Bina P, Agus A, et al. Combined therapy with deferiprone and desferrioxamine in thalassemia major. Haematologica 2005;90(10):1309–14.

[80] Kattamis A, Ladis V, Berdousi H, et al. Iron chelation treatment with combined therapy with deferiprone and deferioxamine: a 12-month trial. Blood Cells Mol Dis 2006;36(1):21–5.

[81] Breuer W, Ermers MJJ, Pootrakul P, et al. Desferrioxamine-chelatable iron, a component of serum non-transferrin-bound iron, used for assessing chelation therapy. Blood 2001;97(3): 792–8.

[82] Link G, Konijn AM, Breuer W, et al. Exploring the "iron shuttle" hypothesis in chelation therapy: effects of combined deferoxamine and deferiprone treatment in hypertransfused rats with labeled iron stores and in iron-loaded rat heart cells in culture. J Lab Clin Med 2001;138(2):130–8.

[83] Tanner MA, Galanello R, Dessi C, et al. A randomized, placebo-controlled, double-blind trial of the effect of combined therapy with deferoxamine and deferiprone on myocardial iron in thalassemia major using cardiovascular magnetic resonance. Circulation 2007; 115(14):1876–84.

[84] Galanello R, Piga A, Alberti D, et al. Safety, tolerability, and pharmacokinetics of ICL670, a new orally active iron-chelating agent in patients with transfusion-dependent iron overload due to beta-thalassemia. J Clin Pharmacol 2003;43(6):565–72.

[85] Nisbet-Brown E, Olivieri NF, Giardina PJ, et al. Effectiveness and safety of ICL670 in iron-loaded patients with thalassaemia: a randomised, double-blind, placebo-controlled, dose-escalation trial. Lancet 2003;361(9369):1597–602.

[86] Porter J, Galanello R, Saglio G, et al. Relative response of patients with myelodysplastic syndromes and other transfusion-dependent anaemias to deferasirox (ICL670): a 1-year prospective study. Eur J Haematol 2008;80(2):168–76.

[87] Cohen AR, Glimm E, Porter JB. Effect of transfusional iron intake on response to chelation therapy in beta-thalassemia major. Blood 2008;111(2):583–7.

[88] Glickstein H, El RB, Link G, et al. Action of chelators in iron-loaded cardiac cells: Accessibility to intracellular labile iron and functional consequences. Blood 2006;108(9):3195–203.

[89] Wood JC, Otto-Duessel M, Gonzalez I, et al. Deferasirox and deferiprone remove cardiac iron in the iron-overloaded gerbil. Transl Res 2006;148(5):272–80.

[90] Porter JB, Tanner MA, Pennell DJ, et al. Improved myocardial T2* in transfusion dependent anemias receiving ICL670 (deferasirox). Blood 2005;106(11):1003a.

[91] Cappellini MD, Bejaoui M, Agaoglu L, et al. Prospective evaluation of patient-reported outcomes during treatment with deferasirox or deferoxamine for iron overload in patients with beta-thalassemia. Clin Ther 2007;29(5):909–17.

[92] Barton JC. Drug evaluation: Deferitrin for iron overload disorders. IDrugs 2007;10(7): 480–90.

[93] Donovan JM, Yardumian A, Gunawardena KA, et al. The safety and pharmacokinetics of deferitrin, a novel orally available iron chelator. Blood 2004;104(11):146a.

[94] Link G, Ponka P, Konijn AM, et al. Effects of combined chelation treatment with pyridoxal isonicotinoyl hydrazone analogs and deferoxamine in hypertransfused rats and in iron-loaded rat heart cells. Blood 2003;101(10):4172–9.

[95] Brittenham GM. Pyridoxal isonicotinoyl hydrazone: an effective iron-chelator after oral administration. Semin Hematol 1990;27(2):112–6.

[96] Cohen AR, Galanello R, Pennell DJ, et al. Thalassemia. Hematology Am Soc Hematol Educ Program 2004;14–34.

[97] Vichinsky E. Consensus document for transfusion-related iron overload. Semin Hematol 2001;38(Suppl 1):2–4.

PEDIATRIC CLINICS

OF NORTH AMERICA

ELSEVIER
SAUNDERS

Pediatr Clin N Am 55 (2008) 483–501

Hydroxyurea for Children with Sickle Cell Disease

Matthew M. Heeney, MD[a,b,*],
Russell E. Ware, MD, PhD[c]

[a]Harvard Medical School, Boston, MA, USA
[b]Division of Hematology/Oncology, Children's Hospital Boston, Fegan 704,
300 Longwood Avenue, Boston, MA 02115, USA
[c]Department of Hematology, St. Jude Children's Research Hospital,
332 North Lauderdale, MS 355, Memphis, TN 38105, USA

Sickle cell disease (SCD) refers to a group of genetic hemolytic anemias in which the erythrocytes have a predominance of sickle hemoglobin (HbS) due to inheritance of a β-globin mutation (β^S). The β^S mutation is the result of a single amino acid substitution (HbS, *HBB Glu6Val*) in the β-globin of the hemoglobin heterotetramer, thus forming HbS. Affected individuals typically are homozygous for the sickle mutation (HbSS) or have a compound heterozygous state (eg, HbSC, HbS β-thalassemia). The β^S mutation creates a hydrophobic region that, in the deoxygenated state, facilitates a noncovalent polymerization of HbS molecules that damages the erythrocyte membrane and changes the rheology of the erythrocyte in circulation, causing hemolytic anemia, vaso-occlusion, and vascular endothelial dysfunction.

SCD is the most common inherited hemolytic anemia in the United States. Approximately 70,000 to 100,000 individuals in the United States are affected, most commonly those who have ancestry from Africa, the Indian subcontinent, the Arabian Peninsula, or the Mediterranean Basin. Worldwide, millions of persons are affected with SCD, especially in regions with endemic malaria, such as Africa, the Middle East, and India. SCD is characterized by a lifelong hemolytic anemia with an ongoing risk for acute

Dr. Heeney is supported by NIH K12 HL087164 and U54 HL070819. Dr. Ware is supported by U54 HL070590, U01 HL078787, N01 HB 07155, and American Syrian Lebanese Associated Charities.

* Corresponding author. Division of Hematology/Oncology, Department of Medicine, Children's Hospital, Boston, Fegan 704, 300 Longwood Avenue, Boston, MA 02115.

E-mail address: matthew.heeney@childrens.harvard.edu (M.M. Heeney).

medical complications and inexorable accrual of organ damage in most affected individuals.

There is wide variability in the phenotypic severity of SCD that is not well understood. This variation can be explained partly by differences in the total hemoglobin concentration, the mean corpuscular hemoglobin concentration, erythrocyte rheology, the percentage of adhesive cells, the proportion of dense cells, the presence or absence of α-thalassemia, and the β-globin haplotype [1–5]. The percentage of fetal hemoglobin (HbF), however, is perhaps the most important laboratory parameter influencing clinical severity in SCD [6,7]. In unaffected individuals, HbF comprises only 5% of the total hemoglobin by age 3 to 6 months and falls to below 1% in adults [8]. In contrast, patients with SCD typically have HbF levels ranging from 1% to 20% [9] and those with genetic mutations leading to hereditary persistence of HbF (HPFH) can have HbF levels that reach 30% to 40% of the total hemoglobin [10].

Based on the observation that infants with SCD have few complications early in life, it was hypothesized that HbF, the predominant hemoglobin in fetal and infant stages of life, might ameliorate the phenotypic expression of SCD [11]. In addition, compound heterozygotes for the sickle mutation and HPFH are relatively protected from severe clinical symptoms [12]. Subsequently, it was shown that increased HbF percentage is associated with decreased clinical severity in SCD, using endpoints, such as the number of vaso-occlusive painful events, transfusions, and hospitalizations [1,13]. HbF does not, however, seem to protect from some complications [14], perhaps because the HbF levels were inadequate to provide protection [3,15]. A potential threshold of 20% HbF is suggested, above which patients experience fewer clinical events [16]. The % HbF also has emerged as the most important predictor of early mortality in patients with SCD [6,17].

Although the genetic and molecular pathophysiology of SCD are well described and understood in considerable detail, there has been disappointing progress toward definitive, curative therapy. Bone marrow transplantation offers a cure but currently requires an HLA-matched sibling donor for best results. This requirement limits the number of patients who can benefit from this approach. Moreover, even using a matched sibling donor, bone marrow transplantation remains associated with considerable morbidity (primarily graft-versus-host disease) and low, but not negligible, mortality.

In lieu of curative therapy, one approach given considerable effort over the past 25 years has been the pharmacologic induction of HbF beyond the fetal and newborn period. Several pharmacologic agents have shown promise, including demethylating agents, such as 5-azacytidine [18] and decitabine [19–21], and short-chain fatty acids, such as butyrate [22–25], but each has limitations in route of administration, safety, or sustained efficacy. Hydroxyurea, in contrast, has a long and growing track record in inducing HbF in patients with SCD. In addition, hydroxyurea has a variety of salutary effects on other aspects of the pathophysiology of SCD, such as increased erythrocyte hydration, improved rheology, and reduced adhesiveness. Hydroxyurea also decreases leukocyte count, and releases nitric oxide. This article reviews the usefulness of hydroxyurea for children with SCD but is not intended to be an exhaustive review of the drug's biochemistry, its therapeutic rationale, or previously published data. Interested readers may read more thorough reviews of hydroxyurea for the management of SCD [26,27]. This article is intended as a practical user's guide for clinicians who wish to know how and why treatment with hydroxyurea should be considered for children with SCD.

An ideal drug for sickle cell disease?

Hydroxyurea may be an ideal therapeutic agent for use in children with SCD. It has excellent bioavailability after oral administration; requires only once-daily dosing, which improves medication adherence; has few if any immediate side effects; has predictable hematologic toxicities that are dose dependent, transient, and reversible; and has potential benefits against multiple pathophysiologic mechanisms of SCD. Although several therapeutic agents currently under development address specific aspects of the pathophysiology of SCD, only hydroxyurea offers a broad range of beneficial effects that collectively can ameliorate the overall clinical severity of disease.

The drug is classified as an antimetabolite and antineoplastic agent. The exact mechanism of its antineoplastic activity is not elucidated fully but believed to be S-phase specific. Hydroxyurea is converted in vivo to a free radical nitroxide that quenches the tyrosyl free radical at the active site of the M2 subunit of ribonucleotide reductase. As a potent ribonucleotide reductase inhibitor, hydroxyurea blocks the conversion of ribonucleotides to deoxyribonucleotides, which interferes with the synthesis of DNA without any effects on RNA or protein synthesis. The drug is used widely in oral doses (ranging from 20 to 80 mg/kg/d) for the long-term treatment of chronic myeloproliferative disorders, such as polycythemia vera and essential thrombocythemia. In combination with reverse transcriptase inhibitors (eg, didanosine), hydroxyurea is finding a role within HIV therapy as a virostatic agent that produces potent and sustained viral suppression [28].

In patients with hemoglobinopathies, the myelosuppressive and cytotoxic effects of hydroxyurea seem to induce erythroid regeneration and the premature commitment of erythroid precursors, with resulting increased production of HbF-containing reticulocytes and total HbF [29]. Additional pharmacologic effects of hydroxyurea that may contribute to its beneficial effects in SCD include increasing erythrocyte HbF through nitric oxide dependent pathways, decreasing the neutrophil count, increasing erythrocyte volume and hydration, increasing deformability of sickle erythrocytes, and altering the adhesion of sickle erythrocytes to the endothelium [29–33].

The release of nitric oxide directly from the hydroxyurea molecule [34,35] should allow beneficial local effects on the endothelium, thereby ameliorating the vaso-occlusive process and limiting vascular dysfunction.

Clinical experience

Preclinical studies in anemic cynomolgus monkeys showed that hydroxyurea increased HbF levels [33]. Pilot trials in patients with SCD demonstrated that hydroxyurea also increased HbF in humans and caused little short-term toxicity [29–32]. These proof-of-principle experiments were critical first steps toward an important multicenter phase I/II trial involving adults with HbSS, which identified the short-term efficacy and toxicities of hydroxyurea used at maximum tolerated dose (MTD) [32].

Developed on the basis of favorable results from the phase I/II trial, the National Heart, Lung, and Blood Institute (NHLBI) sponsored the pivotal Multicenter Study of Hydroxyurea (MSH), a double-blinded, placebo-controlled, randomized control trial conducted from 1992 to 1995 in 21 centers in the United States. and Canada [36]. Two hundred and ninety-nine adult patients with HbSS were randomized (152 on hydroxyurea and 147 received placebo) but because of the beneficial effects observed, the trial was stopped early and only 134 subjects completed the planned 24 months of treatment. The hydroxyurea-treated subjects had a 44% reduction in painful crises per year (2.5 events per year versus 4.5 events per year) and a 58% reduction in median annual hospitalization rate for painful crisis (1.0 versus 2.4). In addition there were significantly fewer hydroxyurea-treated subjects who developed acute chest syndrome (ACS) (25 versus 51) and who received blood transfusions (48 versus 73); the number of units of blood transfused also was significantly less (336 versus 586). The incidence of death and stroke did not differ between the two treatment arms; there were no deaths related to hydroxyurea treatment and none of the patients who had received hydroxyurea developed cancer during the trial. The study did not address long-term safety or potential reversibility or prevention of chronic organ damage [36].

The results of this study led the Food and Drug Administration in 1998 to add to the indications for hydroxyurea, "to reduce the frequency of painful crises and to reduce the need for blood transfusions in adult patients with sickle cell anemia with recurrent moderate to severe painful crises." This additional labeling refers only to adults severely affected by painful events rather than the broader spectrum of patients with SCD. Now, 10 years later, there is no change in the manufacturer's drug labeling for hydroxyurea. Therefore, at this time, all children or patients with mild-to-moderate disease severity or those who do not have painful events but who have ACS or end-organ damage require off-label usage.

The initial success of hydroxyurea in adults led to the first pediatric multicenter phase I/II trial, known as HUG-KIDS, from 1994 to 1996 [37].

Eighty-four children ages 5 to 15 years with severe HbSS disease (defined as three or more painful events within the year before entry, three episodes of ACS within 2 years of entry, or three episodes of ACS or pain within 1 year of entry) were enrolled. Sixty-eight reached MTD and 52 were treated at MTD for 12 months. Similar hematologic effects were seen as in the MSH trial with decreased hemolysis (increased Hb and decreased reticulocytosis, decreased lactate dehydrogenase, and decreased total bilirubin), macrocytosis, improved erythrocyte hydration, myelosuppression, and increased HbF and F cells (Table 1). Laboratory toxicities were mild and reversible with temporary interruption of the medication, and no life-threatening clinical adverse events were observed. Subsequent evaluation of this cohort revealed no adverse effect on height or weight gain or pubertal development [38]. Predictors of HbF response were complex, but a higher treatment HbF was associated with higher baseline HbF, Hb, white blood cell count (WBC), and reticulocytes and compliance [39].

Short-term clinical efficacy in children initially was reported in small open-label studies [40,41]. In a small, randomized study from Belgium, children with HbSS treated with hydroxyurea had significantly fewer hospitalizations for pain, with shorter lengths of stay, compared with those receiving placebo [42]. Additional European data showed improved laboratory and clinical response without significant toxicity and no growth or pubertal delay [43]. Follow-up studies have revealed continued efficacy in association with long-term hydroxyurea use in children [44], including a sustained HbF response greater than 20% using hydroxyurea at MTD [45].

The role of hydroxyurea in preserving organ function in SCD is not yet determined. From a practical standpoint, these beneficial effects are difficult to assess prospectively because organ damage develops broadly over the whole pediatric age range, beginning with splenic and renal changes in infancy and evolving to pulmonary and neurologic deficits with vasculopathy among older children. In the Hydroxyurea Safety and Organ Toxicity (HUSOFT) study, infants with HbSS tolerated open-label liquid hydroxyurea and had preserved splenic filtrative function compared with historical controls

Table 1

Children with homozygous sickle cell anemia have similar laboratory efficacy using hydroxyurea at maximum tolerated dose as adults

	Adults	Children
MTD (mg/kg/d)	21.3	25.6
Δ Hb (g/dL)	+1.2	+1.2
Δ MCV (fL)	+23	+14
Δ HbF (%)	+11.2	+9.6
Δ Reticulocytes (10^9/L)	−158	−146
Δ WBC (10^9/L)	−5.0	−4.2
Δ ANC (10^9/L)	−2.8	−2.2
Δ Bilirubin (mg/dL)	−2.0	−1.0

Data from published phase I/II trials for adults [32] and children [37] with HbSS.

[46]. A follow-up study on this cohort identified preservation of splenic function and apparent gain of function in some cases [47]. In a recent retrospective study, 43 children with HbSS had splenic function measured before and during treatment with hydroxyurea for a median duration of 2.6 years; six patients (14%) completely recovered splenic function and two (5%) had preserved splenic function, suggesting that hydroxyurea might help preserve or recover splenic function [48]. Similar beneficial effects of hydroxyurea are reported anecdotally for children who have proteinuria [49], priapism [50,51], or hypoxemia [52].

The role of hydroxyurea in the prevention of stroke in SCD is an area of active investigation. In a retrospective study, hydroxyurea therapy was associated with lower transcranial Doppler (TCD) flow velocities [53]. In a recent prospective single institution study, hydroxyurea was shown to decrease elevated TCD velocities significantly, often into the normal range [54], suggesting that hydroxyurea might serve as an alternative to chronic erythrocyte transfusions for primary stroke prophylaxis. Hydroxyurea also is reported as an alternative to chronic transfusions for secondary stroke prophylaxis in children for whom transfusions cannot be continued safely (eg, erythrocyte allosensitization) [55,56]. Hydroxyurea in combination with serial phlebotomy effectively prevented secondary stroke and led to resolution of transfusional iron overload in 35 children from a single institution [57]. Based on these encouraging preliminary results, the NHLBI-sponsored Stroke With Transfusions Changing to Hydroxyurea (SWiTCH) trial is underway [58]; this study randomizes children with previous stroke to standard therapy (transfusions and chelation) or alternative therapy (hydroxyurea and phlebotomy) for the prevention of secondary stroke and management of iron overload.

There are limited data regarding the prolonged use of hydroxyurea in SCD, particularly with regard to its long-term risks and benefits, but current clinical experience has not identified any clear detrimental effects or safety concerns. The possibility of hydroxyurea having negative effects on growth and development in children has not been realized [45,47]. Similarly, concerns about DNA damage and leukemogenesis are not validated, with more than 15 years of exposure among adults and more than 12 years of exposure among children; continued vigilance is warranted but current data are encouraging regarding the long-term safety of this therapy. A 9-year observational follow-up study suggests that adults taking hydroxyurea had a significant 40% reduction in overall mortality [59]. During the MSH Patients' Follow-up study, there was little risk associated with the careful use of hydroxyurea; however, it was stated that hydroxyurea must be taken indefinitely to be effective and concerns remain over long-term safety. The teratogenicity of hydroxyurea for SCD is not elucidated fully. Anecdotes of normal offspring of women taking hydroxyurea during pregnancy [60,61] are supported by the lack of birth defects observed in the MSH cohort (Abdullah Kutlar, personal communication, December 2007). Recent reports, however, document abnormal spermatogenesis in men taking hydroxyurea [62,63], so further investigation in this area is needed. A recently opened study at St. Jude Children's Research Hospital, entitled Long Term Effects of Hydroxyurea Therapy in Children with Sickle Cell Disease [64], should provide important data regarding long-term risks and benefits of hydroxyurea in this young patient population.

Practical considerations

Hydroxyurea therapy cannot be prescribed, monitored, and adjusted properly according to exact and specific written guidelines. Instead, optimal treatment with hydroxyurea (as with many other medications) requires careful attention to the details of each patient's treatment response; such individualized therapy often involves as much art as science. The following sections represent the distillation of a combined 25 years of experience with hydroxyurea (>300 treated children), but none of the text should be considered dogma. Instead, these recommendations and suggestions represent a workable and historically successful approach that can serve as a good starting point for health care teams.

Beginning hydroxyurea therapy

The decision to initiate hydroxyurea therapy in a child who has SCD should be made deliberately and thoughtfully. The medical history of a patient should be reviewed carefully to document the number and severity of acute vaso-occlusive events plus any evidence of clinical or laboratory evidence of chronic organ damage, such as hypoxemia, proteinuria, or elevated TCD velocities. Indications for hydroxyurea therapy are not universally agreed upon and each health care team must determine their own threshold; a proposed list is in Table 2. In addition to the laboratory and clinical profile, previous compliance with outpatient clinic visits should be reviewed and the neurocognitive status and psychosocial milieu for the child considered. There are many nonpharmacologic reasons that hydroxyurea therapy can fail in children with SCD, and anticipation of problems with development of creative solutions represents the best way to promote adherence and obtain the optimal drug effects for a child receiving treatment.

Healthcare providers never should make the decision to start hydroxyurea unilaterally; team members must discuss the recommendation openly with patients and families. Ideally, all of a patient's caregivers who might dispense the medication should be present during the initial pretreatment discussions, to ensure that all questions are answered and all concerns addressed. Only if all of the parties involved (patient, parents/guardians, extended family members providing care, and the health care team) are in agreement should hydroxyurea therapy be started. Treatment is likely to fail due to medication nonadherence if any key family member (including

Table 2
Potential indications for hydroxyurea therapy in children with homozygous sickle cell anemia

Acute vaso-occlusive complications	Painful events	
	Dactylitis	
	Acute chest syndrome	
Laboratory markers of severity	Low hemoglobin	
	Low HbF	
	Elevated WBC	
	Elevated LDH	
Organ dysfunction	Brain	Elevated TCD velocities
		Silent MRI or MRA changes
		Stroke prophylaxis
	Lungs	Hypoxemia
	Kidney	Proteinuria
Miscellaneous	Sibling on hydroxyurea	
	Parental request	

Most pediatric hematologists have accepted clinical severity with acute vaso-occlusive complications as an indication for hydroxyurea therapy, but there is little agreement about indications for children with laboratory abnormalities or organ dysfunction. Similarly, the appropriate age for hydroxyurea initiation has not been determined, although clinical trials have demonstrated safety and efficacy for infants, young children, and school-aged children with SCD.

the child) is not fully supportive of the decision to begin treatment. Families are told that 6 to 12 months of therapy with monthly clinic visits for examination and blood draw are needed to establish an optimal dose and dosing regimen, so they should make a commitment to this duration before commencing treatment. This verbal contract emphasizes the importance of the commitment to therapy, which is being made by all involved parties. Two to three pretreatment visits also are advised, to explain the nuances of therapy and answer questions, because the decision to begin an indefinite treatment with monthly visits should not be made quickly by a single person at a single visit. Occasionally, an apparently motivated family member fails to return for a follow-up informational visit with an additional parent/guardian or other family member. This kind of missed visit may reflect some unspoken reluctance to begin treatment by parent or patient, unforeseen psychosocial obstacles, or unidentified financial or transportation barriers but allows an early appraisal of the likelihood of treatment success.

Explaining the rationale

The recommendation to begin hydroxyurea therapy and a description of the potential risks and benefits of taking the drug should be communicated to patients and family members in a straightforward and honest way, using age-appropriate and culturally sensitive language and vocabulary. Some families have access to the Internet and already have acquired detailed information and formed specific questions, whereas others have little knowledge of the drug beyond what is provided by the health care team. Providing a rationale that includes mechanisms of HbF induction or nitric oxide metabolism generally is not helpful or persuasive in the majority of cases. Instead, a general review of the pathophysiology of sickle cell vaso-occlusion typically is sufficient, indicating where hydroxyurea might be beneficial. Most children recognize that sickled erythrocytes have an elongated shape; hence, comments like, "hydroxyurea helps your blood cells stay round" can help motivate even young patients to stay on therapy and serve as easy reminders of the benefits of treatment during subsequent visits. Many families realize that their children were generally healthy during the first few months of life, so the benefits of HbF can be put into this context. The importance of daily medication adherence cannot be overemphasized. To help children understand this principle, hydroxyurea can be likened to a powerful vitamin to be taken daily. Families are reminded that a child will not feel better or worse immediately after each dose, and the beneficial effects occur in the blood cells over time and leading eventually to overall improvement.

Describing risks and benefits

The potential benefits of hydroxyurea therapy are best discussed with patients and families not only in terms of preventing acute clinical complications, such as pain and ACS, but also as helping avoid hospitalizations and transfusions, enhancing growth, and possibly preventing chronic organ damage. Adverse short-term side effects of taking hydroxyurea are described as usually minimal and often none, except for occasional mild gastrointestinal discomfort. The treatment effects of lowering the blood counts to modest neutropenia are described as predictable and actually desired but requiring periodic dose escalation with monthly monitoring to achieve a stable MTD. Potential deleterious effects on hair or skin are mentioned but minimized, except for occasional (<5%) hyperpigmentation and melanonychia; hepatic and renal drug-related toxicity is described as rare, probably no more than approximately 1 in 1000.

The long-term risks for hydroxyurea therapy are discussed as largely unknown, although accumulating evidence of the drug's long-term safety and efficacy (currently > 15 years in adults and > 12 years in children) makes this particular point easier to discuss with each passing year. The risks of hydroxyurea for fertility and offspring are discussed; the potential of hydroxyurea as a teratogen in animals provides the strongest rationale for contraception, but the absence of teratogenicity or sterility observed to date among humans, including adult patients from the MSH study, is emphasized. Among the most important discussion points with families are those related to the potential of long-term hydroxyurea exposure to cause cancer in their child. First, it is noted that hydroxyurea initially was developed as an *anticancer* agent and still is used to treat certain forms of cancer. Next, it is noted that children with SCD, just like other children, can develop leukemia and other pediatric cancers [65]. Third, it is noted that adult patients who have preleukemic conditions, such as myeloproliferative disorders, may have an increased risk for developing cancer after 10 to 20 years of hydroxyurea therapy, but this has not yet been observed in children or adults with SCD. Finally, the theoretic risk of developing cancer in 20 years should be compared with the known natural history of untreated children with SCD and clinical severity, and to the high likelihood of acute and chronic clinical complications, poor quality of life, and increased risk for early death [6,66]. With this approach, the long-term risks of malignancy are not trivialized but are placed into context. A recent National Institutes of Health Consensus Conference concluded that the risk for cancer associated with hydroxyurea therapy in SCD does not appear to be higher than the baseline rate for this patient population [67].

Dose initiation

Before initiating hydroxyurea therapy, baseline laboratory studies should be obtained (Fig. 1). Based on data from the HUG-KIDS [37], HUSOFT [46], Toddler HUG [68], and other studies [45,54], the vast majority of children with HbSS tolerate an initial hydroxyurea dose of 20 mg/kg/d given as a single dose. Earlier studies used a lower initial starting dose of 15 mg/kg/d [32,37], but almost every pediatric patient tolerates hydroxyurea at 20 mg/kg/d unless there is concomitant renal dysfunction. The dose of hydroxyurea does not need to be adjusted for ideal body weight, because obesity is rare among untreated children with SCD. Hydroxyurea capsules are available commercially (200 mg, 300 mg, 400 mg, and 500 mg capsules), allowing fairly precise dosing regimens with accuracy within 2 mg/kg/d. At some centers, dosing is achieved with only 500 mg capsules, using doses such as: one capsule per day (500 mg/d), one capsule alternating with two capsules per day (750 mg/d), two capsules per day (1000 mg/d), and so forth. Adherence is improved, however, when the same dose is administered every day. Giving the entire daily dose at once, as opposed to a twice or three times daily dosing, improves adherence and offers some pharmacokinetic advantages [69].

For young children or those who cannot tolerate swallowing capsules, a liquid hydroxyurea formulation often can be prepared by a local or institutional pharmacy. Hydroxyurea capsule contents or bulk hydroxyurea powder can be dissolved in water with vigorous stirring and sweetener can be added for flavoring palatability; such liquid formulations are stable for weeks to months with refrigeration or at room temperature [70]. The initial hydroxyurea slurry should not be heated to speed up dissolution, however, because structural and functional activity is diminished. Liquid hydroxyurea formulations are easy to dose (usually to 0.2 mL precision), allowing fine tuning of daily doses before and after MTD is achieved.

It is recommended that the hydroxyurea dose be administered at a time of day that is most convenient for patients and families. In many instances, this is

Laboratory Studies Before Initiation
Complete blood count with WBC differential and reticulocyte count
Hemoglobin electrophoresis with quantitative % HbF
Chemistry profile (eg, LDH, total & direct bilirubin, AST / ALT, BUN / Cr)
Pregnancy test for post-menarchal females
*Serum B-12 and RBC Folate, serum Iron, TIBC, Ferritin
    (to help interpret Hydroxyurea related-macrocytosis)
*Viral serologies (Hepatitis A, B, C; Parvovirus, HIV)
    (to help interpret transaminitis or unexpected cytopenia)

Initiation Dose
Approximately 20 mg/kg/d in a single daily oral dose
Timing of administration to be convenient for patient and family
Ideally use single formulation (eg, 500 mg capsules)

Dose Escalation to MTD
Increase dose by approximately 5 mg/kg/d q8weeks until MTD reached
    Typical MTD dose 25 - 30 mg/kg/d
    Target ANC 2000 - 4000 / μL or other hematologic toxicity
    Maximum dose 35 mg/kg/d or 2000 mg/d

Laboratory Monitoring during Dose Escalation
Monthly visits with review of toxicities and medication adherence
Monthly complete blood count with WBC differential and reticulocyte count
Bimonthly chemistry profile (LDH, total & direct bilirubin, AST / ALT, BUN / Cr)
Periodic hemoglobin electrophoresis

Subsequent Dose Modification
Hematologic toxicity:
    Neutrophils   ANC < 1.0 x 10^9/L (1000 per μL)
    Hemoglobin   < 7.0 gm/dL with low reticulocytes
                       eg ARC < 100 x 10^9/L (100K per μL)
                       Decrease > 20% from baseline with low reticulocytes
    Reticulocytes   < 80 x 10^9/L (80K per μL)
                       unless the hemoglobin >8.0 gm/dL
    Platelets   < 80 x 10^9/L (80K per μL)

If hematologic toxicity occurs
    Discontinue medication until counts recover (usually within 1 week)
    Restart at previous dose or reduce dose by 2.5 – 5.0 mg/kg/d

Monitoring After Reaching MTD
Monthly visits can extend to bimonthly if:
    a stable MTD has been reached and
    adherence is judged unlikely to suffer with decreased visit frequency

Each visit: Complete blood count with WBC differential and reticulocyte count
                 Assessment of clinical toxicity
                 Reinforcement of adherence using peripheral smear or lab trends

Alternate visits: Chemistry profile (LDH, total & direct bilirubin, AST / ALT, BUN / Cr)
                  Hemoglobin electrophoresis

Fig. 1. Guideline for initiating, modifying, and monitoring hydroxyurea therapy (see text for further details). Asterisk indicates prehydroxyurea laboratory studies that are performed to help determine the etiology of potential treatment related laboratory changes or toxicities (eg, transaminitis, macrocytosis, and reticulocytopenia).

in the morning or before school or the workday but can be in the afternoon, early evening, or before bedtime. The exact timing should not be regimented or overly emphasized; the critical feature is reliable dosing once each day. Families may worry about "missing a dose" by several hours but this is not a problem; it should be emphasized, however, that the daily dose just needs to be swallowed at some time during each day. Occasional patients (approximately 5%) mention gastrointestinal symptoms, such as stomachache or nausea, after taking hydroxyurea in the morning; in these instances, changing to evening dosing almost always leads to resolution of symptoms.

Dose escalation to maximum tolerated dose

Beneficial effects of hydroxyurea can begin in the first few weeks after commencing therapy [71], which can lead to some reluctance by medical providers to increase the dose beyond that needed for subjective clinical improvement. Because the salutary laboratory effects of hydroxyurea, especially induction of HbF and diminution of WBC and absolute neutrophil count (ANC), are dose dependent [32,45], however, it seems logical and advisable to increase the daily hydroxyurea dose to achieve the MTD. Based on comparative data documenting superior laboratory effects when hydroxyurea is prescribed at MTD [45], the goal of hydroxyurea should be to achieve modest marrow suppression without undue hematologic toxicity.

After initiating hydroxyurea therapy (approximately 20 mg/kg/d), the child is seen in the outpatient clinic setting approximately every 4 weeks. At each interval visit, medical history is obtained and physical examination performed along with a discussion of dosing issues and emphasis on daily adherence. A complete blood cell count with WBC differential and reticulocyte count should be performed at each interval visit, and the next month's dose should not be ordered or dispensed until that day's weight and blood counts are available. The daily dose should be increased by approximately 5 mg/kg/d every 8 weeks if no toxicity occurs. The 4-week interval is too short for most dose adjustments, because hematologic toxicity can accumulate and not manifest fully until 8 weeks after a dose increase. It is critical to examine the trends in peripheral blood counts at each visit—sometimes toxicity is slowly cumulative and can be anticipated based on changes identified over 8 to 16 weeks.

Hydroxyurea is titrated most easily according to the peripheral blood counts and typically is limited by neutropenia, occasionally by reticulocytopenia, and more rarely by thrombocytopenia. The target ANC for MTD should be approximately 2 to $4 \times 10^9/L$ (2000–4000 per μL), although other hematologic toxicity may limit dose escalation. Based on published data [45,55,57], most children with HbSS require a dose of 25 to 30 mg/kg/d to reach this MTD. The maximum daily dose of hydroxyurea should not exceed 35 mg/kg/d or 2000 mg/d; failure to achieve marrow suppression at these doses strongly suggests medication nonadherence. The MTD, measured in mg/kg/d, typically is established within 4 to 8 months of initiating hydroxyurea therapy but should be assigned only after a child tolerates a particular dose for at least 8 weeks. The MTD then usually remains relatively stable unless there is substantial weight gain, development of splenomegaly, or change in renal function. Once a child reaches MTD, the dose in mg/kg/d, should not be modified frequently, because multiple dose changes and blood count checks are unnecessary and may incorrectly suggest a narrow therapeutic window. Periodic increases in absolute daily dose due to weight gain are appropriate. When a stable MTD is reached, it may be appropriate to decrease the frequency of clinic visits to bimonthly, depending on patient response and family reliability. Extension to quarterly visits usually is associated, however, with a decline in adherence, likely because of lack of frequent reminders from medical providers.

Dose modification

Hematologic toxicity is by far the most common reason to modify the hydroxyurea dose, usually before reaching the MTD. Although early studies on children with SCD used conservative thresholds for medication stoppage and subsequent dose modifications (eg, ANC < 2000 in HUG-KIDS) [37], a more liberal approach can be used safely in the majority of children. Practical toxicity definitions and thresholds for erythrocytes, reticulocytes, neutrophils, and platelets are listed in Table 3. Traditionally, hydroxyurea toxicity guidelines also include thresholds for hepatic or renal toxicity (eg, alanine aminotransferase increase $> 3–5 \times$ the upper limit of normal or a doubling of creatinine) but such organ toxicity almost never is associated with hydroxyurea treatment. An increase in alanine aminotransferase or creatinine should never be assumed to be drug related, and additional investigations with ultrasonography or other tests should be strongly considered.

When a hematologic toxicity occurs on hydroxyurea therapy, the medication should be discontinued to allow the counts to recover. Almost all hematologic toxicities are transient, reversible, and dose dependent and recover within 1 week of drug interruption, although severe toxicities may feature pancytopenia and take 2 to 3 weeks until recovery. If the counts recover in 1 week, then the dose can either be resumed at the previous amount or decreased

Table 3
Hematologic toxicity thresholds requiring hydroxyurea dose modifications

Neutrophils	ANC $< 1.0 \times 10^9$/L (1000 per µL)
Hemoglobin	<7.0 g/dL with low reticulocytes (eg, absolute reticulocyte count $< 100 \times 10^9$/L [100 K per µL]) Decrease by $> 20\%$ from previous value, with low reticulocytes (as previously)
Reticulocytes	$<80 \times 10^9$/L (80 K per µL) unless the hemoglobin concentration is >8.0 g/dL
Platelets	$<80 \times 10^9$/L (80 K per µL)

modestly (eg, reduced by 2.5–5 mg/kg/d). Conversely, if laboratory values suggest that a dose increase would be tolerated after 2 months at a stable dose, the MTD dose can be increased by a small amount (such as 2.5 mg/kg/d). Before increasing a hydroxyurea dose beyond a previously established stable MTD, however, the likelihood of diminished medication adherence should be strongly considered.

Increasing adherence

Medication adherence is "perhaps the best documented but least understood health-related behavior" [72]. Children and their family members are much more likely to be adherent to hydroxyurea therapy and the frequent clinic visits if they believe that treatment will be beneficial. At each clinic visit, the importance of daily medication should be emphasized; specific questions should be asked regarding who gives the dose, what time it is administered, how many doses are missed per week, and so forth. Visualization of the peripheral blood smear is an effective way to illustrate the benefits of hydroxyurea therapy. The de-identified peripheral blood smears of several patients, which were obtained pre- and post-treatment MTD, can be shown to children and family members. The authors use a multiheaded microscope before initiating hydroxyurea therapy to demonstrate the obvious changes that occur with good adherence and a good treatment response (Fig. 2), including anisocytosis, macrocytosis, decreased polychromasia,

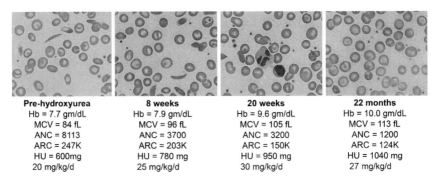

Pre-hydroxyurea	8 weeks	20 weeks	22 months
Hb = 7.7 gm/dL	Hb = 7.9 gm/dL	Hb = 9.6 gm/dL	Hb = 10.0 gm/dL
MCV = 84 fL	MCV = 96 fL	MCV = 105 fL	MCV = 113 fL
ANC = 8113	ANC = 3700	ANC = 3200	ANC = 1200
ARC = 247K	ARC = 203K	ARC = 150K	ARC = 124K
HU = 600mg	HU = 780 mg	HU = 950 mg	HU = 1040 mg
20 mg/kg/d	25 mg/kg/d	30 mg/kg/d	27 mg/kg/d

Fig. 2. Changes in complete blood cell count parameters and erythrocyte morphology in association with hydroxyurea therapy, from dose initiation through escalation to MTD. The initial panel shows blood counts and the peripheral blood smear at dose initiation, with hemolytic anemia and leukocytosis evident along with sickled forms. The second panel is after 8 weeks of hydroxyurea therapy (at approximately 20 mg/kg/d) with some macrocytes and anisocytosis present, along with reductions in the ANC and ARC; the dose was escalated (to approximately 25 mg/kg/d). The third panel is after 20 weeks of hydroxyurea therapy, with less anemia and sickling, more macrocytosis, and modest myelosuppression; the dose was escalated (to approximately 30 mg/kg/d). The fourth panel is after 22 months of hydroxyurea therapy (at MTD of 27 mg/kg/d); there is improved Hb with pronounced macrocytosis and no sickled forms, along with modest neutropenia and reticulocytopenia. ARC, absolute reticulocyte count; Hb, hemoglobin; HU, hydroxyurea.

and fewer sickled forms. This viewing and explanation should be performed by an experienced medical provider who can emphasize that adherence also can be monitored by review of the blood counts and the peripheral blood smear.

When explanations of risks and benefits of hydroxyurea therapy are given to patients and family members, it is emphasized that a parent must be in charge of ensuring that the medication actually is swallowed each day. It is imperative to anticipate that occasionally children miss a dose of hydroxyurea without any ill effect, and therefore be tempted to miss several days, wondering if they somehow have been cured. Explaining that blood cells are produced every day, hence the medication must be taken every day, is logical even for young patients. Parents must be reminded at each interval visit that they must be sure to give the medication; teenagers are especially notorious for embellishing adherence. In some instances, patients can be remarkably adherent and even remind parents about dosing.

The use of a "medication score card" can be helpful for improving hydroxyurea adherence. Serial listing of monthly blood counts according to various blood count parameters can be used to show beneficial changes, such as increased hemoglobin concentration, mean corpuscular volume (MCV), and HbF; concomitant decreases in WBC and ANC also easily can be seen. Additional strategies to improving hydroxyurea adherence include providing a calendar to mark off days after medicine has been swallowed, preloading a weekly/biweekly/monthly pill container with prescribed capsules, keeping the pill bottle in plain sight (eg, the kitchen table) to minimize forgotten doses, and counting leftover or unused pills. Whatever the mnemonic devices used, among the best strategies for successful treatment are a thorough understanding of the rationale for treatment, a limited number of health care providers for continuity to patients and family, and regular clinic visits on a 1 to 2 month basis, to engender trust and loyalty with emphasis on the beneficial treatment effects and the need for daily adherence.

Summary

Hydroxyurea is a powerful therapeutic agent with proved laboratory and clinical efficacy for children with SCD. Although there are important questions regarding its long-term efficacy and safety, hydroxyurea has the potential to ameliorate many of the signs and symptoms of the disease. Ongoing clinical trials will help answer questions about the proper clinical indications for its use and, in particular, its ability to prevent organ damage and preserve organ function and long-term safety.

Acknowledgments

The authors thank Nicole A. Mortier, MHS PA-C, and William H. Schultz, MHS PA-C, for years of experience and dedication to treating children with SCD. We appreciate their insights and advice regarding the optimal use of hydroxyurea in this patient population.

References

[1] Platt OS, Thorington BD, Brambilla DJ, et al. Pain in sickle cell disease. Rates and risk factors. N Engl J Med 1991;325(1):11–6.

[2] Steinberg MH, Rosenstock W, Coleman MB, et al. Effects of thalassemia and microcytosis on the hematologic and vasoocclusive severity of sickle cell anemia. Blood 1984;63(6): 1353–60.

[3] Baum KF, Dunn DT, Maude GH, et al. The painful crisis of homozygous sickle cell disease. A study of the risk factors. Arch Intern Med 1987;147(7):1231–4.

[4] Phillips G Jr, Coffey B, Tran-Son-Tay R, et al. Relationship of clinical severity to packed cell rheology in sickle cell anemia. Blood 1991;78(10):2735–9.

[5] Powars DR. Sickle cell anemia: beta s-gene-cluster haplotypes as prognostic indicators of vital organ failure. Semin Hematol 1991;28(3):202–8.

[6] Platt OS, Brambilla DJ, Rosse WF, et al. Mortality in sickle cell disease. Life expectancy and risk factors for early death. N Engl J Med 1994;330(23):1639–44.

[7] Charache S. Fetal hemoglobin, sickling, and sickle cell disease. Adv Pediatr 1990;37:1–31.

[8] Wood WG. Increased HbF in adult life. Baillieres Clin Haematol 1993;6(1):177–213.

[9] Serjeant GR. Fetal haemoglobin in homozygous sickle cell disease. Clin Haematol 1975;4(1): 109–22.

[10] Wood WG, Stamatoyannopoulos G, Lim G, et al. F-cells in the adult: normal values and levels in individuals with hereditary and acquired elevations of Hb F. Blood 1975;46(5): 671–82.

[11] Watson J, Stahman AW, Bilello FP. Significance of paucity of sickle cells in newborn negro infants. Am J Med Sci 1948;215:419–23.

[12] Steinberg MH. Compound heterozygous and other hemoglobinopathies. In: Steinberg MH, Forget BG, Higgs DR, editors. Disorders of hemoglobin: genetics, pathophysiology, and clinical management. Cambridge (UK): Cambridge University Press; 2001. p. 786–810.

[13] Odenheimer DJ, Sarnaik SA, Whitten CF, et al. The relationship between fetal hemoglobin and disease severity in children with sickle cell anemia. Am J Med Genet 1987;27(3):525–35.

[14] Gladwin MT, Sachdev V, Jison ML, et al. Pulmonary hypertension as a risk factor for death in patients with sickle cell disease. N Engl J Med 2004;350(9):886–95.

[15] Powars DR, Schroeder WA, Weiss JN, et al. Lack of influence of fetal hemoglobin levels or erythrocyte indices on the severity of sickle cell anemia. J Clin Invest 1980;65(3):732–40.

[16] Powars DR, Weiss JN, Chan LS, et al. Is there a threshold level of fetal hemoglobin that ameliorates morbidity in sickle cell anemia? Blood 1984;63(4):921–6.

[17] Leikin SL, Gallagher D, Kinney TR, et al. Mortality in children and adolescents with sickle cell disease. Cooperative Study of Sickle Cell Disease. Pediatrics 1989;84(3):500–8.

[18] Ley TJ, DeSimone J, Noguchi CT, et al. 5-Azacytidine increases gamma-globin synthesis and reduces the proportion of dense cells in patients with sickle cell anemia. Blood 1983; 62(2):370–80.

[19] DeSimone J, Koshy M, Dorn L, et al. Maintenance of elevated fetal hemoglobin levels by decitabine during dose interval treatment of sickle cell anemia. Blood 2002;99(11):3905–8.

[20] Koshy M, Dorn L, Bressler L, et al. 2-Deoxy 5-azacytidine and fetal hemoglobin induction in sickle cell anemia. Blood 2000;96(7):2379–84.

[21] Saunthararajah Y, Hillery CA, Lavelle D, et al. Effects of 5-aza-2′-deoxycytidine on fetal hemoglobin levels, red cell adhesion, and hematopoietic differentiation in patients with sickle cell disease. Blood 2003;102(12):3865–70.

[22] Atweh GF, Sutton M, Nassif I, et al. Sustained induction of fetal hemoglobin by pulse butyrate therapy in sickle cell disease. Blood 1999;93(6):1790–7.

[23] Dover GJ, Brusilow S, Charache S. Induction of fetal hemoglobin production in subjects with sickle cell anemia by oral sodium phenylbutyrate. Blood 1994;84(1):339–43.

[24] Resar LM, Segal JB, Fitzpatric LK, et al. Induction of fetal hemoglobin synthesis in children with sickle cell anemia on low-dose oral sodium phenylbutyrate therapy. J Pediatr Hematol Oncol 2002;24(9):737–41.

[25] Sher GD, Ginder GD, Little J, et al. Extended therapy with intravenous arginine butyrate in patients with beta-hemoglobinopathies. N Engl J Med 1995;332(24):1606–10.

[26] Davies SC, Gilmore A. The role of hydroxyurea in the management of sickle cell disease. Blood Rev 2003;17(2):99–109.

[27] Halsey C, Roberts IA. The role of hydroxyurea in sickle cell disease. Br J Haematol 2003; 120(2):177–86.

[28] Lori F, Foli A, Groff A, et al. Optimal suppression of HIV replication by low-dose hydroxyurea through the combination of antiviral and cytostatic ('virostatic') mechanisms. AIDS 2005;19(11):1173–81.

[29] Dover GJ, Humphries RK, Moore JG, et al. Hydroxyurea induction of hemoglobin F production in sickle cell disease: relationship between cytotoxicity and F cell production. Blood 1986;67(3):735–8.

[30] Platt OS, Orkin SH, Dover G, et al. Hydroxyurea enhances fetal hemoglobin production in sickle cell anemia. J Clin Invest 1984;74(2):652–6.

[31] Charache S, Dover GJ, Moyer MA, et al. Hydroxyurea-induced augmentation of fetal hemoglobin production in patients with sickle cell anemia. Blood 1987;69(1):109–16.

[32] Charache S, Dover GJ, Moore RD, et al. Hydroxyurea: effects on hemoglobin F production in patients with sickle cell anemia. Blood 1992;79(10):2555–65.

[33] Letvin NL, Linch DC, Beardsley GP, et al. Augmentation of fetal-hemoglobin production in anemic monkeys by hydroxyurea. N Engl J Med 1984;310(14):869–73.

[34] Gladwin MT, Shelhamer JH, Ognibene FP, et al. Nitric oxide donor properties of hydroxyurea in patients with sickle cell disease. Br J Haematol 2002;116(2):436–44.

[35] Huang J, Yakubu M, Kim-Shapiro DB, et al. Rat liver-mediated metabolism of hydroxyurea to nitric oxide. Free Radic Biol Med 2006;40(9):1675–81.

[36] Charache S, Terrin ML, Moore RD, et al. Effect of hydroxyurea on the frequency of painful crises in sickle cell anemia. Investigators of the Multicenter Study of Hydroxyurea in Sickle Cell Anemia. N Engl J Med 1995;332(20):1317–22.

[37] Kinney TR, Helms RW, O'Branski EE, et al. Safety of hydroxyurea in children with sickle cell anemia: results of the HUG-KIDS study, a phase I/II trial. Pediatric Hydroxyurea Group. Blood 1999;94(5):1550–4.

[38] Wang WC, Helms RW, Lynn HS, et al. Effect of hydroxyurea on growth in children with sickle cell anemia: results of the HUG-KIDS Study. J Pediatr 2002;140(2):225–9.

[39] Ware RE, Eggleston B, Redding-Lallinger R, et al. Predictors of fetal hemoglobin response in children with sickle cell anemia receiving hydroxyurea therapy. Blood 2002;99(1):10–4.

[40] Scott JP, Hillery CA, Brown ER, et al. Hydroxyurea therapy in children severely affected with sickle cell disease. J Pediatr 1996;128(6):820–8.

[41] Jayabose S, Tugal O, Sandoval C, et al. Clinical and hematologic effects of hydroxyurea in children with sickle cell anemia. J Pediatr 1996;129(4):559–65.

[42] Ferster A, Vermylen C, Cornu G, et al. Hydroxyurea for treatment of severe sickle cell anemia: a pediatric clinical trial. Blood 1996;88(6):1960–4.

[43] de Montalembert M, Belloy M, Bernaudin F, et al. Three-year follow-up of hydroxyurea treatment in severely ill children with sickle cell disease. The French Study Group on Sickle Cell Disease. J Pediatr Hematol Oncol 1997;19(4):313–8.

[44] Ferster A, Tahriri P, Vermylen C, et al. Five years of experience with hydroxyurea in children and young adults with sickle cell disease. Blood 2001;97(11):3628–32.

[45] Zimmerman SA, Schultz WH, Davis JS, et al. Sustained long-term hematologic efficacy of hydroxyurea at maximum tolerated dose in children with sickle cell disease. Blood 2004; 103(6):2039–45.

[46] Wang WC, Wynn LW, Rogers ZR, et al. A two-year pilot trial of hydroxyurea in very young children with sickle-cell anemia. J Pediatr 2001;139(6):790–6.

[47] Hankins JS, Ware RE, Rogers ZR, et al. Long-term hydroxyurea therapy for infants with sickle cell anemia: the HUSOFT extension study. Blood 2005;106(7):2269–75.

[48] Hankins JS, Helton KJ, McCarville MB, et al. Preservation of spleen and brain function in children with sickle cell anemia treated with hydroxyurea. Pediatr Blood Cancer 2008;50(2): 293–7.

[49] Fitzhugh CD, Wigfall DR, Ware RE. Enalapril and hydroxyurea therapy for children with sickle nephropathy. Pediatr Blood Cancer 2005;45(7):982–5.

[50] Saad ST, Lajolo C, Gilli S, et al. Follow-up of sickle cell disease patients with priapism treated by hydroxyurea. Am J Hematol 2004;77(1):45–9.

[51] Maples BL, Hagemann TM. Treatment of priapism in pediatric patients with sickle cell disease. Am J Health Syst Pharm 2004;61(4):355–63.

[52] Singh S, Koumbourlis A, Aygun B. Resolution of chronic hypoxemia in pediatric sickle cell patients after treatment with hydroxyurea. Pediatr Blood Cancer;[epub ahead of print].

[53] Kratovil T, Bulas D, Driscoll MC, et al. Hydroxyurea therapy lowers TCD velocities in children with sickle cell disease. Pediatr Blood Cancer 2006;47(7):894–900.

[54] Zimmerman SA, Schultz WH, Burgett S, et al. Hydroxyurea therapy lowers transcranial Doppler flow velocities in children with sickle cell anemia. Blood 2007;110(3):1043–7.

[55] Ware RE, Zimmerman SA, Schultz WH. Hydroxyurea as an alternative to blood transfusions for the prevention of recurrent stroke in children with sickle cell disease. Blood 1999; 94(9):3022–6.

[56] Sumoza A, de Bisotti R, Sumoza D, et al. Hydroxyurea (HU) for prevention of recurrent stroke in sickle cell anemia (SCA). Am J Hematol 2002;71(3):161–5.

[57] Ware RE, Zimmerman SA, Sylvestre PB, et al. Prevention of secondary stroke and resolution of transfusional iron overload in children with sickle cell anemia using hydroxyurea and phlebotomy. J Pediatr 2004;145(3):346–52.

[58] ClinicalTrials.gov. Stroke with transfusions changing to hydroxyurea (SWiTCH). Available at: http://clinicaltrials.gov/ct2/show/NCT00122980. Accessed March 1, 2008.

[59] Steinberg MH, Barton F, Castro O, et al. Effect of hydroxyurea on mortality and morbidity in adult sickle cell anemia: risks and benefits up to 9 years of treatment. JAMA 2003;289(13): 1645–51.

[60] Pata O, Tok CE, Yazici G, et al. Polycythemia vera and pregnancy: a case report with the use of hydroxyurea in the first trimester. Am J Perinatol 2004;21(3):135–7.

[61] Byrd DC, Pitts SR, Alexander CK. Hydroxyurea in two pregnant women with sickle cell anemia. Pharmacotherapy 1999;19(12):1459–62.

[62] Grigg A. Effect of hydroxyurea on sperm count, motility and morphology in adult men with sickle cell or myeloproliferative disease. Intern Med J 2007;37(3):190–2.

[63] Masood J, Hafeez A, Hughes A, et al. Hydroxyurea therapy: a rare cause of reversible azoospermia. Int Urol Nephrol 2007;39(3):905–7.

[64] ClinicalTrials.gov. Long term effects of hydroxyurea therapy in children with sickle cell disease. Available at: http://clinicaltrials.gov/ct2/show/NCT00305175. Accessed March 1, 2008.

[65] Schultz WH, Ware RE. Malignancy in patients with sickle cell disease. Am J Hematol 2003; 74(4):249–53.

[66] Miller ST, Sleeper LA, Pegelow CH, et al. Prediction of adverse outcomes in children with sickle cell disease. N Engl J Med 2000;342(2):83–9.

[67] NIH. National Institutes of Health Consensus Development Conference statement: hydroxyurea treatment for sickle cell disease; 2008. Available at: http://consensus.nih.gov/2008/Sickle%20Cell%20Draft%20Statement%2002-27-08.pdf. Accessed March 1, 2008.

[68] Thornburg CD, Dixon N, Burgett S, et al. Efficacy of hydroxyurea to prevent organ damage in young children with sickle cell anemia. Blood 2007;110(11):3386.

[69] Yan JH, Ataga K, Kaul S, et al. The influence of renal function on hydroxyurea pharmacokinetics in adults with sickle cell disease. J Clin Pharmacol 2005;45(4):434–45.

[70] Heeney MM, Whorton MR, Howard TA, et al. Chemical and functional analysis of hydroxyurea oral solutions. J Pediatr Hematol Oncol 2004;26(3):179–84.

[71] Bridges KR, Barabino GD, Brugnara C, et al. A multiparameter analysis of sickle erythrocytes in patients undergoing hydroxyurea therapy. Blood 1996;88(12):4701–10.

[72] Becker MH, Maiman LA. Sociobehavioral determinants of compliance with health and medical care recommendations. Med Care 1975;13(1):10–24.

PEDIATRIC CLINICS

OF NORTH AMERICA

Pediatr Clin N Am 55 (2008) 503–519

Partial Splenectomy for Hereditary Spherocytosis

Elisabeth T. Tracy, MD[a], Henry E. Rice, MD[b],*

[a]*Division of General Surgery, Department of Surgery, Duke University Medical Center, Box 3654, Durham, NC, 27710, USA*
[b]*Division of Pediatric Surgery, Department of Surgery, Duke University Medical Center, Durham, Box 3815, NC, 27710, USA*

Total splenectomy is an effective but challenging therapeutic option to recommend for children who have various forms of congenital hemolytic anemia [1]. In children who are affected severely, total splenectomy can alleviate anemia, reduce the rate of hemolysis, lower the risk for splenic sequestration, and eliminate symptoms of splenomegaly [2,3]. The surgical procedure itself is not without risks, however, and the use of total splenectomy in children is limited by concerns of assorted peri- and postoperative complications, most notably the lifelong risk for overwhelming postsplenectomy sepsis [4–11].

These ill-defined but clinically significant risks associated with total splenectomy have led to recent interest in the use of partial splenectomy as an alternative surgical therapy for children who have congenital hemolytic anemia. Partial splenectomy is designed to remove enough spleen to gain the desired hematologic outcomes while preserving splenic immune function [2,12–16]. Although preliminary data from small studies from North America and Europe have demonstrated successful laboratory and clinical outcomes after partial splenectomy in children who have various congenital hemolytic anemias, conclusive data comparing the efficacy of partial splenectomy to total splenectomy are not reported to date. Based on preliminary data, however, a definitive clinical trial for partial splenectomy in children who have severe congenital hemolytic anemia may be warranted.

This article reviews the current status of partial splenectomy for treatment of the most common congenital red blood cell (RBC) membrane disorder in children, namely hereditary spherocytosis (HS), also known as

* Corresponding author.
E-mail address: rice0017@mc.duke.edu (H.E. Rice).

doi:10.1016/j.pcl.2008.02.001
pediatric.theclinics.com

congenital spherocytosis. Concerns with the use of total splenectomy, methods for evaluating the laboratory and clinical effects of total and partial splenectomy, and preliminary experience with partial splenectomy are described. The rationale and options for design of a clinical trial that would compare partial splenectomy to total splenectomy for the management of children who have HS also are described.

Total splenectomy in hereditary spherocytosis

HS is the most common inherited RBC membrane disorder in Northern Europe and North America, with a reported incidence of 1 in 5000 births [17]. More recent studies of osmotic fragility in blood donors, however, suggest the existence of mild forms, raising the prevalence of HS to 1 in 2000 [18]. The majority of patients have HS have European ancestry, but HS also occurs in African Americans and persons of Hispanic and Asian ancestry. Although some children and adults who have HS have a mild clinical phenotype, many patients develop clinically significant and eventually severe clinical consequences, such as anemia, hemolytic crises, splenic sequestration, and gallstones, which traditionally have led to the recommendation of total splenectomy.

The shortened lifespan of RBCs in HS is related to a deficiency or dysfunction of constituents within the RBC cytoskeleton [1,19,20]. The erythrocyte cytoskeleton is a spectrin-based 2-D network of cell membrane proteins, with each spectrin moiety (α- or β-subunit) consisting of repeating polypeptide domains that fold into repeating helices. Paired α/β-spectrin heterodimers form tetramers, whereas the other end of the spectrin heterodimer is physically associated with protein 4.1 and actin that anchors the cytoskeleton to the lipid bilayer. This attachment of the spectrin latticework to the lipid bilayer involves the transmembrane proteins band 3 and glycophorin C. Band 3 interacts with ankyrin that binds to β-spectrin and protein 4.1 and interacts with protein 4.2 to provide additional stability. Glycophorin C interacts with protein p55 and protein 4.1, which in turn binds to β-spectrin. Defects in erythrocyte ankyrin are among the most common causes of typical, autosomal dominant HS [21]. Dysfunction in any one of these membrane components, however, can destabilize the cytoskeleton, resulting in a shortened RBC lifespan and variable clinical phenotype.

Most children who have HS do not have signs or symptoms that require surgical intervention early in life. For children who have severe anemia and substantial splenomegaly, a total splenectomy is considered "curative" based on laboratory and clinical effects. Splenectomy is not truly curative but does remove the primary "graveyard" for spherocytes and, thus, has a normalizing effect on the hemolytic anemia. Total splenectomy results in higher hemoglobin concentrations, reduced rates of hemolysis, elimination of splenic sequestration, and alleviation of symptoms associated with splenomegaly [1]. The major disadvantage of total splenectomy, however, in this setting is the concern for developing overwhelming postsplenectomy infection (OPSI), which is sepsis from encapsulated bacterial organisms and often is fatal, particularly in young children. Unfortunately, total splenectomy occasionally is recommended erroneously for young children who have a mild clinical phenotype.

Contrary to the common misconception that total splenectomy rarely is used in children who have HS, the incidence and public health impact of children who have HS requiring total splenectomy is substantial. The 2003 Healthcare Cost and Utilization Project (HCUP) Kids Inpatient Database, a robust and widely used measure of pediatric disorders, demonstrated that the number of children who have HS ages 0 to17 who received total splenectomy was estimated at 373 children per year (HCUP Kids' Inpatient Database, *International Classification of Diseases, Ninth Revision, Clinical Modification* category) [22]. In addition to HS, total splenectomy is performed in children for a variety of other indications, including other hematologic disorders, such as sickle cell anemia or thalassemia, trauma, and various acquired illnesses. In children less than 18 years of age, nearly 2000 splenectomy procedures are performed annually in the United States, with aggregate hospital charges (a "national bill") for these procedures exceeding $71,000,000 annually [22].

Considering the high incidence and potentially serious complications associated with total splenectomy in children, the routine use of splenectomy in children who have HS has an extensive financial and public health impact. Therefore, examination of alternative surgical approaches, such as partial splenectomy, has important and widespread implications for improving the clinical care of children who have hematologic disorders, such as HS.

Immunologic complications of splenectomy and role of memory B cells

Total splenectomy leads to a wide range of immunologic deficits and complications. The role of the spleen in protecting against infections is based on complex and interrelated phagocytic and immune functions, including filtration and phagocytosis of bacteria from the blood, removal of foreign material, and production of opsonins: antigen-specific IgM, alternate complement components, properdin, and tuftsin [23]. Therefore, an intact and functioning spleen seems to have critical protective effects against common childhood infections. Given the complexity of splenic-dependent and splenic-independent immune responses involved in bacterial clearance, determining whether or not and how much immune function is preserved after partial splenectomy is essential before widespread acceptance of this procedure.

Recently, a population of surface $IgM^{bright}IgD^{dull}CD22^+CD27^+$ human peripheral blood B cells, termed IgM memory B cells, has been described that is similar to the murine B-1a B-cell subset producing natural antibodies

and antibodies against T-independent antigens, such as pneumococcal poly-
saccharides [24–26]. Natural antibodies primarily are IgM, are independent
of previous immunization, bind antigens with low affinity, and limit infections before generation of specific antibody [27,28]. IgM memory B cells
correspond to circulating splenic marginal zone B cells and are lacking in
patients who do not have a spleen [25,29]. The absence of IgM memory
B cells correlates with diminished serum antipneumococcal polysaccharide
IgM antibody responses in splenectomized patients [24].

The specific clinical benefits of splenic-mediated immune function are
demonstrated in children who have common variable immunodeficiency
(CVID), a heterogeneous immune disorder of unknown pathogenesis characterized by the inability to mount protective antibody responses in the presence of normal numbers of circulating B cells. Recent studies of CVID and
related conditions have demonstrated further the critical function of splenic-
mediated IgM memory B cells. In these children, IgM memory B cells seem
essential for prevention and control of common childhood infections, such
as those of the respiratory tract caused by encapsulated bacteria [24].
Memory B cells are lacking in infants and children who have CVID and
in children who are asplenic. It seems, therefore, that surgical interventions
for the management of HS that avoid rendering patients asplenic would
have far-ranging implications not only in reducing the incidence of the
rare but lethal cases of OPSI but also possibly in reducing the more common
infections that affect children.

Complications of total splenectomy and risks for overwhelming postsplenectomy infection

Total splenectomy carries significant risks for children and adults. The
most well-known and feared complication of total splenectomy is OPSI,
characterized by multisystem organ failure after invasive infection with
encapsulated bacteria, such as *Streptococcus pneumoniae*. OPSI is lethal in
the majority of affected children. The risk for OPSI is higher for children
compared with adults and may be as high as 20% for children who undergo
splenectomy before the age 5 [3–6]. The rate of sepsis in children less than
5 years of age who have undergone total splenectomy is 60-fold to 100-fold
higher than for children who have not had a splenectomy [5].

Although the risk for OPSI is reduced by the use of immunizations
against *Streptococcus pneumoniae*, *Neisseria meningitidis*, *Haemophilus influenzae* type b, and postoperative antibiotic prophylaxis, its risk never is
eliminated fully. Despite the frequent belief that older children and adults
are not affected adversely by asplenia, patients who undergo splenectomy
remain at lifelong increased risk for overwhelming infection [6,23]. The
risk is compounded by the fact that vaccinations do not provide complete
protection, antibiotic resistance may emerge, and poor compliance with recommended antibiotic prophylaxis often is observed [6,30].

Intravascular hemolysis and its complications after total splenectomy

In addition to decreased immune competence, total splenectomy seems to lead to a broad range of additional clinical pathology, including severe vascular and endothelial derangements. After removal of the spleen, the main site of extravascular RBC clearance, there is an obligate increase in intravascular hemolysis. This leads to increased levels of intravascular hemoglobin, which triggers widespread deleterious effects on vascular tone and homeostasis. This disruption of vascular integrity seems to be mediated by nitric oxide (NO), a regulator of vasodilatation, because interactions of NO with hemoglobin are critical for maintenance of vascular tone [31]. NO produced by endothelium is scavenged by free plasma hemoglobin and then is incapable of diffusion from endothelium to vascular smooth muscle. Under normal physiologic conditions, the ability of hemoglobin to react with NO is limited by compartmentalization of hemoglobin inside the erythrocyte. In conditions of increased intravascular hemolysis and higher levels of free hemoglobin, however, such as the postsplenectomy state, these homeostatic mechanisms may be compromised.

An increase in intravascular hemolysis and subsequent vascular derangement may lead to increased long-term risks of hypertension, vascular thrombosis, pulmonary hypertension, and cardiovascular disease [32,33]. Hemoglobin also exerts direct cytotoxic, inflammatory, and pro-oxidant effects that affect endothelial function adversely [34]. Therefore, use of total splenectomy is implicated as one factor in the development of severe chronic clinical conditions with substantial morbidity and public health consequences.

Role of partial splenectomy for hereditary spherocytosis

Given the substantial morbidity and potential mortality associated with the use of total splenectomy for HS, especially when performed in young children, recent interest has developed in alternative surgical approaches that can preserve splenic function. In other clinical settings, such as trauma, splenic salvage already has replaced total splenectomy as the standard of care for children and adults. This evolution in clinical care is based on several animal studies, in which preservation of approximately one third of the normal spleen volume seems to protect against bacterial infections [35,36]. The challenge in determining the exact role of partial splenectomy in the management of HS and related conditions is the identification of useful clinical parameters to assess the risks and benefits of this surgical procedure.

Technique of partial splenectomy

Partial splenectomy is a technically challenging surgical procedure designed to resect enough spleen to achieve the desired hematologic effect while preserving splenic immune function. Based on animal models suggesting that limited splenic volume can preserve the splenic phagocytic response to *Streptococcus pneumoniae*, several groups (including the authors) have adopted a goal of removing 80% to 90% of the enlarged spleen for most conditions [16,37–39]. The residual 10% to 20% volume is equivalent to approximately one third of the normal splenic volume, estimated as sufficient for immune preservation.

Preoperative considerations include assessing splenic volume by ultrasonography and ensuring that patients are vaccinated adequately, in case during surgery the need to convert to total splenectomy is determined. Because some children have a splenic anatomy that is not amenable to partial splenectomy, all children undergoing partial splenectomy should be prepared preoperatively for potential total splenectomy. Immunizations against encapsulated bacteria, including polyvalent pneumococcal vaccination (Pneumovax, Prevnar) and meningococcal vaccination (Meningovax, Menactra) should be administered, and *H influenzae* type b vaccination if prior administration cannot be confirmed.

Partial splenectomy can be performed using an open laparotomy or by a laparoscopic approach, and the choice of approach is dependent a surgeon's experience and preference. In cases of massive splenomegaly (> 500 mL volume), the authors prefer the open approach, although further refinement of surgical techniques may allow for good clinical outcomes by laparoscopy. With either approach, the spleen first is exposed carefully. The splenic vasculature is examined and vessels ligated to ensure adequate perfusion of the splenic remnant. The authors generally prefer to preserve the upper pole of the spleen given the risk for torsion associated with nonfixation of the lower pole, although other groups prefer preservation of the lower pole with associated splenopexy, similar to treatment for a wandering spleen [40]. Before proceeding with splenic transection, adequate flow is confirmed to the upper pole via one or two short gastric vessels. If vessels to the upper pole are absent or if severe intraoperative bleeding is encountered, the authors convert to a total splenectomy. In the authors' experience, intraoperative conversion to total splenectomy is required in less than 5% of cases.

After assessing the vessels, the spleen is devascularized partially to maintain flow from the short gastric arcades to the upper pole, and the ischemic portion of the spleen is allowed to demarcate visually between the pink vascularized tissue and the dark devascularized portion. Before splenic transection, the devascularized spleen then can be compressed manually for two reasons: first, to autotransfuse a substantial volume of blood back into the patient, and second, to enable an easier surgical transaction of this 3-D mass. The splenic parenchyma then is divided using a surgical stapler (for small or normal spleens) or with electrocautery, TissueLink device, or LigaSure (for cases of massive splenomegaly). After parenchyma transection, bleeding from the splenic bed can be controlled with an argon beam coagulator, suture ligation of vessels, and topical hemostatic agents (Fig. 1).

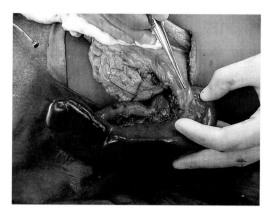

Fig. 1. Intraoperative photograph of spleen after selective devascularization of lower pole and main body. Upper pole remains perfused from short gastric vessels, allowing for resection of 85% of the splenic parenchyma.

The authors' goal of performing partial splenectomy, retaining approximately 30% of normal splenic volume, can require 90% to 95% resection in patients who have massive splenomegaly. Their previous published experience has shown that intraoperative surgeons' estimates of retained splenic volume correlate closely with sonographic measurements of postoperative retained splenic parenchyma [12].

After the procedure, ultrasonography should be performed periodically to assure blood flow to and from the splenic remnant and to estimate the residual splenic volume. The authors routinely perform an ultrasonography measurement in the early postoperative period (ie, before discharge) and then at 1 month and 2 months and thereafter at 6- to 12-month intervals. Along with regular sonographic assessment of the splenic remnant, the authors prescribe postoperative antibiotic prophylaxis with oral penicillin (or a suitable alternative) for at least 1 year and continue long-term prophylaxis at the discretion of the hematologist. With the laparoscopic or open approach, the authors also advise activity restrictions for 6 weeks after surgery to minimize the risk for postoperative bleeding.

Evaluation of splenic function after partial splenectomy

Demonstration that splenic function is preserved after partial splenectomy is critically important in assessing its role in the management of children who have clinically severe HS. The gold standard for evaluating splenic immunologic function is the liver-spleen radionuclide scan, which detects the ability of the splenic macrophages to phagocytose technetium-99m sulfur colloid. Uptake of the radionuclide within the spleen remnant is an indicator of functioning splenic tissue, although concerns about radioactive exposure limits its frequent use in children. The quantitation of circulating erythrocytes with vesicles, which normally are removed by splenic filtration, constitutes the pitted cell measurement that correlates well with the radionuclide liver-spleen scan. Pit count measurement is technically laborious, however, and requires special equipment, including Nomarski optics, so is not available routinely for clinical practice.

In addition to liver-spleen scan and pitted cell measurement, there are other measures of splenic function used commonly, including measurement of overall immunoglobulin levels, delineation of lymphocyte subsets and immunoglobulin subtypes, and specific antibody response to pneumococcal or other immunizations. In toto, these measures provide a broad assessment of various aspects of splenic phagocytic and immune function. Ideally, any critical evaluation of partial splenectomy would include quantitative assessment of the incidence of OPSI/sepsis compared with the incidence observed in patients undergoing total splenectomy. Given the low incidence of OPSI, however, any significant risk reduction in OPSI after partial splenectomy compared with total splenectomy would require an exceedingly large patient population with decades of follow-up. This is unlikely to happen; thus, alternative laboratory and clinical parameters of splenic function must serve as surrogates to help answer these important questions.

Recently, a novel method of assessing splenic function by the quantification of Howell-Jolly bodies (HJB)-containing erythrocytes (micronuclei) has been developed based on flow cytometry. This technique is a reproducible and inexpensive method for detecting chromosome fragments within circulating erythrocyte subpopulations and offers an alternative method of assessing splenic phagocytic function [41]. This technique of micronuclei enumeration is shown to correlate with splenectomy status in children who have sickle cell disease [42] and currently is used in the National Institutes of Health–sponsored phase III hydroxyurea trial (BABY HUG) for infants who have sickle cell anemia. Preliminary analysis suggests that flow cytometry–based enumeration of HJB is comparable to other traditional measures of splenic function, such as a liver-spleen scan and pitted erythrocyte counts [43]. The enumeration of micronuclei using flow cytometry may become an alternative measure of splenic function after partial splenectomy in HS, but to date no data have been gathered prospectively in this patient population.

Partial splenectomy and vascular thrombosis

Another potentially serious clinical complication after total splenectomy is that of thromboembolic events, which occur in up to 10% patients [44]. Clinical thrombotic complications after splenectomy range from portal vein thrombosis to deep vein thrombosis and pulmonary embolism [45]. Improved diagnostic modalities suggest that the true incidence of thrombosis may be higher than can be appreciated clinically. Ikeda and colleagues [46] reported that the incidence of portal or splenic vein thrombosis after laparoscopic splenectomy was 55% as determined by abdominal CT.

Similarly, Soyer and colleagues [47] demonstrated an elevated rate of thrombosis in a cohort of children who had hematologic conditions and were undergoing splenectomy. At this time, it is unclear whether or not there is a decreased risk for thrombosis after partial splenectomy compared with the risk noted after total splenectomy. A demonstrable risk reduction for thrombosis would further support the use of partial splenectomy not only for children who have HS but also in other common conditions requiring splenic resection.

Clinical studies of partial splenectomy in hereditary spherocytosis

For children who have HS, the role of partial splenectomy has been evaluated in several nonrandomized clinical studies in Europe and North America [7,13,48]. The following section summarizes the experience gained to date [7,13,14,16,48–51].

French experience

The resurgence of and recent interest in using partial splenectomy was stimulated by Tchernia and colleagues from the Hôpital Bicètre in Paris, France [2,7,13]. This group advocates an 80% to 90% partial splenectomy in children who have HS. In their most recent summary, 40 children who had HS and underwent partial splenectomy were monitored for 1 to 14 years. In this nonrandomized trial, partial splenectomy resulted in a sustained decrease in hemolytic anemia with a significantly increased hemoglobin concentration, which improved from 9.2 ± 2.6 g/dL at baseline to 12.3 ± 1.9 g/dL at 3 to 4 years after surgery ($P < .01$). The increased hemoglobin concentration was maintained for up to 10 years after surgery.

This group also demonstrated preserved phagocytic function of the splenic remnant using radionuclide liver-spleen imaging in most children. Furthermore, they demonstrated in a subset of children an increased red cell lifespan averaging 6.5 days (range: 5 to 14.5 days). Tchernia and colleagues [2,7,13] have shown that partial splenectomy does not abolish the risk for aplastic crisis or the formation of gallstones, documenting that a moderate degree of hemolysis persists in some children. Furthermore, they have shown that the remnant spleen grew in some patients, although there was no clear correlation between splenic regrowth and recurrent hemolytic anemia. The authors have made this same fascinating observation.

In addition to the French group, a group in the Czech Republic recently published their initial experience with a cohort of 14 children who had HS and were undergoing partial splenectomy by a similar technique to that used by Tchernia. In this nonrandomized study, the mean hemoglobin concentration increased from 9.9 to 13.8 g/dL [52]. After 5 years of follow-up, no child required late conversion to total splenectomy.

German experience

An alternative and more extensive approach to partial splenectomy in children who have HS has been advocated by Stoehr and colleagues [49,50] from Göttingen, Germany. In response to the concerns of persistent hemolysis after partial splenectomy as noted by the French and the authors' groups, Stoehr and colleagues have advocated a more radical spleen resection. This technique is termed, near-total splenectomy (NTS), and is designed to preserve a residual spleen volume of approximately 10 mL, the equivalent of an approximately 98% resection.

In their most recent summary, 30 children who had HS received a NTS. At follow-up, the mean hemoglobin concentration increased by 2.9 to 5.0 g/dL, whereas the serum bilirubin level decreased significantly by 15.4 to 56.4 mol/L (approximately 1–3 mg/dL). Although a NTS seems to result in improved hemoglobin levels and decreased hemolysis compared with baseline, preserved splenic function is not demonstrated clearly in this patient cohort and is a point of concern for many clinicians. Therefore, the authors' group continues to advocate a less radical splenic resection, because an acceptable hematologic result and preserved splenic function are essential to validate and support the use of a partial splenectomy.

North American experience

Several investigators in North America have reported the use of partial splenectomy in children who have not only HS but also a range of other congenital hemolytic anemias [14,51,53,54]. The authors' initial experience was with 25 children from Duke University or the Children's Hospital of Wisconsin [14]. In this initial report, the underlying diagnoses included HS (n = 16), pyruvate kinase deficiency (n = 2), congenital nonspherocytotic hemolytic anemia of unknown etiology (n = 1), HbSC disease (n = 2), HbSS disease (n = 2), HbCC disease (n = 1), and combined HbS/β-thalassemia (n = 1). Since the authors' original publications, combined experience at these two centers alone is more than 60 children [14,54]. Similar numbers of children have undergone partial splenectomy at other pediatric centers in North America. The results of these studies are summarized later.

Splenic regrowth

One concern often cited regarding partial splenectomy is regrowth of the splenic remnant and the potential for recurrent hematologic signs and symptoms. In the authors' experience, there almost always is mild to moderate splenic regrowth after partial splenectomy, as measured by sonographic splenic volume. Regrowth initially is slow, as the splenic remnant usually grows only 15% to 30% above the baseline volume during the first 2 years of follow-up, thus remains significantly below the preoperative size ($P < .05$). Although the rate of splenic regrowth is variable among children, by 4 years of follow-up, the splenic regrowth can be more pronounced, averaging 40% of the original splenic size. Regrowth of the spleen after partial splenectomy, however, is not associated with recurrent hemolysis, similar to the French experience. These findings suggest that although moderate regrowth may occur in some children, the clinical importance of these findings is unclear, because few children, even those who have a high rate of regrowth, have recurrent hematologic symptoms. Therefore, surveillance of splenic regrowth and correlation with clinical status are critical to understanding the long-term outcomes of partial splenectomy.

Effect on anemia and hemolysis

In the authors' initial experience, children who had HS and underwent partial splenectomy achieved significantly increased hemoglobin concentrations, similar to the findings of the European investigators. On average, the mean hemoglobin increased by 2 to 3 gm/dL within 3 months of surgery. In some children, this increase persisted for up to 10 years (Fig. 2) [14,54]. Sustained control of hemolysis also was observed, as reticulocyte counts decreased from 12.7% ± 4.2% preoperatively to 4.9% ± 2.9% at 2.3 ± 1.5 years of follow-up (mean ± SD, $P < .05$). Mean serum bilirubin levels decreased from a level of 2.6 ± 1.1 mg/dL preoperatively to 1.3 ± 0.7 mg/dL at similar follow-up (mean ± SD, $P < .05$). Partial splenectomy eliminates almost all symptoms of hypersplenism and control of splenic sequestration (Table 1).

As suggested initially in the French experience, the authors also showed that partial splenectomy does not eliminate hemolysis completely. Two of

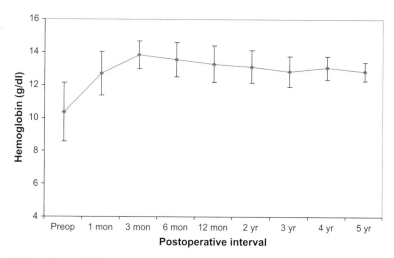

Fig. 2. Mean hemoglobin concentration after partial splenectomy for 12 recent children who had HS and underwent partial splenectomy at Duke University. Hemoglobin concentration increased compared with preoperative values throughout 4 to 6 years of follow- up ($P < .05$ by paired Student t test). Error bars show standard deviation.

Table 1
Effect of partial splenectomy on clinical findings in 25 children who had congenital hemolytic anemia, including 16 who had hereditary spherocytosis

Signs and symptoms	Preoperative hereditary spherocytosis (N = 16)		Postoperative hereditary spherocytosis (N = 15)		Preoperative non–hereditary spherocytosis (N = 9)		Postoperative non–hereditary spherocytosis (N = 9)	
Red blood cell transfusions	10	63%	1	7%	8	88%	1	11%
Sequestration crisis	8	50%	1	7%	7	77%	0	–
Abdominal pain	6	38%	0		6	66%	0	–
Jaundice	10	63%	1	7%	9	100%	2	22%

Red blood cell transfusions indicates need for one or more transfusion; sequestration crisis, hospitalization for sequestration crisis; abdominal pain, complaint of left upper quadrant abdominal pain; and jaundice, bilirubin level ≥ 2.0 mg/dL.

the children developed gallstones after partial splenectomy, requiring cholecystectomy. The importance of these findings relative to those seen after total splenectomy is unclear, however, as ongoing hemolysis often is seen with a severe HS phenotype even after total splenectomy [55]. Therefore, the clinical importance of splenic regrowth after partial splenectomy remains poorly defined and requires further evaluation.

Measures of splenic function after partial splenectomy

Splenic function as measured by liver-spleen radionuclide imaging is preserved in almost all children after partial splenectomy [14,54]. In the first three of 16 children who had HS in the authors' initial cohort, technetium 99m sulfur colloid scans were performed postoperatively and all three had evidence of radionuclide uptake. Also demonstrated was that after partial splenectomy, splenic phagocytic function was preserved in most children as assessed by the sustained clearance of HJB. During the first month postoperatively, many children have detectable circulating HJB. This finding is transient, however, and only one child in the authors' experience had detectable HJB beyond 6 months after surgery. Of five children who were tested postoperatively for pitted RBC, three had normal pit counts (<2%) and two had only mildly elevated levels (3%–6%), indicating preservation of splenic filtrative function.

In terms of immune function, the available data suggest that partial splenectomy does not impair nonspecific measures of the immune response. The authors measured serum immunoglobulin levels in seven children 3 years post surgery, and all retained normal immunoglobulin profiles, with normal levels of IgG and IgM (IgG 977 $\pm$ 266 mg/dL at baseline and 1193 $\pm$ 405 mg/dL measured 3 years after surgery; IgM 99 $\pm$ 32 mg/dL at baseline and 89 $\pm$ 33 mg/dL measured 3 years after surgery) [14]. Five of six children retained normal specific antibody titers to Streptococcus pneumoniae. In this small cohort, no child has developed a severe postoperative infection or sepsis. In summary, in the authors' experience and that of the French group, there seems to be preservation of splenic phagocytic and an intact immune response after partial splenectomy.

Effect of partial splenectomy on IgM memory B cells

As discussed previously, IgM memory B cells seem critical for control of many common childhood infections, and these cells usually are absent in asplenic children. The authors recently examined one patient who had HS who underwent partial splenectomy. Four weeks after surgery. this patient had retained IgM memory cells (Fig. 3). This intriguing observation indicates that memory B cells are detectable to at least 4 weeks after partial splenectomy and offers the possibility that the splenic remnant can provide sustained immunologic function. This is in contrast to data published previously on the lack of these cells in children after total splenectomy [24]. If this finding can be substantiated in other patients and for a longer period of time after surgery, the use of partial splenectomy may become more attractive for these patients.

Partial splenectomy in the setting of massive splenomegaly

To evaluate the safety and efficacy of partial splenectomy in children who had various congenital hemolytic anemias and had massive splenomegaly (defined as measured splenic volume >500 mL), the authors examined 29 children who underwent partial splenectomy [54]. The main technical difference for children who had massive splenomegaly compared with children who had normal-size spleens was that for safety reasons the laparoscopic approach was not used in the setting of massive splenomegaly. Furthermore, to preserve a splenic remnant representing 20% to 30% of normal spleen volume, as much as 90% to 95% of the massively enlarged spleens had to be resected.

The authors found that children who had and who did not have massive splenomegaly had successful outcomes from partial splenectomy. Both groups demonstrated decreased transfusion requirements, increased hematocrit,

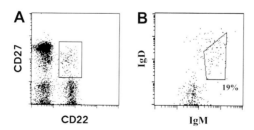

Fig. 3. IgM memory B-cell staining demonstrates the persistence of IgM memory B cells in a child who had HS 4 weeks after partial splenectomy (B). The selected CD22$^+$CD27$^+$ gate is shown in (A).

decreased bilirubin levels, decreased reticulocyte counts, and elimination of splenic sequestration [54]. From this experience, the authors conclude that partial splenectomy is a safe, effective, and technically feasible option for children who have various congenital hemolytic anemias, even in the setting of massive splenomegaly [54].

Rationale for a clinical trial

As discussed previously, retrospective clinical studies suggest that children who have HS and require splenectomy benefit from partial splenectomy. Given the small patient numbers and the fact that these studies were nonrandomized, however, the true benefits of partial splenectomy over total splenectomy remain poorly defined. It perhaps is not surprising, therefore, that several medical centers throughout North America and Europe have expressed strong enthusiasm for partial splenectomy whereas others are reluctant to accept the use of partial splenectomy, citing a lack of adequate clinical data to alter what they continue to consider standard therapy.

Leading national and international hematology organizations recognize the need to study the best surgical approach in patients who have HS who require splenectomy. For example, the General Haematology Task Force of the British Committee for Standards in Haematology has identified the need for further studies of surgical management of HS [20]. Specifically, they have suggested that "collaborative studies of the surgical management of HS" would be helpful, including evaluation of the role and mode of splenic resection. Additionally, this panel has stated the clear need for a national audit of the thromboembolic risk after splenectomy in children who have HS, suggesting that a national database be established to acquire this information. Finally, this panel emphasized the clinical importance of surgical issues, stating that, "from a patient perspective, the research priorities [should] center on surgical intervention[s]" [19].

Elements of a clinical trial for partial splenectomy in spherocytosis

The authors currently are developing a clinical trial for children who have HS. This trial will test the hypothesis that a partial splenectomy results in an acceptable alleviation of anemia compared with total splenectomy and preservation of splenic function. The exact design of the trial (ie, randomized prospective trial versus observational study) remains to be determined. Specific study endpoints include measurement of hemoglobin concentration, surgical morbidity/outcomes, hematologic events, hemolysis, splenic phagocytic and immune function, immune competence, infectious events, thrombosis, and splenic regrowth.

For proper design of this trial, it is critical to recognize that a partial splenectomy may not improve the hemoglobin concentration to an equivalent degree as a total splenectomy, because there is not the same degree of parenchymal resection after partial splenectomy. An equivalent resolution of anemia may not be clinically significant, however. Therefore, a head-to-head trial of total splenectomy versus partial splenectomy should not simply compare the hemoglobin response of these two surgical interventions. Because splenic function is not preserved after total splenectomy, many clinicians agree that an acceptable hematologic outcome with preserved splenic function in children is a more desirable goal, even though the improvement in hematologic status may be slightly less after a partial splenectomy than with a total splenectomy. Therefore, hematologic improvement and preservation of splenic function must be addressed in a study of partial splenectomy; only the opportunity to examine these dual outcomes makes the study of value.

In summary, the limitations of current care of children who have HS coupled with the ability to coordinate a multicenter pediatric clinical trial consortium and make meaningful quantitative measurements of hematologic and immunologic function make HS an ideal condition to use as a model disease to study the role of partial splenectomy. The authors' proposed study to compare partial splenectomy to total splenectomy in HS not only may lead to direct and immediate improvement in care for children who have HS but also may have a far-reaching impact on the large number of children worldwide who may benefit from splenic salvage therapies.

References

[1] Delaunay J. Genetic disorders of the red cell membrane. Crit Rev Oncol Hematol 1995;19: 79–110.
[2] Tchernia G, et al. Effectiveness of partial splenectomy in hereditary spherocytosis. Curr Opin Hematol 1997;4(2):136–41.
[3] King H, Shumacker HB Jr. Susceptibility to infection after splenectomy performed in infancy. Ann Surg 1952;136(2):239–42.
[4] Lynch AM, Kapila R. Overwhelming postsplenectomy infection. Infect Dis Clin North Am 1996;10(4):693–707.
[5] Leonard AS, et al. The overwhelming postsplenectomy sepsis problem. World J Surg 1980;4: 423–32.
[6] Brigden ML, Pattullo AL. Prevention and management of overwhelming postsplenectomy infection—an update. Crit Care Med 1999;27(4):836–42.
[7] Tchernia G, et al. Initial assessment of the beneficial effect of partial splenectomy in hereditary spherocytosis. Blood 1993;81(8):2014–20.
[8] Styrt B. Infection associated with asplenia: risks, mechanisms, and prevention. Am J Med 1990;88(5N):33N–42N.
[9] Green JB, et al. Late septic complications in adults following splenectomy for trauma: a prospective analysis in 144 patients. J Trauma 1986;26(11):999–1004.
[10] Brigden ML. Overwhelming postsplenectomy infection still a problem. West J Med 1992; 157(4):440–3.
[11] Holdsworth RJ, Irving AD, Cuschieri A. Postsplenectomy sepsis and its mortality rate: actual versus perceived risks. Br J Surg 1991;78(9):1031–8.
[12] Freud E, et al. Should repeated partial splenectomy be attempted in patients with hematological diseases? Technical pitfalls and causes of failure in Gaucher's disease. J Pediatr Surg 1997;32(9):1272–6.

[13] Bader-Meunier B, et al. Long-term evaluation of the beneficial effect of subtotal splenectomy for management of hereditary spherocytosis. Blood 2001;97:399–403.

[14] Rice HE, et al. Clinical and hematological benefits of partial splenectomy for congenital hemolytic anemias in children. Ann Surg 2003;237(2):281–8.

[15] Svarch E, et al. Partial splenectomy in children with sickle cell disease and repeated episodes of splenic sequestration. Hemoglobin 1996;20(4):393–400.

[16] Rescorla FJ, et al. Laparoscopic splenic procedures in children: experience in 231 children. Ann Surg 2007;246(4):683–7.

[17] Morton N, et al. Genetics of spherocytosis. Am J Hum Genet 1962;14:170–84.

[18] Eber SW, et al. Prevalence of increased osmotic fragility of erythrocytes in German blood donors: screening using a modified glycerol lysis test. Ann Hematol 1992;64:88–92.

[19] Tse WT, Lux SE. Red blood cell membrane disorders. Br J Haematol 1999;104:2–13.

[20] Bolton-Maggs PH, et al. Guidelines for the diagnosis and management of hereditary spherocytosis. Br J Haematol 2004;126(4):455–74.

[21] Edelman EJ, et al. A complex splicing defect associated with homozygous ankyrin-deficient hereditary spherocytosis. Blood 2007;109(12):5491–3.

[22] Agency for Healthcare Research and Quality. HCUP Kids' inpatient database. Rockville (MD): Agency for Healthcare Research and Quality; 2003.

[23] Price VE, et al. The prevention and treatment of bacterial infections in children with asplenia or hyposplenia: practice considerations at the Hospital for Sick Children, Toronto. Pediatr Blood Cancer 2006;46(5):597–603.

[24] Kruetzmann S, et al. Human immunoglobulin M memory B cells controlling Streptococcus pneumoniae infections are generated in the spleen. J Exp Med 2003;197(7):939–45.

[25] Weller S, et al. Human blood IgM "memory" B cells are circulating splenic marginal zone B cells harboring a prediversified immunoglobulin repertoire. Blood 2004;104:3647–54.

[26] Forster I, Rajewsky K. Expansion and functional activity of Ly-1 + B cells upon transfer of peritoneal cells into allotype-congenic, newborn mice. Eur J Immunol 1987;17:521–8.

[27] Ochsenbein AF, et al. Control of early viral and bacterial distribution and disease by natural antibodies. Science 1999;286:2156–9.

[28] Ochsenbein AF, Zinkernagel RM. Natural antibodies and complement link innate and acquired immunity. Immunol Today 2000;21:624–30.

[29] Weller S, et al. CD40-CD40L independent Ig gene hypermutation suggests a second B cell diversification pathway in humans. Proc Natl Acad Sci U S A 2001;98:1166–70.

[30] Gold HS, Moellering RC Jr. Antimicrobial drug resistance. N Engl J Med 1996;335:1445–53.

[31] Rother RP, et al. The clinical sequelae of intravascular hemolysis and extracellular plasma hemoglobin: a novel mechanism of human disease. JAMA 2005;293(13):1653–62.

[32] Hoeper MM, et al. Pulmonary hypertension after splenectomy? Arch Intern Med 1999;130:506–9.

[33] Robinette CD, Farumeni JF Jr. Splenectomy and subsequent mortality in veterans of the 1939-1945 war. Lancet 1977;2:127–9.

[34] Wagener FA, Eggert A, Boerman OC. Heme is a potent inducer of inflammation in mice and is counteracted by heme oxygenase. Blood 2001;98:1802–11.

[35] Hebert JC. Pulmonary antipneumococcal defenses after hemisplenectomy. J Trauma 1989;29(9):1217–20.

[36] Maruyama A. Immunologic function against infection in splenic autotransplanted mice. Nippon Geka Gakkai Zasshi 1991;92(5):567–76.

[37] Goldthorn JF, et al. Protective effect of residual splenic tissue after subtotal splenectomy. J Pediatr Surg 1978;13:587–90.

[38] Malangoni MA, et al. Splenic phagocytic function after partial splenectomy and splenic autotransplantation. Arch Surg 1985;120:275–8.

[39] Witte MH, et al. Preservation of the spleen. Lymphology 1983;16:128–37.

[40] Soleimani M, et al. Surgical treatment of patients with wandering spleen: report of six cases with a review of the literature. Surg Today 2007;37(3):261–9.

[41] Dertinger SD, et al. Micronucleated CD71-positive reticulocytes: a blood-based endpoint of cytogenetic damage in humans. Mutation Research/Genetic Toxicology and Environmental Mutagenesis 2003;542:77–87.

[42] Harrod VL, et al. Quantitative analysis of Howell-Jolly bodies in children with sickle cell disease. Exp Hematol 2007;35:179–83.

[43] Rogers ZR, et al. Evaluation of splenic function in infants with sickle cell anemia in the BABY HUG trial [abstract]. Blood 2004;104:975.

[44] Cappellini MD, et al. Coagulation and splenectomy: an overview. Ann N Y Acad Sci 2005; 1054:317–24.

[45] Mohren M, et al. Thromboembolic complications after splenectomy for hematologic diseases. Am J Hematol 2004;76:143–6.

[46] Ikeda M, et al. High incidence of thrombosis of the portal venous system after laparoscopic splenectomy: a prospective study with contrast-enhanced CT scan. Ann Surg 2005;241: 208–16.

[47] Soyer T, et al. Portal vein thrombosis after splenectomy in pediatric hematologic disease: risk factors, clinical features, and outcome. J Pediatr Surg 2006;41:1899–902.

[48] Freud E, et al. Splenic "regeneration" after partial splenectomy for Gaucher disease: histological features. Blood Cells Mol Dis 1998;24(6):309–16.

[49] Stoehr GA, et al. Near-total splenectomy for hereditary spherocytosis: clinical prospects in relation to disease severity. Br J Haematol 2006;132:791–3.

[50] Stoehr GA, Stauffer UG, Eber SW. Near-total splenectomy: a new technique for the management of hereditary spherocytosis. Ann Surg 2005;241:40–7.

[51] Dutta S, et al. A laparoscopic approach to partial splenectomy for children with hereditary spherocytosis. Surg Endosc 2006;20:1719–24.

[52] Jabali Y, et al. Ten-year experience with partial splenectomy (PSX) for hereditary spherocytosis (HS) in children [abstract]. Haematologica 2007;92(Suppl 1):289.

[53] Hall JG, et al. Partial splenectomy prior to hematopoietic stem cell transplantation in children. J Pediatr Surg 2005;40:221–7.

[54] Diesen DL, et al. Partial splenectomy for children with congenital hemolytic anemia and massive splenomegaly. J Pediatr Surg, in press.

[55] Agre P, et al. Inheritance pattern and clinical response to splenectomy as a reflection of erythrocyte spectrin deficiency in hereditary spherocytosis. N Engl J Med 1986;315:1579–83.

ELSEVIER
SAUNDERS

Pediatr Clin N Am 55 (2008) 521–528

PEDIATRIC CLINICS

OF NORTH AMERICA

Index

Note: Page numbers of article titles are in **boldface** type.